PHYSIOLOGY OF EXERCISE

for Physical Education
and Athletics

PHYSIOLOGY

Second Edition

OF EXERCISE

for Physical Education and Athletics

HERBERT A. DEVRIES

University of Southern California

WM. C. BROWN COMPANY PUBLISHERS
Dubuque, Iowa

PHYSICAL EDUCATION

Consulting Editor
Aileene Lockhart
Texas Woman's University

HEALTH

Consulting Editor
Robert Kaplan
The Ohio State University

PARKS AND RECREATION

Consulting Editor
David Gray
California State University, Long Beach

Printed in the United States of America

Contents

Contents

Preface

During the years of working with undergraduate and graduate students in the physiology of exercise laboratory, it has become apparent that theory and practice are not always related in the student's mind. Too often, the scientific method remains an *ivory tower* concept. Unfortunately, some coaches base their practices on methods of the highly successful athlete, whose success may be totally unrelated to the "fads" used in his training. Because of such practices and conditions, this author has made an effort to bring theory and practice into a closer and more meaningful relationship—to add the *how to* approach while at the same time developing respect for scientific investigations that provide the *why* for the *how to*.

Physiology of Exercise for Physical Education and Athletics is concerned with human functions under stress of muscular activity. The text provides a basis for the study of physical fitness and athletic training. Because this is a basic text, the information contained within is directly applicable to the needs of many specialists. The text is written primarily for the upper division *undergraduate student* who has a background in basic anatomy and general physiology. Physics, chemistry, or mathematics beyond that of the high school level are not necessary for comprehension. In addition, those who aspire to be *athletic coaches* will find within these pages the scientific basis for their profession. Since emphasis is placed upon the "holes" in our patchwork quilt of knowledge and since a substantially updated and expanded bibliography is provided at the end of each chapter, the *graduate student,* who wishes to "chip away" at the frontiers of knowledge in this discipline will be aided. Those who use exercise as one of the *modalities for medical treatment* will also find guiding principles in this text.

Physiology of Exercise is organized on the knowledge that students enter this field with very diverse backgrounds in general physiology. Therefore, this text is organized into three parts. Part one selectively reviews the most pertinent areas of basic physiology. For classes where the background in general physiology is strong the emphasis may be shifted toward part two which relates this knowledge directly to practice in physical education, and part three which relates the principles of physiology directly to the problems of the athletic coach.

Emphasis is on areas that are of practical importance, many of which have been neglected in the past. Whole chapters are devoted to muscle soreness, therapeutic and prophylactic effects of exercise, and the female in sports. Neurophysiology is also presented in sufficient detail so that its principles may be applied to the everyday procedures of physical education.

The research horizons in exercise physiology have greatly expanded in recent years by the advent of the electron microscope and new techniques in microbiology and histochemistry. Use of these tools in the hands of a new generation of highly trained exercise physiologists has created an increasing body of knowledge in cellular and molecular biology applied to human performance. Since much of the emerging material resulting from these new directions of investigation is very pertinent to and of direct practical value in physical education and athletics, no exercise physiology text could be complete without this new material. Unfortunately, very few physical education majors are exposed to courses in organic chemistry and biochemistry without which complete understanding of the theoretical aspects of this new phase is difficult if not impossible. For these reasons, a new chapter is provided—*Energetics of Muscular Contraction and Adaptations to Training at the Cellular Level*—treating such material in a fashion designed for students having little or no background in chemistry.

There has also been a gradual increase in the use of electromyography by physical educators in the effort to better understand muscle physiology. Consequently, the well-prepared physical educator needs sufficient exposure to these procedures to be able to read his professional literature critically. Chapter fourteen provides this background, simply but in sufficient depth to allow comprehension.

Just as each chapter ends with a summary, so in the second edition a final chapter has been added to enable the coach and athlete to synthesize the first twenty-six chapters. *The Unified Athlete: Monitoring Training Progress* is designed to encourage the young coach to take his exercise physiology background to the athletic field instead of leaving it behind in the ivory tower of his college days.

The author has benefitted greatly from the constructive critiques with respect to the first edition. The author values most highly the comments from you—his colleagues—who use this text on the firing line—the classroom—and he solicits your continuing help to make this text more valuable to you and your students.

Grateful appreciation is extended to the author's associates at the University of Southern California, particularly to Dr. J. Tillman Hall.

Part One

BASIC PHYSIOLOGY
UNDERLYING THE
STUDY OF PHYSIOLOGY
OF EXERCISE

1 Structure of Muscle Tissue

All human activity, whether in work or sport, depends ultimately on the contraction of muscle tissue for its driving forces. There are three types of muscle tissue in the human body:

1. Smooth, nonstriated muscle, which is found in the walls of the hollow viscera and blood vessels.
2. Striated, skeletal muscle, which provides the force for movement of the bony, leverage system.
3. Cardiac muscle, which is found only in the heart.

Smooth muscle receives its innervation from the autonomic nervous system, and ordinarily contracts independently of voluntary control. The fibers of smooth muscle are usually long, spindle-shaped bodies, but their external shape may change somewhat to conform to the surrounding elements. Each fiber usually has only one nucleus.

Skeletal muscle, which is innervated by the voluntary or somatic nervous system, consists of long, cylindrical muscle fibers. Each fiber is a large multinucleated cell, with as many as several hundred nuclei and it is structurally independent of its neighboring fiber or cell. Skeletal, or striated, muscle, as the name implies, is most easily distinguished by its cross-striations of alternating light and dark bands.

Cardiac muscle in all vertebrates is a network of striated muscle fibers. It differs structurally from the other two types of muscle tissue mainly in the interweaving of its fibers to form a network, called a *syncytium*, which differentiates it from skeletal muscle which is also striated. It further differs from smooth muscle in that it has cross striations, which smooth muscle does not have. Cardiac muscle contracts rhythmically and automatically, without outside stimulation. Whereas in skeletal muscle each fiber is a discrete entity, and can contract individually (but with other members of its motor unit) tissue innervation in cardiac muscle results in a wavelike contraction that passes through the entire network of fibers.

GROSS STRUCTURE OF SKELETAL MUSCLE

If we dissected a limb such as the upper arm, and removed the skin, subcutaneous adipose tissue, and the superficial fascia, we would lay bare the biceps brachii muscle and note that it is covered in its entirety by a deep layer of fascia that binds the muscle into one functional unit. This outermost sheath of connective tissue is called the *epimysium*, and it merges at the ends of the muscle with the connective tissue material of the tendon. Thus the force of muscular contraction is transmitted through the connective tissues, binding the muscle to the tendon, then through the tendon to the bony structures, to bring about movement.

In cross-section, it may be seen that the interior of the muscle is subdivided by septa into bundles of muscle fibers (fig. 1.1). Each bundle contains upwards of a dozen, possibly as many as 150, fibers. Each bundle is called a *fasciculus,* and it has a more or less complete connective tissue

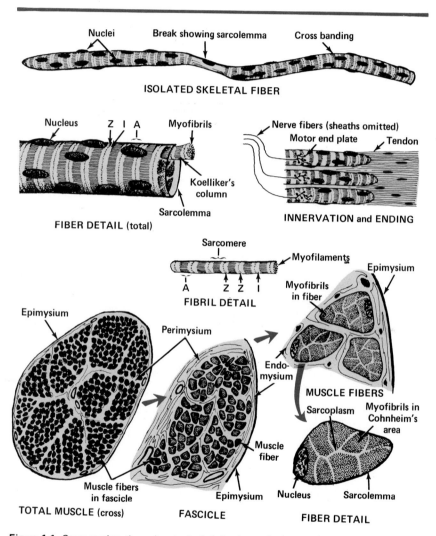

Figure 1-1. Cross section through a typical skeletal muscle showing (below) the breakdown from the gross muscle to the single muscle fiber and (above) relationships of the microscopic structures to the muscle fiber. (From Arey, L.B. *Human Histology,* 1968. Courtesy of W.B. Saunders Company, Philadelphia.)

sheath that is called the *perimysium*. The structures discussed so far are visible with the naked eye.

MICROSCOPIC STRUCTURE OF SKELETAL MUSCLE

More detailed study requires the aid of a microscope, so that the structure of an individual fiber and its relationships to other fibers, to form fasciculi, may be seen (fig. 1.2). Each fiber is surrounded by a connective sheath called the *endomysium*. The need for these connective tissue sheaths—endomysium around the single fiber, perimysium around the fasciculus, and epimysium about the whole muscle—can better be understood when it is realized that one fiber may not run through the whole length of a muscle, or even through a fasciculus (fig. 1.3). Therefore it becomes necessary to transmit the force of contraction from fiber to fiber

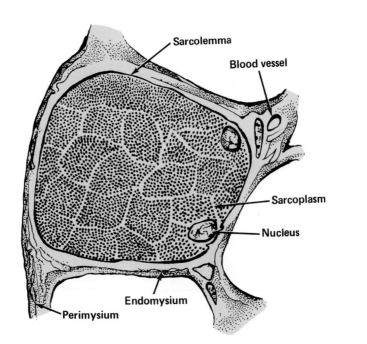

Figure 1-2. Cross section of human skeletal muscle fiber drawn with camera lucida. Each dot represents a myofibril (x 1500). (From Copenhaver, W.M.; Bunge, R.P.; and Bunge, M.B. *Bailey's Textbook of Histology,* 1971. Courtesy of Williams and Wilkins Company, Baltimore.)

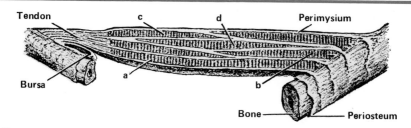

Figure 1-3. Diagram of attachment of muscle to skeleton and relation of fibers to each other within a fasciculus, (a) fiber extends the length of fasciculus, (b) fiber begins at periosteum but ends in muscle, (c) fiber begins at tendon but ends in muscle, (d) both ends of fiber within the muscle (redrawn from Braus). (From Copenhaver, W.M.; Bunge, R.P.; Bunge, M.B. *Bailey's Textbook of Histology,* 1971. Courtesy of Williams and Wilkins Company, Baltimore.)

to fasciculus, and from fasciculus to fasciculus (since these ordinarily do not run through the length of a large muscle either), to the tendons, which act upon the bones. This function is provided by the connective tissues described above.

The dimensions of individual fibers may vary, according to most investigators, from ten to 100 microns (1,000 microns = 1 mm) in diameter and from 1 mm to the length of the whole muscle. Thus the thickness of a large fiber is roughly comparable to that of a fine human hair, although the smaller fibers can not be seen by the unaided eye.

Each fiber constitutes one muscle cell. Each muscle has fibers of characteristic size, and the thickness of each fiber is related to the forces involved in the function of the muscle. Thus the fibers of the extrinsic ocular muscles are small in diameter whereas those of the quadriceps femoris are large.

STRUCTURE OF THE MUSCLE CELL OR FIBER

The cell membrane of the muscle cell is called the *sarcolemma*. This membrane is extremely thin, and seems almost structureless, even under the electron microscope. Inside the sarcolemma are the many nuclei, mainly situated peripherally, close to the sarcolemma. Corresponding to the cytoplasm of other cells, is the *sarcoplasm*, which is the more fluid part of the cell. Running longitudinally within the sarcoplasm are slender column-like structures called *myofibrils*, which have alternating segments of light and dark color. The presence of the myofibrils impart to the fiber as a whole the appearance of lengthwise striations. The cross-striations, however, are far more obvious because the dark segments of the many myofibrils are arranged in lateral alignment. All light segments are likewise aligned with each other.

For many years, anatomists and histologists have classified muscles as red or white according to whether red or white fibers predominated in the make up of the gross muscle structure. In this classification the red fibers were considered to be better suited to long-term, slow contractions as was required of postural, antigravity muscles, while the white fibers were considered to be differentiated for speed of contraction and thus were to be found predominantly in the flexor muscles.

More recent work involving new staining techniques and electron microscopy suggests the need for a three way classification: (1) fast twitch red, (2) fast twitch white, and (3) slow twitch intermediate fibers (2). Available evidence supports such a classification on the basis that muscles which are both red and white in appearance show fast contraction

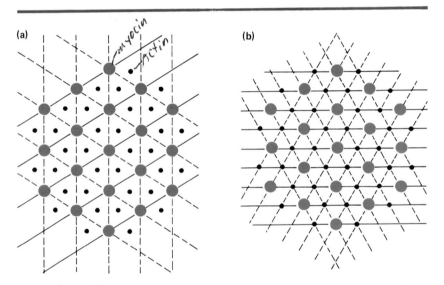

Figure 1-4. (a) End-on view of double hexagonal lattice of thick and thin filaments, characteristic of overlap region in A bands of vertebrate striated muscle, showing the three sets of lattice planes in the crystallographic directions. The actin filaments at the trigonal points of the lattice will tend to fill in the space between the dense planes of filaments at the hexagonal lattice points, thereby decreasing the intensity of the X-ray reflexions given by the thick filaments on their own. (b) Similar view, showing lattice planes in crystallographic directions. In this case, both the actin and myosin filaments lie in the same lattice planes and so their contributions to the intensity of the corresponding X-ray reflexion are additive. Hence, as the amount of material at the trigonal points is increased, the intensity of the reflexions decreases and that of the reflexions increases. (From Huxley, H.E. "The Structural Basis of Muscular Contraction." Proc. of Royal Society of London 178:131, 1971.)

times; and *actomyosin adenosine-triphosphatase activity* (muscle enzyme which is important in determination of speed of contraction) is low in the intermediate fiber and high in both the red and white fibers (5).

STRUCTURE OF THE MYOFIBRIL AND THE CONTRACTILE MECHANISM

The advent of the electron microscope and its wide usage in recent years has provided greater insight into both the structure and function of the myofibril. Though the story is not complete in all details, the sliding filament model of muscle contraction is now widely accepted as best explaining all the experimental data (Huxley 1971).

The *sarcomere* is the functional unit of the myofibril, and it extends from Z line to Z line, as shown in figures 1.4 and 1.5. Each sarcomere is composed of two types of interdigitating parallel filaments that run lengthwise of the myofibril. One type is about twice as thick as the other, and its length is equal to the length of the A band (the dark band seen as part of the striation effect). The second and thinner type of filament is longer, and extends inward from both Z membranes, almost to the center of the sarcomere. The amount by which the two ends of the thin

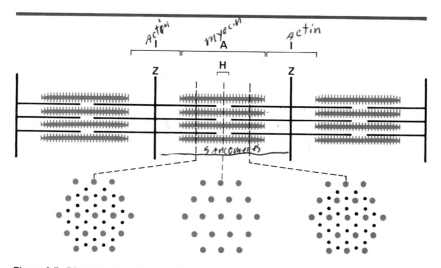

Figure 1-5. Diagrammatic representation of the structure of striated muscle, showing overlapping arrays of actin- and myosin-containing filaments, the latter with projecting crossbridges on them. For convenience of representation, the structure is drawn with considerable longitudinal foreshortening; with filament diameters and side-spacings as shown, the filament lengths should be about five times the lengths shown. (From Huxley, H.E. "The Structural Basis of Muscular Contraction." Proc. of Royal Society of London 178:131, 1971.)

filament fail to meet constitutes a lighter band, within the dark *A* band which is called the *H* zone. The area between the ends of the thick filaments is less dense, and therefore gives the light band appearance of the striation effect, which is known as the *I* band. Thus the light and dark striped effect of striated muscle rests on a rational basis of bands of greater and lesser optical density, as can be seen in figure 1.5. The cross-sectional views show the relationship of each thick filament to a hexagon of six thin filaments, each hexagon, however, being shared by three thick filaments.

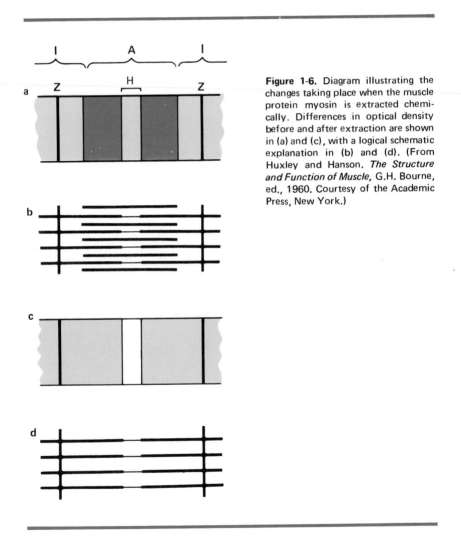

Figure 1-6. Diagram illustrating the changes taking place when the muscle protein myosin is extracted chemically. Differences in optical density before and after extraction are shown in (a) and (c), with a logical schematic explanation in (b) and (d). (From Huxley and Hanson. *The Structure and Function of Muscle,* G.H. Bourne, ed., 1960. Courtesy of the Academic Press, New York.)

Chemical extraction of the muscle protein, myosin, results in the disappearance of the dark A band (fig. 1.6), and extraction of the muscle protein, actin, similarly affects the I band. These facts are very strong evidence that the thick filaments consist of myosin and the thin filaments are composed of actin and, also tropomyosin.

A sliding movement of the actin and myosin filaments during contraction of the myofibril has been well demonstrated and it seems that the A bands remain the same length while the I bands change only in shortening below ninety percent of the myofibrils' resting length (fig. 1.7). The exact nature of the changes in the H zone are not as yet clearly understood, although its disappearance during contraction is well established. The contractile process depends upon the presence of adenosine triphosphate (ATP) and its splitting by dephosphorylation into ADP (adenosine diphosphate) and phosphate. This splitting of an ATP bond furnishes large amounts of energy.

Earlier in vitro experiments (11, 13) had shown that three necessary elements of muscle function—relaxation, contraction, and rigor mortis—could be explained as follows:

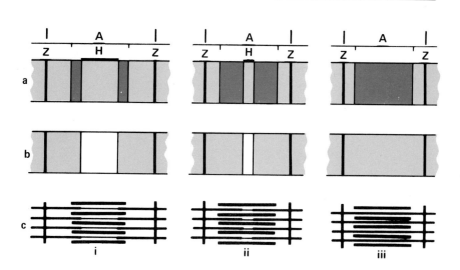

Figure 1-7. Diagram illustrating the structural changes associated with contraction (iii) and extension (i) from resting length (ii). The top row (a) shows the band patterns of intact fibrils. The next (b) shows the band patterns after extraction of myosin. The bottom row (c) shows the positions of the filaments. (From Huxley and Hanson. *The Structure and Function of Muscle,* G.H. Bourne, ed., 1960. Courtesy of the Academic Press, New York.)

1. In the presence of ATP (unsplit), actomyosin breaks down into a non-contractile state of dissociated actin and myosin, thus causing relaxation.
2. When ATP splits to form ADP + P, actomyosin threads reform, and the reformed threads contract in the presence of more ATP.
3. If the reformed actomyosin thread is removed from the presence of ATP, it resists extension.

These in vitro observations seem to explain the necessary facts observed in vivo:

1. Relaxation, in the presence of unsplit ATP.
2. Contraction, in the presence of unspit ATP, when some ATP is undergoing dephosphorylation.
3. Rigor mortis, caused by total dissipation of ATP after its splitting has already caused the precipitation of inextensible actomyosin threads.

Now we must account for the mechanics involved in bringing about the sliding of the filaments and the biochemical events which initiate and provide the energy for this interdigitation of the actin and myosin filaments. The most acceptable explanation for the process of contraction at the cellular level is as follows:

1. An electrical impulse conducted by the motor nerve, activates the motor end-plate of the muscle fiber which in turn brings about the release of a substance which depolarizes the resting muscle membrane. This depolarization is what is recorded and measured by electromyographic methods as muscle action potentials.
2. The action potential in turn sets off two independent electrical currents, one of which is a weak longitudinal current; the other is transverse and moves inward into the fiber along a system of tubules (see fig. 1.8).
3. The inwardly invading current releases internal tightly bound calcium (7).
4. In the fiber's resting state, inactivity is maintained because a complex of two other proteins, *troponin* and *tropomyosin*, when in combination with actin prevents the normal course of interaction between actin and myosin filaments. When the calcium ions are released because of the electrical excitation, they bind strongly to the troponin-tropomyosin complex and thus suppress the inhibitory action upon the actinmyosin interaction which is then free to combine.
5. The combination of actin-myosin acts as an enzyme (*catalyst*) which is called actomyosin adenosine-triphosphatase or *actomyosin ATPase*

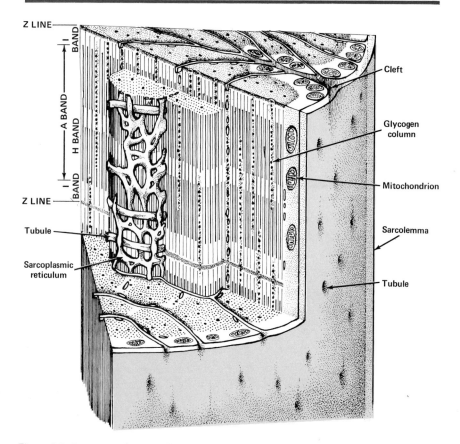

Figure 1-8. Structure of muscle fiber consists of a number of fibrils, which in turn are made up of orderly arrays of thick and thin filaments of protein. A system of transverse tubules opens to the exterior of the fiber. The sarcoplasmic reticulum is a system of tubules that does not open to the exterior. The two systems, which are evidently involved in the flow of calcium ions, meet at a number of junctions called dyads or triads. Mitochondria convert food to energy. The sarcolemma is a membrane surrounding the fiber. (From Graham Hoyle. *How Is Muscle Turned On and Off?* Copyright © 1970 by Scientific American, Inc. All rights reserved.)

which catalyzes the breakdown of ATP to ADP + P which in turn furnishes the energy for contraction (4).

6. Having the contractile structure and its source of energy defined we now need to explain the mode of action of the cross bridges in making the filaments slide to shorten the sarcomere and thus the myofibril—the fiber and the whole muscle. The most plausible explanation

is offered by H. E. Huxley (10) who was involved in the original formulation of the sliding filament theory (6) along with the independent work of A. F. Huxley (8). Figure 1.9 illustrates the process which is referred to as the swinging cross bridge model.

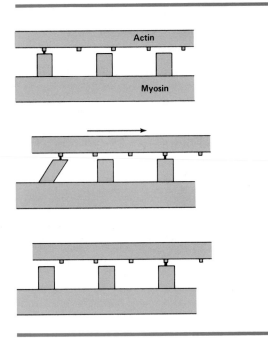

Figure 1-9. Diagram showing, very schematically, possible mode of action of cross-bridges. A cross-bridge attaches to a specific site on the actin filament, then undergoes some configurational change which causes the point of attachment to move closer to the centre of the A band pulling the actin filament along in the required manner. At the end of its working stroke, the bridge detaches and returns to its starting configuration, in preparation for another cycle. During each cycle, probably one molecule of ATP is dephosphorylated. Asynchronous attachment of other bridges maintains steady force. (From Huxley, H.E. "The Structural Basis of Muscular Contraction." Proceedings of the Royal Society of London 178:131, 1971.)

BLOOD SUPPLY AND LYMPHATICS

In keeping with the high level of metabolic activity of muscle tissue, it is extremely well supplied with capillaries; each muscle fiber is supplied with several capillaries. To furnish this rich vascularization, larger branches of arteries penetrate the muscle by following the paths of the septa between fasciculi (in the perimysium). The arteries furnish arterioles to the fasciculi, and the arterioles give off capillaries at sharp angles to individual fibers. The veins follow the arteries, typically, and even the smallest veins have valves. Lymphatic capillaries are found only at the fascicular level of organization.

NERVE SUPPLY

Because each muscle fiber represents a single cell and is a discrete functioning unit, it must be innervated individually. This is not to say, however, that one nerve cell may not innervate more than one muscle cell, by sending twigs from the same nerve fiber to several or many muscle fibers. The cell bodies of the neurons (nerve cells) lie in the ventral horns of the spinal cord. The axons of these cells form the nerve fibers of the efferent fibers of the peripheral nerves, which innervate the muscles. Each nerve, as seen grossly in dissection, represents the association of many axons or nerve fibers, just as a gross muscle also represents many muscle fibers. The nerve fibers, as do the arterioles, travel in the perimysium, and branch several times, thus permitting one neuron to innervate more than one muscle fiber.

The ratio of nerve fibers to muscle fibers varies with the degree of precision that is required of the muscle. In one of the muscles that moves the eye, a ratio of one nerve fiber to one muscle fiber has been found. However, one nerve cell may innervate as many as 150 or more muscle fibers.

The neuron and its axon (or nerve fiber) with its twigs plus the muscle fibers supplied by all the twigs, form the basic neuromuscular unit: the *motor unit*. After the repeated branchings, referred to above, the nerve fibers (or their branches) lose their myelin sheaths and enter individual muscle fibers. The neurolemma sheath of the nerve fiber apparently becomes continuous with the sarcolemma of the muscle fiber, and the nerve fiber branches into several club-like *terminal endings*. These terminal endings are embedded in sarcoplasm, just under the sarcolemma, and are called the *motor end-plate* or the *myoneural junction*.

The muscle fibers making up one motor unit do not lie contiguously; they are usually scattered throughout a considerable volume of the gross muscle structure (3, 12). This fact has important implications for our discussion of electromyography in a later chapter.

SUMMARY

1. Three types of muscle tissue are present in the human body
   a. Smooth, nonstriated: usually found in viscera and blood vessels
   b. Skeletal, striated: found in the somatic muscles
   c. Cardiac, striated syncytium: found only in the heart
2. Gross structure of skeletal muscle is at three levels.
   a. Whole muscle, surrounded by epimysium
   b. Muscle bundle or fasciculus, surrounded by perimysium, which constitutes the septae seen grossly in cross-section
   c. Muscle fiber, surrounded by endomysium
3. In the microscopic structure of skeletal muscle, fiber diameter is roughly related to the load of work the muscle ordinarily performs.

4. Each skeletal muscle fiber represents one multinucleated cell, in which the sarcolemma is the cell membrane and the sarcoplasm roughly corresponds to the cytoplasm of other cells.
5. The supply of capillaries to muscle tissue is very abundant in order to support the large metabolic demands of exercise.
6. When a neuron in the ventral horn of the spinal cord is stimulated, its axon, all of the axon's branches, and all the muscle fibers supplied by the branches function together, simultaneously, as a motor unit.
7. A motor unit may consist of one neuron, with its axon (nerve fiber), innervating one muscle fiber; or it may consist of one neuron, with its axon branching, and innervating as many as 150 or more muscle fibers.
8. Although the muscle fibers of one motor unit function together they do not constitute a unified structure. In fact they are distributed throughout a considerable volume of muscle tissue in many cases.

REFERENCES

1. Bailey, Kenneth. 1956. Muscle protein, *British Medical Bulletin* 12:183-87.
2. Barnard, R. J.; Edgerton, V. R.; Furukawa, T.; and Peter, J. B. 1971. Histochemical, biochemical, and contractile properties of red, white and intermediate fibers. *American Journal of Physiology* 220:410-14.
3. Buchthal, F.; Guld, C.; and Rosenfalck, P. 1957. Multi-electrode study of the territory of a motor unit. *Acta Physiologica Scandinavica* 39:83-103.
4. Ebashi, S., and Endo, M. 1968. Calcium ion and muscular contraction. *Progress in Biophysical and Molecular Biology* 18:125-83.
5. Guth, L., and Samaha, F. J. 1969. Qualitative differences between actomyosin ATPase of slow and fast mammalian muscle. *Experimental Neurology* 25:138-52.
6. Hanson, J., and Huxley, H. E. 1955. The structural basis of contraction in striated muscle. *Symp. Society for Experimental Biology and Medicine* 9:228-64.
7. Hoyle, G. 1970. How is muscle turned on and off? *Scientifc American* 222:84-93.
8. Huxley, A. F. 1957. Muscle structure and theories of contraction. *Progress in Biophysical Chemistry* 7:257-318.
9. Huxley, H. E. 1956. The ultra structure of striated muscle. *British Medical Bulletin* 12:171-73.
10. Huxley, H. E. 1971. The structural basis of muscular contraction. *Proceedings of the Royal Society of Medicine* 178:131-49.
11. Needham, D. M. 1956. Energy production in muscle. *British Medical Bulletin* 12:194-98.
12. Norris, F. H., Jr., and Irwin, R. L. 1961. Motor unit area in a rat muscle. *American Journal of Physiology* 200:944-46.
13. Perry, S. V. 1956. Interactions of actomyosin and adenosine-triphosphate. *British Medical Bulletin* 12:188-93.

2 Energetics of Muscular Contraction and Adaptations to Training at the Cellular Level

As described in the first chapter the breakdown of adenosine triphosphate (ATP) to adenosine diphosphate (ADP)

$$ATP \rightarrow ADP + P + \text{approximately 8000 calories of energy (or 8 Kcal)}$$

furnishes the immediate source of energy for the contractile mechanism. It is the purpose of this chapter to discuss the processes by which ingested food energy is converted and utilized to regenerate the energy of the high energy bonds of the ATP which ultimately make the muscle cell (fiber) contract.

In the past, considerations in depth of the biochemistry of muscular contraction did not seem justified because no practical application of these theoretical concepts could be applied to "down to earth" physical education and athletic training principles. However, there are now several compelling, reasons for the physical educator and coach to become familiar with at least the rudiments of muscle contraction at the cellular level.

1. There is recent evidence that some very important effects of athletic training occur at the cellular level of organization in terms of modification of intracellular structure and the enzyme systems which are so important to energy supply.
2. There is now excellent laboratory data bearing upon the need for diet modification to maximize the athletes cellular energy supply.
3. Researchers in physical education have become sophisticated in the use of the electron microscope and biochemical procedures and their research reports will require more background on the part of our professional readership.

In short, the material in this chapter is now essential to conduct a scientifically based program of physical education and athletic training.

The metabolic processes that supply the energy needs of muscle contraction ordinarily take place in the presence of adequate O_2 to oxidize the carbohydrate sources of energy completely to CO_2 and H_2O. This constitutes *aerobic* muscle activity which in general is exercise whose intensity is low enough that it can be carried on for at least five minutes or longer. On the other hand if the intensity of exercise is very high so that exhaustion ensues within one to two minutes or less, the energy must be supplied largely by *anaerobic* processes (without O_2), because O_2 cannot be transported via the lungs and cardiovascular system rapidly enough to supply such a demand.

In general, four processes all occurring within the muscle cell are concerned with the chemistry of muscle contraction and three of them are common to aerobic and anaerobic contraction. It will be noted that the first three reactions are reversible. That is to say, the reactions are such that as some molecules of ATP are being broken down to provide energy for muscle fiber contraction, other molecules of ADP and P are being regenerated (at a cost of energy provided by the next reaction down, CP → C + P). A balance must obviously be struck between the rate of breakdown and the rate of regeneration or the muscle effort would run out of gas. Thus each reaction shown depends upon energy supply from below in order that it may remain in balance while supplying energy to the reaction above. Or we may say that each succeeding reaction supplies energy for the reversal of the preceding reaction as follows:

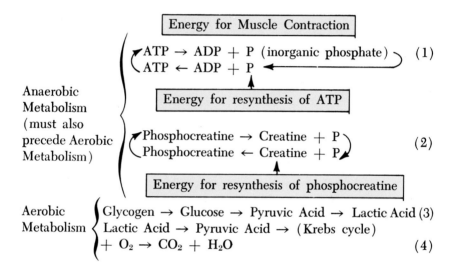

This diagram is, of course, a great oversimplification in that it does not show the intermediary reactions and enzyme systems that are necessary. Figure 2.1 (p. 21) provides the details.

It will be noted that aerobic and anaerobic metabolism share the common paths of *glycogenolysis* and *glycolysis*. Glycogenolysis is defined as the breakdown of the large glycogen molecule to many glucose molecules and glycolysis is defined as the splitting of the glucose molecule into two pyruvic acid molecules. In the absence (or relative shortage) of O_2 the reactions can only proceed through equation #3 with the production of lactic acid as the end product plus the freeing of small amounts of energy. The fourth reaction with its oxidative (therefore called aerobic) pathway provides for greater amounts of energy.

REGENERATION OF ATP ENERGY FROM CARBOHYDRATE FOOD

We may think of the overall conversion of the carbohydrate in our food to energy in terms of the following simple equation which summarizes all of the diagram found on page 19.

$$C_6H_{12}O_6 + 6O_2 \rightarrow 6CO_2 + 6H_2O + Energy$$
Glucose   Oxygen   Carbon   Water
dioxide

While this is indeed straight forward it could only happen in such direct fashion by raising the temperature very high and actually *burning* the carbohydrate in a very hot flame not consistent with living tissue. To bring about the conversion of food energy to ATP energy for muscle contraction at body temperature many intermediate steps catalyzed by enzyme systems are necessary. The above equation is quite correct in that it summarizes the whole process, but it tells us nothing about how this process is actually accomplished. It is the enzyme systems which promote the stepwise chemical breakdown of the food stuffs at body temperature to provide the energy for muscle contraction. Enzymes are proteins which have the ability to promote a specific chemical reaction without themselves being degraded or changed in the process. Thus the same enzyme protein can function over and over again in the same metabolic process.

The final products of carbohydrate digestion in the alimentary tract are the *monosaccharides* (6 carbon atom sugars) *glucose, fructose,* and *galactose*. These are the results of the breakdown of such larger carbohydrate molecules as starch and the usual sugars included in the diet (*disaccharides*). The three monosaccharides are interconvertible and as they pass through the liver they are converted almost entirely to glucose for transport in the blood to the muscle cells and other tissues of the body.

As the glucose molecule enters the muscle cell through the sarcolemma, a process greatly aided by the presence of insulin, it is immediately phosphorylated. That is to say the 6 carbon atom monosaccharide picks up a phosphate radical on its number 6 carbon atom and becomes glucose-6-phosphate. Note in figure 2.1 (p. 21) that this process of phosphorylation requires the presence of the enzyme *hexokinase* as well as the breakdown of one ATP to form ADP + P. Since our discussion has to do with formation of ATP, this first step would seem to be in the wrong direction but we will wait for the whole story.

Once phosphorylated, the glucose molecule is trapped in the muscle cell because it requires the enzyme *phosphatase* to dephosphorylate the glucose and the muscle cell has no phosphatase although the liver cells

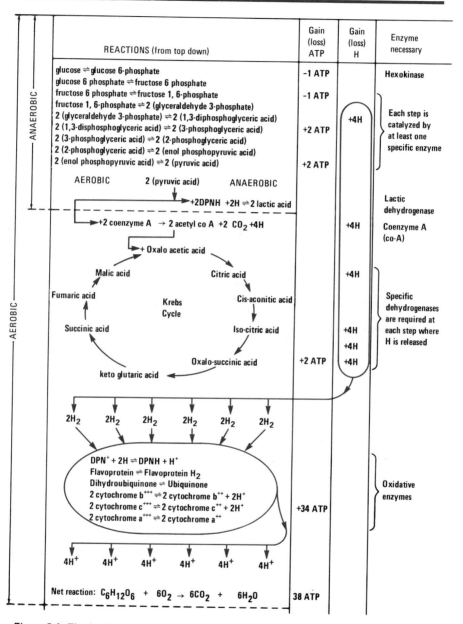

		Gain (loss) ATP	Gain (loss) H	Enzyme necessary
	glucose ⇌ glucose 6-phosphate	-1 ATP		Hexokinase
	glucose 6 phosphate ⇌ fructose 6 phosphate			
ANAEROBIC	fructose 6 phosphate ⇌ fructose 1, 6-phosphate	-1 ATP		
	fructose 1, 6-phosphate ⇌ 2 (glyceraldehyde 3-phosphate)			Each step is catalyzed by at least one specific enzyme
	2 (glyceraldehyde 3-phosphate) ⇌ 2 (1,3-diphosphoglyceric acid)		+4H	
	2 (1,3-disphosphoglyceric acid) ⇌ 2 (3-phosphoglyceric acid)	+2 ATP		
	2 (3-phosphoglyceric acid) ⇌ 2 (2-phosphoglyceric acid)			
	2 (2-phosphoglyceric acid) ⇌ 2 (enol phosphopyruvic acid)			
	2 (enol phosphopyruvic acid) ⇌ 2 (pyruvic acid)	+2 ATP		

AEROBIC 2 (pyruvic acid) ANAEROBIC

+2DPNH +2H ⇌ 2 lactic acid — Lactic dehydrogenase

+2 coenzyme A → 2 acetyl co A +2 CO_2 +4H — +4H — Coenzyme A (co-A)

+ Oxalo acetic acid

Malic acid   Citric acid   +4H

Fumaric acid   Krebs Cycle   Cis-aconitic acid

Succinic acid   Iso-citric acid   +4H

Oxalo-succinic acid   +2 ATP   +4H

keto glutaric acid

Specific dehydrogenases are required at each step where H is released

$2H_2$ $2H_2$ $2H_2$ $2H_2$ $2H_2$ $2H_2$

$DPN^+ + 2H \rightleftharpoons DPNH + H^+$
Flavoprotein ⇌ Flavoprotein H_2
Dihydroubiquinone ⇌ Ubiquinone
2 cytochrome b^{+++} ⇌ 2 cytochrome b^{++} + $2H^+$
2 cytochrome c^{+++} ⇌ 2 cytochrome c^{++} + $2H^+$
2 cytochrome a^{+++} ⇌ 2 cytochrome a^{++}

+34 ATP — Oxidative enzymes

$4H^+$ $4H^+$ $4H^+$ $4H^+$ $4H^+$ $4H^+$

Net reaction: $C_6H_{12}O_6$ + $6O_2$ → $6CO_2$ + $6H_2O$ 38 ATP

Figure 2-1. The breakdown of glucose (basic building block of all carbohydrate) to furnish the energy for regeneration of ATP.

and some other tissues do. This is immediately important from the practical standpoint in that we now know that the energy stored away in one muscle is not available to another which may be in the process of exhaustion due to locally heavy work. We will return to this concept later in the consideration of muscular endurance.

The glucose-6-phosphate once in the cell, can either be utilized directly for energy as shown in figure 2.1 (p. 21) or it can be stored depending upon cell activity levels. In order to be stored it must be converted to glycogen which is a large chain or network of glucose molecules called a *polymer.* The polymerization process involves several steps and requires several enzymes. The glycogen is deposited as granules in glycogen columns as shown in figure 1.8 (p. 13). Storage in the form of large polymerized molecules is necessary in order not to unduly raise the intracellular osmotic pressure which storage as glucose units would do. The amount of glycogen stored in the muscle cell determines its endurance for exercise under certain conditions as we will discuss later in this chapter. The breakdown products of protein and fat digestion and lactic acid can also be converted to glucose and thence to glycogen for storage. We shall now direct our attention to the more detailed pathways by which carbohydrate can be broken down to produce the energy necessary for rebuilding the ATP which is what is needed by the myofilaments to bring about muscle contraction. Basically, we are concerned with aerobic and anaerobic sources of energy. It is important, however, to resist the temptation to think of muscular activity as *either* aerobic or anaerobic. Even light exercise brings both mechanisms into play as will be described in the chapter, *Exercise Metabolism.*

Figure 2.1 (p. 21) illustrates the whole process of carbohydrate metabolism schematically. While it is not suggested that the student commit this to memory, a level of understanding is necessary. Glucose becomes available as an energy substrate either by the glycogenolysis of glycogen stored in the muscle fiber, or by blood glucose transported into the muscle fiber. The glucose molecule first undergoes glycolytic breakdown into two pyruvic acid molecules as shown in figure 2.1. The enzyme hexokinase is necessary to add a phosphate (PO_4 or P) radical to make glucose-6-phosphate. This process costs the breakdown of one ATP to ADP + P. Each of the further steps of glycolysis is also catalyzed by at least one enzyme specific to that step and one more ATP is broken down to add the second P to form fructose-1, 6-phosphate (the 1, 6 means that there are two phosphates in the molecule, one at the number 1 carbon atom and one at the number 6 carbon atom). Note however that this cost of two ATPs broken down is recouped with a net total gain of two ATP molecules during the process of glycolysis which results in formation of two molecules of pyruvic acid. In the absence of O_2 (or insufficient O_2), the end products of glycolysis, pyruvic acid and H-atoms combine to form lactic acid. This last step is important because if the end products of a reaction accumulate, the reaction is ended before all of the energy substrate can be used. Since the lactic acid diffuses freely into the tissue fluids and blood, it is removed and thus anaerobic metabolism can proceed until the energy substrate is used up.

In the presence of sufficient O_2, the system does not back up at the pyruvic acid step because pyruvic acid can now continue on its aerobic course by entering a metabolic system called the *Krebs cycle* (also called *citric acid cycle* or *tricarboxylic acid cycle*). The course of aerobic metabolism is much more advantageous, because up to this point the anaerobic route has netted us only two ATP molecules generated from one molecule of glucose. As will be seen, complete aerobic breakdown will provide at least thirty-eight molecules of ATP per molecule glucose.

The next stage in glucose breakdown requires the conversion of the two pyruvic acid molecules into two molecules of acetyl coenzyme A (acetyl Co-A). Acetyl Co-A combines with oxaloacetic acid to become citric acid and the Krebs cycle is underway. The net result of the Krebs cycle is to degrade the acetyl portion of the acetyl Co-A to CO_2 and H atoms. The steps of the Krebs cycle depend upon specific enzymes called *dehydrogenases* to break off the H atoms which are subsequently oxidized with resulting large amounts of energy liberated for formation of ATP molecules. Note that although only two ATP molecules are regenerated in the Krebs cycle itself, twenty H atoms are released.

The H atoms which are released must be converted to H ions, written H^+ before they can react with O_2 to form water and large amounts of energy. This is accomplished by the oxidative enzymes of the respiratory chain. (These enzymes and those of the Krebs cycle reside in the mitochondria of the cell). This is schematized as the bottom of figure 2.1 in which the final breakdown of the glucose molecule is completed and the net chemical reaction for the whole aerobic process depicted in figure 2.1 is as follows:

$$C_6H_{12}O_6 + 6\ O_2 + 38ADP + 38\ P \rightarrow 6\ CO_2 + 6\ H_2O + 38\ ATP$$

Since each high energy phosphate bond represents about 8 Kcal and since each gram molecular weight of glucose (180 gm) has an ultimate energy value of about 4 Kcal/gm the efficiency of this process of storage

of energy as ATP is about $\dfrac{38 \times 8}{180 \times 4} = \dfrac{304}{720} = 42\%$.

REGENERATION OF ATP ENERGY FROM FAT AND PROTEIN

As will be seen in later discussion, exercise of intensities up to about seventy percent of maximum proceeds largely by way of energy gained from fat metabolism. Thus the regeneration of *ATP* energy from fat is quite important in exercise physiology. Energy can also be provided for work by protein metabolism but becomes important in exercise physiology only in a state of negative balance (starvation or the semistarvation of rigorous weight reduction).

Use of Fat for Energy. Fat is basically a combination of three fatty acids, each of which is attached to one of the three carbon atoms of a glycerol molecule. Chemically this combination (fat) is called a *triglyceride.*

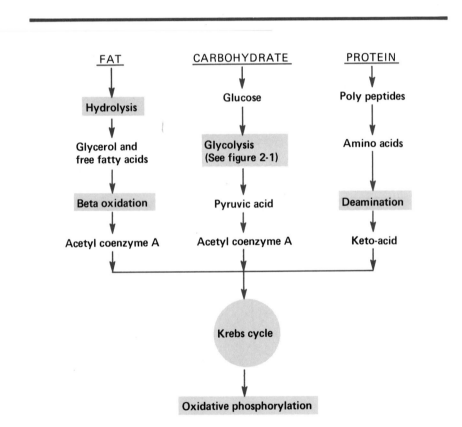

Figure 2-2. Derivation of energy from the metabolism of the three basic foodstuffs by way of the final common path: the Krebs cycle and oxidative phosphorylation.

The first step in the utilization of fat for energy is the hydrolysis into the original components, glycerol plus three fatty acids. The glycerol is easily changed by enzymic action into glyceraldehyde which can be used for energy via the phosphogluconate pathway which occurs in the liver or in the fat cells but not in muscle. The fatty acids undergo a process called *Beta Oxidation* which involves a stepwise breakdown of the long chain fatty acid molecule into acetyl Co-A molecules which then enter the Krebs cycle and proceed just as the acetyl Co-A from carbohydrate.

Use of Protein for Energy. Proteins are very large complex molecules and consist of from twenty to 100,000 amino acids which are the basic building blocks of all proteins. The digestive enzymes of the stomach start the breakdown of protein and it is carried further in the small intestine to the polypeptide level (combination of several amino acids) and completed to the amino acid level in passage through the wall of the small intestine into the blood. The amino acids are then deaminated in the liver (removal of the ammonia radical) becoming keto acids. These resulting keto acids are then converted into substances which can enter the Krebs cycle and thence proceed to complete degradation and energy formation as has been described for carbohydrate.

It is important to recognize that just as all three foodstuffs can be utilized for energy, they are also convertible into fat for storage when the food ingested exceeds the need. In the case of protein, some amino acids must first go through gluconeogenesis to become carbohydrate before deposition on the hips, etc., as fat pads.

IMPLICATIONS FOR TRAINING OF ATHLETES

One can see that lactic acid would build up in the tissues under either of two conditions: (1) hypoxia (insufficient O_2 supply by the blood to keep the respiratory chain functioning in oxidizing the H atoms to form ATP energy), or (2) insufficient enzyme activity in either the Krebs cycle or in the respiratory chain enzymes to fully utilize the O_2 which is supplied by the blood.

It has long been known that a trained individual has a much lower rate of rise in lactic acid than the untrained individual working at the same load. Until recently it has been assumed that this was due to better O_2 transport in the trained. While the trained individual's *capacity* for *maximum transport* is indeed better (better max $\dot{V}O_2$) recent evidence shows that he neither uses more O_2 at submaximal levels nor does he do a better job of supplying the working muscle through better distribution (5, 7, 30).

Thus the greater rise of lactate in the untrained at submaximal work loads needs an explanation other than the improved cardiorespiratory function which is a well-documented result of physical conditioning.

STRUCTURAL CHANGES AT THE CELLULAR LEVEL FROM TRAINING

When a muscle is required to work at higher intensity than that to which it is accustomed (*overload principle*) the well-known phenomenon of *hypertrophy* occurs. That this increase in size is due to enlarged fibers and not the result of an increased number of muscle fibers was first shown by Morpurgo in 1897 (26). The question of just how the muscle fiber enlarges has only recently been answered. It has been shown in animal studies that hypertrophy is accompanied by a several fold increase in the number of the myofibrils (6, 9).

The total increase in the muscle protein has been shown to be the result of proportional increases in sarcoplasm, myofilaments, and mitochondria (8). The myofilaments increase only in number while the mitochondria increase both in number and size.

Another interesting change resulting from training experiments in guinea pigs was reported by Barnard, Edgerton, and Peter who found a significant increase in the percentage of red fibers in the gastrocnemius after treadmill running. The increase in red fibers was at the expense of a decrease in white fibers with no change in the intermediate (3).

Probably the most important training effect is the increase in mitochondrial protein which has been reported by several different groups of investigators (3, 11, 23). Both the size and the number of mitochondria in the muscle cell are increased as the result of training if the intensity of the training stimulus is sufficiently severe. It will be recalled from the preceding discussion of muscle metabolism that the very important enzymes of both the Krebs cycle and the repiratory chain reside in the mitochondria of the muscle cell. Holloszy (13) has shown that training rats on a treadmill results in a twofold increase in the capacity to oxidize pyruvate. Oxidation of pyruvate represents the entire aerobic portion of the muscle cells metabolic process and thus tells us that the cell is now able to work at double the load since the gycolytic pathway is probably not a limiting factor.

ENERGY SUBSTRATE AND TRAINING

Until quite recently our only evidence regarding the energy substrate utilized by working muscles was indirect-by calculation of respiratory quotients (RQ) as described in the later chapter on exercise metabolism.

In 1962 Bergstrom introduced a biopsy needle which he and Hultman and their coworkers subsequently used to good advantage in making direct observations of the level of various energy substrates remaining in an active muscle after various types, intensities and duration of muscle work. From such studies, rates of utilization and various very practical implications for athletes and coaches have become available.

Figure 2.3 shows the rate of glycogen depletion in working muscle cells when they are fatigued by bicycle exercise at various work loads (29). When the individual is working at seventy to eighty percent of his maximal aerobic capacity (max $\dot{V}O_2$) then exhaustion occurs when the muscle fiber's glycogen supply is depleted. This suggests that at such work loads, the muscle can utilize only glycogen stored in the muscle cells for its energy substrate, although at lighter loads glucose and free fatty acids transported by the blood form the source of energy. At maximal work loads, the load cannot be sustained long enough to bring about glycogen depletion. Since it has also been shown that neither ATP nor CP are limiting factors under maximal loads (21) it is likely that

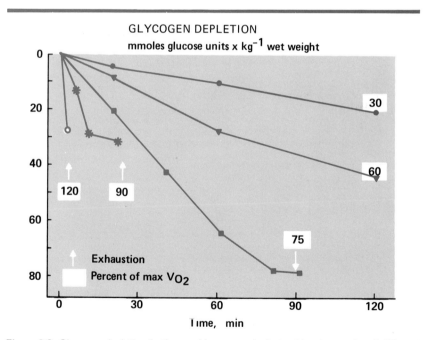

Figure 2-3. Glycogen depletion in the quadriceps muscle during bicycle exercise of different intensities. (From Saltin, B., and Karlsson, J. *Muscle Metabolism during Exercise,* Pernow, B., and Saltin, B., eds., 1971. Courtesy of Plenum Press, New York.)

endurance under these conditions depends upon lactic acid accumulation (and the ability to buffer it and withstand the pain of the pH change). The lactic acid formed is in turn dependent upon the level of O_2 transport. At lighter loads of sixty percent or less of aerobic capacity, the limiting factor is probably the availability of blood borne glucose and free fatty acids (FFA). Under the conditions of lighter loading, the liver store of carbohydrate may become an important factor (28). It must be understood that only the duration of the effort is set by the energy stores available; the rate of work that can be maintained depends upon O_2 transport.

The situation is quite different with respect to isometric exercise. It has been calculated that the actual utilization of glycogen under maximum isometric contraction is only about one-tenth that available to the muscle and consequently glycogen stores cannot be a limiting factor in isometric contraction (17). Indeed, fatigue occurring isometrically at any load above twenty percent of maximum cannot be explained on the basis of glycogen depletion and loads below that are unimportant in human athletic performance (1). A more definitive answer regarding the question of isometric muscle fatigue must await further research.

Training Effects on Cellular Energy Substrate Level.   Using the muscle biopsy technique, Karlsson et al. (22) have shown increased levels of ATP concentration in muscle to result from seven months of military training which included distance running two to three times per week. This of course would be very important during periods of anaerobic work where work load intensity is too heavy to permit O_2 transport to keep up with tissue demand.

With respect to carbohydrate energy sources, the percentage of energy which is supplied by glycogen is apparently affected to some extent by the relative availability to the muscle cell as a result of diet. Pruett (27) has shown the percentage contribution of carbohydrate to vary with diet and work load as follows:

Work load	Standard Diet	High Fat	High Carbohydrate
50% max VO_2	40%	35%	50%
70% max VO_2	53%	50%	60%

Hultman working with Bergstrom and others has reported some findings which are of importance to all concerned with endurance type athletics (16, 17, 18, 19). Most importantly he has shown that endurance under heavy aerobic work loads is determined largely by the level of glycogen storage in the muscle cells. Thus for such work, the rate or intensity is set by O_2 transport capacity (to be discussed in following chapters) but the duration or total work which can be accomplished is set by the level of glycogen stored within the cell.

Of even greater practical interest are the data found in figure 2.4. Here one can see first the very important *overshoot phenomenon* that is, when a muscle is worked hard enough to bring about glycogen depletion, then it develops the ability to store greater than normal amounts of glycogen. Secondly, it can also be seen that recharging of the glycogen stored depends greatly upon the type of diet. On a carbohydrate rich diet glycogen resynthesis was complete in twenty-four hours, whereas on a carbohydrate free diet of the same caloric content, resynthesis was complete only after eight to ten days. It was also shown that the glycogen content

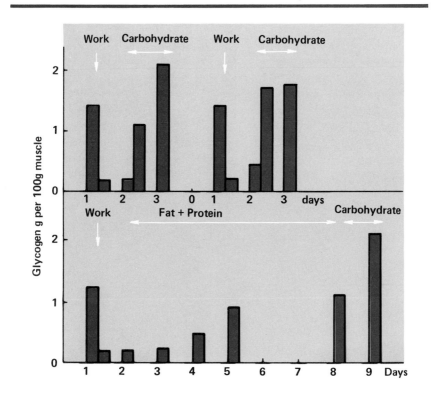

Figure 2-4. Muscle glycogen before and after work. Two subjects (upper graph) fasted for one day and got carbohydrate diet on day two; the third subject (lower graph) got fat and protein diet during eight days and thereafter one day carbohydrate. (From Hultman, E. *American Heart Association Monograph, no. 15,* 1967, p. 106. Courtesy of the American Heart Association, New York.)

of the liver was dependent upon diet. If CHO is not supplied in the diet, liver glycogen can decrease rapidly to values which will not sustain work for more than about one hour (by glycogenolysis after muscle glycogen has been depleted).

Unfortunately, the overshoot phenomenon works only for the muscle which has been worked and the glycogen storage level varies considerably from muscle to muscle. A short fast of up to six hours was found to have no effect on glycogen level, so that a long wait for an athletic competition after a meal will have no adverse effects, unless stomach growls annoy teammates.

The exact mechanism by which the overshoot phenomenon occurs is not yet fully understood. Jeffress, Peter, and Lamb (20) have reported an increase in glycogen synthetase, an enzyme necessary to the storage of glycogen, to result from training but this alone cannot fully explain the overshoot.

Training also has a *glycogen sparing* effect in that the better trained individual can supply more blood borne energy substrate, primarily free fatty acids which supply the bulk of the energy for resting and low level long duration exercise (12).

Cellular Oxidative Capacity—Enzyme Systems. The most impressive cellular changes reported thus far to result from training reside in the aerobic pathway. Holloszy and coworkers have reported training changes in rats which doubled the cellular oxidative capacity. Underlying this change were twofold increases in activity levels of the respiratory enzymes involved in the oxidation of DPNH and succinate (13) and of some of the enzymes of the citric acid cycle (15). The rise in activity is the result of increased enzyme protein rather than an increase in activity per unit protein. Barnard and Peter (4) also found significant improvement of the respiratory enzymes cytochrome a and c. Interestingly, they found a strong correlation between cytochrome c concentration and the performance of the *isolated* guinea pig muscle but not with the *running time to exhaustion.*

Holloszy et al. (14) have shown that while the constituents of the respiratory chain (oxidative phosphorylation in figure 2.1, (p. 21) increase in proportion with one another in response to training, this is not true with the enzymes of the citric acid cycle which also reside in the mitochondria and therefore there is a change in mitochondrial composition as a result of training.

In contrast with the well-defined changes of the aerobic pathway described above, only transitory changes which probably have no training significance have been found in the glycolytic pathway (anaerobic part of figure 2.1). Barnard and Peter (2) and Lamb et al. (24) found significant increases in hexokinase activity in guinea pigs which were later confirmed by Holloszy et al. (15) in rats. *free fatty acids*

We have alluded earlier to the glycogen-sparing effect of FFA utilization as an energy source and it is of interest to note that Mole, Oscai and Holloszy (25) have reported a significant rise in the capacity of rat gastrocnemius muscle to oxidize free fatty acids after a heavy training regimen.

Finally, it has also been reported that the activity of myosin ATP-ase, the enzyme which catalyzes the reaction of the actin-myosin myofilament shortening, is increased if the exercise is sufficiently severe (31).

Significance of Cellular Training Changes. Since the training changes in enzyme activity and consequent oxidative capacity of the muscle cell have been shown to be twofold or even greater and since training changes in the total human organism for maximal O_2 consumption usually fall between ten to 30 percent, an explanation is needed. Experimental data regarding causation are lacking, but the increase in total body work capacity in terms of maximal O_2 consumption is usually accompanied by equivalent increases in maximum cardiac output and A-V O_2 difference. Thus it seems that changes in the O_2 transport system can explain all of the improvement of total physical working capacity. This is borne out by the observation of no correlation between concentration of cytochrome c in the cell and run time to exhaustion reported by Barnard and Peter (4).

It seems likely that the major importance of the improvement in cellular oxidative capacity lies in the fact that less dependence upon the anaerobic pathway results with a lowered level of lactic acid production at submaximal work loads.

It would seem that the effect of training in delaying the end point of a workbout due to fatigue depends upon the rate of work done. In very heavy work, which can be maintained only for ten to twenty minutes, the improvement is probably due to a combination of improved O_2 transport and the improved cellular oxidative capacity which results in a slower build-up of lactic acid to the point where further work becomes impossible or too painful. In work of an intensity which can be supported for sixty to 180 minutes, improvement in the endurance time will depend largely upon the overshoot of cellular glycogen storage. Duration of work of lighter loads which can be maintained for longer than three hours may be limited in duration at least in some cases by hypoglycemia resulting from depletion of both muscle and liver glycogen. Such fatigue (as in marathon events) can be delayed by feeding of sugar in various forms.

For the reader who would like greater detail on the subject of cellular adaptations to exercise an excellent review by Gollnick is available (10).

SUMMARY

1. ATP energy which is the immediate source of energy at the acto myosin filament level is replenished by the break down of phosphocreatine. The energy for regeneration of phosphocreatine is in turn supplied by *glycolysis,* the breakdown of glucose to pyruvic acid. Under *anaerobic* conditions the pyruvic acid is converted to lactic acid whose accumulation eventually brings about cessation of exercise. Under *aerobic* conditions the first three reactions are in turn refueled by energy gained from the complete oxidation of the pyruvic acid to carbon dioxide and water.

2. Both fat and protein can also be used for energy but only fat is important in exercise metabolism.

3. The chemical breakdown of foodstuffs to supply energy for the regeneration of ATP from ADP and P is accomplished by a complex process in which many protein enzymes are necessary as catalysts. The overall reaction describing the entire chain of events can be written as follows:

$$C_6H_{12}O_6 + 6O_2 + 38ADP + 38P \rightarrow 6CO_2 + 6H_2O + 38ATP$$

in which the synthesis of 38 ATP molecules represents the accumulation of about 304 Kcal of energy from the oxidation of some 720 Kcal of glucose (1 gram molecular weight).

4. *Muscular hypertrophy* which results from overload exercise is the result of an increase in the total protein material of the muscle due to increased size of the muscle fibers, with no increase in number. The increased size of the fiber is in turn due to increased numbers of myofibrils with concommitant increases in sarcoplasm, myofilaments, and mitochondria. The filaments increase in number but not in size, and the mitochondria increase in both number and size.

5. At heavy work loads of seventy to eighty percent of capacity glycogen stored in the muscle cell provides the energy for contraction and endurance time depends upon the level of glycogen storage in the muscle at the beginning of exercise. This is not true, however, for isometric exercise.

6. At maximal work loads the work cannot be sustained long enough to deplete the stored glycogen and the endpoint is probably determined by the level of lactic acid accumulation.

7. Increased concentrations of ATP result from heavy endurance train-

ing and this should be effective in improving the capacity for anaerobic work.

8. When muscular work is such that glycogen depletion is brought about, the muscle responds by large increases of glycogen storage. This response is complete within twenty-four hours on a carbohydrate rich diet, but may take eight to ten days on a carbohydrate free diet of equal caloric content.

9. Training also has a *glycogen sparing* effect in that better trained individuals are able to utilize more free fatty acid as energy substrate.

10. If a training program is sufficiently intense, the mitochondria increase up to twofold in total protein material with accompanying increases of oxidative capacity. The glycolytic pathway is apparently unaffected.

11. It may be hypothesized that the major significance of the increased cellular oxidative capacity is in allowing submaximal exercise work loads to proceed with lower rates of lactic acid accumulation.

REFERENCES

1. Ahlborg, B.; Bergstrom, J.; and Hultman, E. 1972. Muscle metabolism during isometric exercise performed at constant force. *Journal of Applied Physiology* 33:224-28.

2. Barnard, R. J., and Peter, J. B. 1969. Effect of training and exhaustion on hexokinase activity of skeletal muscle. *Journal of Applied Physiology* 27:691-95.

3. Barnard, R. J.; Edgerton, V. R.; and Peter, J. B. 1970. Effect of exercise on skeletal muscle: I. Biochemical and histological properties. *Journal of Applied Physiology* 28:762-66.

4. Barnard, R. J., and Peter, J. B. 1971. Effect of exercise on skeletal muscles: III. Cytochrome changes. *Journal of Applied Physiology* 31:904-8.

5. Clausen, J. P.; Larsen, O. A.; and Trap-Jensen, J. 1969. Physical training in the management of coronary artery disease. *Circulation* 40:143-54.

6. Denny-Brown, D. 1964. Experimental studies pertaining to hypertrophy, regeneration, and degeneration. In *Neuromuscular Disorders,* eds. R. P. Adams, L. M. Eaton, and A. M. Shy, pp. 147-196. Proceedings of the Association for Research in Nerve and Mental Disorders. Baltimore: Williams & Wilkins.

7. Frick, M. H., and Katila, M. 1968. Haemodynamic consequences of physical training after myocardial infarction. *Circulation* 37:192-202.

8. Goldberg, A. L. 1968. Protein synthesis during work-induced growth of skeletal muscle. *Journal of Cellular Biology* 36:653-58.

9. Goldspink, G. 1964. The combined effects of exercise and reduced food intake on skeletal muscle fibers. *Journal of Cellular and Comparative Physiology* 63:209-16.

10. Gollnick, P. D. 1971. Cellular adaptations to exercise. In *Frontiers of Fitness*, ed. R. J. Shepherd. Springfield: Charels C Thomas.

11. Gollnick, P. D.; Ianuzzo, C. D.; and King, D. W. 1971. Ultrastructural and enzyme changes in muscles with exercise. In *Muscle Metabolism during Exercise*, eds. B. Pernow and B. Saltin, pp. 69-71. New York: Plenum Press.

12. Havel, R. J. 1971. Influence of intensity and duration of exercise on supply and use of fuels. In *Muscle Metabolism during Exercise*, eds. B. Pernow and B. Saltin, pp. 315-25. New York: Plenum Press.

13. Holloszy, J. O. 1967. Effects of exercise on mitochondrial oxygen uptake and respiratory enzyme activity in skeletal muscle. *Journal of Biological Chemistry* 242:2278-82.

14. Holloszy, J. O.; Oscai, L. B.; Don, I. J.; and Mole, P. A. 1970. Mitochondrial citric acid cycle and related enzymes: adaptive response to exercise. *Biochemical and Biophysical Research Communications* 40:1368-73.

15. Holloszy, J. O.; Oscai, L. B.; Mole, P. A.; and Don, I. J. 1971. Biochemical adaptations to endurance exercise in skeletal muscle. In *Muscle Metabolism during Exercise*, eds. B. Pernow and B. Saltin, pp. 51-61. New York: Plenum Press.

16. Hultman, E. 1967. Physiologlical role of muscle glycogen in man with special reference to exercise. In *American Heart Association Monograph* #15, pp. 99-112.

17. Hultman, E. 1971. Muscle glycogen stores and prolonged exercise. In *Frontiers of Fitness*, ed. R. J. Shephard, pp. 37-60. Springfield: Charles C Thomas.

18. Hultman, E. and Nilsson, L. H. 1971. Liver glycogen in man. Effect of different diets and muscular exercise. In *Muscle Metabolism during Exercise*, eds. B. Pernow and B. Saltin, pp. 143-51. New York: Plenum Press.

19. Hultman, E.; Bergstrom, J.; and Roch-Norlund, A. E. 1971. Glycogen storage in human skeletal muscle. In *Muscle Metabolism during Exercise*, eds. B. Pernow and B. Saltin, pp. 273-88. New York: Plenum Press.

20. Jeffress, R. N.; Peter, J. B.; and Lamb, D. R. 1968. Effects of exercise on glycogen synthetase in red and white skeletal muscle. *Life Sciences* 7: 957-60.

21. Karlsson, J., and Saltin, B. 1970. Lactate, ATP and CP in working muscles during exhaustive exercise in man. *Journal of Applied Physiology* 29:598-602.

22. Karlsson, J.; Nordesjo, L. O.; Jorfeldt, L.; and Saltin, B. 1972. Muscle lactate, ATP, and CP levels during exercise after physical training in man. *Journal of Applied Physiology* 33:199-203.

23. Kressling, K. H.; Piehl, K.; and Lundquist, C. G. 1971. Effect of physical training on ultrastructural features in human skeletal muscle. In *Muscle Metabolism during Exercise*, ed. B. Pernow and B. Saltin, pp. 97-101. New York: Plenum Press.

24. Lamb, D. R.; Peter, J. B.; Jeffress, R. N.; and Wallace, H. A. 1969. Glycogen, hexokinase, and glycogen synthetase adaptations to exercise. *American Journal of Physiology* 217:1628-32.
25. Molé, P. A.; Oscai, L. B.; and Holloszy, J. O. 1971. Adaptation of muscle to exercise. *Journal of Clinical Investigations* 50:2323-30.
26. Morpurgo, B. 1897. Ueber aktivitäts-hypertrophie der willkurlichen muskeln. *Virchows Archiv für Pathologische Anatomie und Physiologie und für Kinische Medizin* 150:522-54.
27. Pruett, E. D. R. 1970. Glucose and insulin during prolonged work stress in men living on different diets. *Journal of Applied Physiology* 28:199-208.
28. Rowell, L. B. 1971. The liver as an energy source in man during exercise. In *Muscle Metabolism during Exercise,* eds. B. Pernow and B. Saltin, pp. 127-41. New York: Plenum Press.
29. Saltin, B., and Karlsson, J. 1971. Muscle glycogen utilization during work of different intensities. In *Muscle Metabolism during Exercise,* eds. B. Pernow and B. Saltin, pp. 289-99. New York: Plenum Press.
30. Varnauskas, E.; Bergman, H.; Houk, P.; and Bjorntorp, P. 1966. Haemodynamic effects of physical training in coronary patients. Lancet 2:8-12.
31. Wilkerson, J. E., and Evonuk, E. 1971. Changes in cardiac and skeletal muscle myosin ATPase activities after exercise. *Journal of Applied Physiology* 30:328-30.

3 The Physiology of Muscle Contraction

Muscle tissue is specifically differentiated for the purpose of contraction, thus its most important physiological property is *contractility*. However, it also possesses other properties common to protoplasm in general: *irritability* and *conductivity*. Irritability indicates that muscle tissue responds to adequate stimuli with its typical response, contraction; and conductivity means that an adequate stimulus will be propagated throughout any one muscle fiber in skeletal muscle, and from fiber to fiber in smooth and cardiac muscles for reasons described in chapter one.

Excised muscle may be stimulated electrically, chemically, and mechanically. The intact muscle is normally stimulated by its motor nerve only, but it can also be stimulated electrically through the skin, as is frequently done by physicians and physical therapists, and mechanically, as when a bruise elicits a contracture (charley horse).

THE MUSCLE TWITCH AND ITS MYOGRAM

It has been customary in elementary physiology textbooks to describe the simple muscle twitch as the basis for understanding the process of muscle contraction. This concept is likely to be helpful only if the student realizes from the outset that this is not typical of muscle contraction either in the intact body, or even in an excised muscle that is normally innervated.

In the typical laboratory experiment, the gastrocnemius muscle of a frog is excised and hung from a ringstand so that its contraction, in terms of the movement of its free end, is recorded on the rotating drum of a kymograph. The muscle is then stimulated electrically by a single shock to the entire sciatic nerve trunk, or to the muscle itself, and it responds under these conditions by a single twitch. The record of the events occurring during this contraction is called a *myogram* (fig. 3.1).

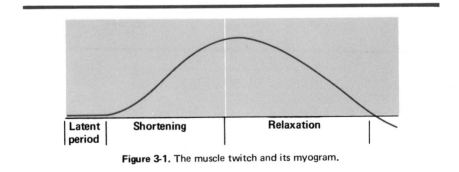

| Latent | Shortening | Relaxation | |
| period | | | |

Figure 3-1. The muscle twitch and its myogram.

At this point the student must understand the two basic differences between the laboratory preparation and normal stimulation and contraction processes as they occur in the intact animal; otherwise, difficulty will arise in conceptualizing other aspects of neuromuscular function.

1. In the laboratory preparation, nearly all of the nerve fibers for the whole muscle are innervated simultaneously because all the fibers of the sciatic nerve are shocked at the same time, but the innervation of normal human muscle is asynchronous, motor unit by motor unit or we might say each nerve fiber is stimulated individually at varying points in time.

2. In the laboratory preparation, the twitch is the response to a single stimulation (shock), and this probably never occurs in the intact organism, for we know that innervation of human muscle is accomplished by volleys of nerve impulses, ranging from five or six per second to as many as eighty or ninety.

Having recognized the foregoing artifacts, there is still much we can learn from the myogram of the muscle twitch. After the stimulus is applied, approximately 0.01 second elapses before contraction of the frog muscle begins. This interval is called the *latent period,* and it has been found to be much shorter—0.001 second—if the muscle is completely unloaded (recording by optics). The shortening of the muscle is called the *contraction phase,* which typically takes approximately 0.04 seconds in the frog gastrocnemius. The lengthening of the muscle back to its resting length occupies about 0.05 seconds, and this is called the *relaxation phase.* These values, of course, vary from species to species and from muscle to muscle within the same species, as was discussed in chapter one in regard to fast and slow twitch muscle fibers.

wave summation

SUMMATION OF CONTRACTIONS AND TETANUS

With the same muscle preparation discussed above, and by application of a second stimulus to the nerve trunk within the period of the single twitch, tension can be increased considerably (fig. 3.2, p. 40). The best results are usually gained when the stimulus for the second contraction occurs at the high point of the first. The second contraction is very similar to the first, but it starts with the elevated level of tension (or shortening) supplied by the first contraction. The explanation for this phenomenon, *summation of contractions,* seems to be that the short duration of the single twitch does not allow sufficient time for the structural rearrangements within fibers (discussed in chapter one) to go to completion (19).

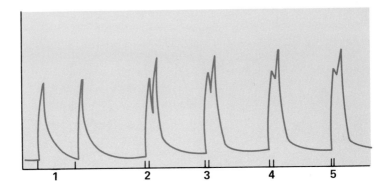

Figure 3-2. Summation of twitches. (From Zoethout. *Introduction to Human Physiology,* 1948. Courtesy of The C.V. Mosby Company, St. Louis.)

If the same preparation is stimulated repeatedly with a series of shocks too closely spaced to allow a complete relaxation phase, a prolongation of the contraction occurs, which is called *tetanus* (fig. 3.3). If a relaxation phase persists, as is shown in the curves A, B, C, D of the illustration, it is termed a *partial* or *incomplete tetanus*. If the relaxation

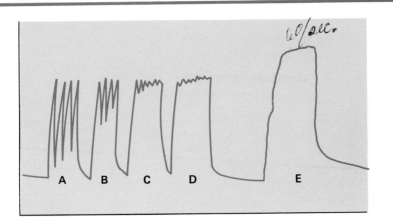

Figure 3-3. Muscle curves showing the genesis of tetanus: A, B, C, D, incomplete tetani; E, complete tetanus. Faradic shocks of the same intensity were used throughout. (From Zoethout. *Introduction to Human Physiology,* 1948. Courtesy of The C.V. Mosby Company, St. Louis.)

phases are completely eliminated, as in the curve *E,* it is called a *complete tetanus*. In a complete tetanus the developed tension may be three to four times that of the single twitch.

STAIRCASE OR TREPPE PHENOMENON

Although this phenomenon has little practical significance, it has achieved a place in the physiological literature related to muscle contraction, and consequently is discussed briefly here. If, in the fresh, rested muscle preparation previously discussed, shocks are presented repetitively, but at intervals that allow complete relaxation to occur for each twitch, each successive twitch or contraction will develop greater tension, until a maximum is reached after some five to ten contractions (fig. 3.4). This increment in tension for the first several contractions is called the *staircase* or *treppe phenomenon* because of the appearance of the kymograph record. This is best explained in terms of a lessening internal resistance factor in the muscle, since it occurs only immediately after rest. It should be pointed out that the entire effect is over in a very short period of time—a fraction of a second, or two or three seconds at most.

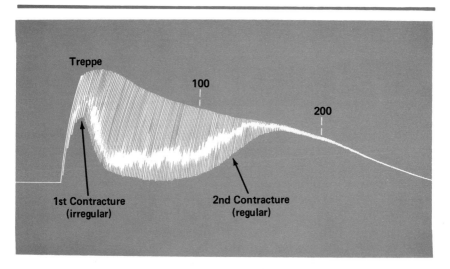

Figure 3-4. Effect of repeated stimulation. The muscle was stimulated electrically at intervals of one second. Note (1) the treppe effect, and (2) the effect of fatigue on the ability of the muscle to "relax." (From Howell. *A Textbook of Physiology,* 11th ed., 1930. Courtesy of W.B. Saunders Company, Philadelphia.)

TEMPERATURE EFFECTS UPON MUSCLE CONTRACTION

The effects of temperature upon intact human muscle have been well demonstrated (17, 18). The contraction time for the human gastrocnemius muscle increases, with cooling by as much as twenty-one to eighty-two percent, depending upon the length of time the muscle is cooled and the temperature drop. The relaxation time under comparable conditions of cooling increases from fifty-one to 150 percent. Heating the muscle, on the other hand, causes small but significant improvements in the speed of contraction (twelve percent) and in the speed of relaxation (twenty-two percent). It should be pointed out that the important factor here is the deep-muscle temperature.

More recent work has corroborated the early work in this area and has provided further elucidation which has practical significance. Petijan and Eagan (12) have shown that exercise induced heating is more effective than is the same amount of passive heating in improving the rate of muscular relaxation after stimulation. Furthermore, they also provided evidence that training induces an increased rate of muscle relaxation after exercise.

It may also be noted that if the gastrocnemius muscle is cooled, the relaxation phase is slowed down two to three times as much as the contraction phase. It has been postulated that this difference may explain poor performance or muscle injury after improper or insufficient warm-up. The rationale for this hypothesis indicates the possibility that a slowly relaxing antagonist may be driven into its relaxation phase by a relatively faster contracting agonist. Thus there would be an opposition of forces of the paired muscles around any given joint, which might result in sore muscles or impaired performance—certainly a reasonable hypothesis.

The author would like to present another equally reasonable hypothesis in this vein. A representative time for one stride in sprinting is approximately 0.4 second, and Tuttle's work (17) indicated a slowing of the total twitch (gastrocnemius) in cooling down to 0.54 second after five minutes and to 0.88 second after twenty minutes of cooling. This indicates the possibility that contraction of the agonist, or prime mover, may occur while the muscle is still in a somewhat contracted condition from the previous stimulation; this results in a summation of contractions without a relaxation phase for the muscle concerned. That this condition may very likely result in contracture or sore muscles will be discussed in detail in a later chapter.

The words of A. V. Hill summarize the effects of temperature. "The speed of everything that can be measured in muscle is diminished two or three times by a fall in temperature of 10° C (7)." Hill also points out that mammalian muscle can be quickened approximately twenty percent by elevating body temperature 2° C., and he suggests that a good runner might do the 100 yards in eight seconds under these conditions.

THE ALL OR NONE LAW

If a muscle fiber (or motor unit) is stimulated by a single impulse at or above threshold value, it responds by a contraction, or twitch, that is maximal for any given set of conditions of nutrition, temperature, etc. In other words, stimulation by impulses much larger than threshold value will result in no increase in either the shortening or the force of contraction. The muscle fiber contracts maximally or it does not contract at all, and this fact is referred to as the *all or none law* of muscle contraction. Obviously, this law applies to the motor unit since all its component fibers are innervated by the same nerve fiber and impulse (it does not, of course, apply to whole muscles).

GRADATION OF RESPONSE

Because of the all or none law for the contraction of motor units and fibers, other explanations must be sought for the fact that whole muscles are capable of exquisitely fine gradation in speed and in force of contraction. The ability of a large muscle to function in providing the force necessary for lifting a maximal weight in weight training and also to thread a needle requires explanation. There are two explanations or methods by which the nervous system brings this about.

First, and probably most importantly, the gradation of muscular effort is brought about by the innervation of varying numbers of the motor units within the whole muscle. A skeletal muscle may consist of several hundred (or well over a thousand in a large muscle) motor units. The size of the impending task is evaluated through sensory channels and an appropriate number of motor units is stimulated to respond to the task. Occasionally an error is made in evaluating the severity of the job, as in lifting a mock bar-bell whose real weight is far less than its size and apparent material indicate. In this event an embarrassingly large number of motor units is brought into play. A similar situation occurs when a weight slips out of grasp in the act of throwing, and the arm is "thrown out" because of the imbalance between the resistance and the muscular effort brought to bear.

The second factor known to operate in grading muscular response is the variation of the frequency of stimulation. Thus innervation in any motor unit is usually in volleys of stimuli or nervous impulses, ranging from several to eighty or ninety per second. In reference to the principle of tetanic contraction, it will be recalled that frequent stimulation, which results in complete tetanus, may increase the tension by as much as four times that of a single twitch. This, then, is the second factor operative in bringing about graded responses. It may seem that this second factor violates the all or none law, but the law applies only to the response of a motor unit to a single stimulus.

These two factors appear to act simultaneously and cooperatively to bring about the very fine gradation in response seen in even the large skeletal muscles.

MUSCLE FATIGUE

It has long been known that when a muscle is caused to contract repeatedly and with very short rest intervals (one to two seconds), a decrement in response can be seen both in the intact muscle and in the excised muscle. Figure 3.4, p. 41, illustrates this fatigue phenomenon in the excised muscle. The first few contractions demonstrate the treppe effect (in a rested muscle); then, after a period of normal contractions, the response of the muscle grows less—both in the contraction and the relaxation phase—until, finally, no visible reaction to further stimulation is obtained.

This should denote several factors of practical importance to the physical educator and the coach. First, the effect upon the relaxation phase is earlier, and larger in magnitude, than the effect upon the contraction phase. This lack of relaxation is referred to as *contracture*, which plays an important role in the discussion of muscle soreness. Second, there is good evidence (11) that at the point of complete fatigue, where no further visible response results from the stimulation, the muscle action potentials are undiminished. This indicates that the nervous transmission of the impulse through the myoneural junction can be absolved of the blame for fatigue. Furthermore, nerve fibers have been found to be practically indefatigable, and thus the site of fatigue would seem to be either in the muscle contractile mechanism or in the coupling of the action potential to the contraction process. Although older work seemed to indict the myoneural junction as the site of fatigue, at least in excised muscle, the finding of undiminished action potentials by Merton (when the muscle is no longer capable of response) is strong evidence to the contrary.

Our discussion refers only to *local muscular fatigue* in one muscle or in one functional muscle group. General fatigue of the entire organism must be considered from a different vantage point, much greater in scope. This will be discussed at greater length in succeeding chapters which will consider fatigue in relation to work load, physical fitness, accumulation of metabolites, and depletion of energy stores.

TYPES OF CONTRACTION

Muscular contraction is an unfortunate term in that it implies shortening. In actuality, innervation of a muscle often results in an expenditure of energy to produce force that is used either in maintaining a held position or in opposing lengthening as a muscle resists a superior force or slows down the effect of gravity. The nomenclature for these various types of muscular contraction is not standard; and therefore, at least three pairs of terms are necessary for the study of exercise physiology.

Isotonic Versus Isometric Contraction. This is the most widely used terminology for differentiating between the shortening contraction, *isotonic* (one level of tension throughout the contraction), and the contraction of holding a position, *isometric* (one length throughout the contraction).

Phasic Versus Static (or Tonic) Contraction. *Phasic* and *static* serve the same purpose and are virtually synonymous with isotonic and isometric.

Concentric Versus Eccentric Contraction. This pair of terms differentiates between shortening and lengthening types of contraction. *Concentric* is synonymous with isotonic contraction. *Eccentric contraction*, however, refers to a situation in which a muscle is innervated and responds with an expenditure of energy to produce force that is less than the opposing outside force; although the muscle tries to shorten, it is actually lengthened during its contraction phase. Examples of this are (*A*) use of the biceps brachii in letting the body down slowly from a chin-up, and (*B*) use of the inward rotators of the humerous in arm wrestling. The loser's inward rotators, although attempting to shorten, have been forced to lengthen by the superior force of the opponent.

It is customary to measure the work output of muscular contraction by the method of the physicist: $W = F \times D$; W is the work done, and F is the force acting through a distance, D. Thus the computation of the workload for isotonic or concentric contraction in lifting a 100-pound weight two feet is $W = 100 \times 2$, or $W = 200$ foot-pounds of work done. In isometric or static contraction, however, since no movement is involved and $D = 0$, no work is done, and all of the energy of muscular contraction goes into the development of heat. In eccentric contraction, where the 100-pound weight is slowly lowered two feet—through the forced stretching of muscles resisting the force of gravity—it is suggested that the same formula be used, and that this work load of 200 foot-pounds be termed negative work.

MECHANICAL FACTORS IN MUSCULAR ACTIVITY

For any given strength and nutritive condition of a muscle, there are at least three very practical considerations for physical educators and coaches regarding the external force that can be produced from that muscle:

1. The angle of pull of the muscle
2. The length of the muscle at any given time
3. The velocity of muscle shortening

Angle of Pull.   This may be described as the angle between the lengthwise axis of the muscle and the lengthwise axis of the bone it is causing to move, angle *a*. In the diagram (fig. 3.5), force triangles are drawn to show the relationship of the internal muscular force exerted (side *B*)

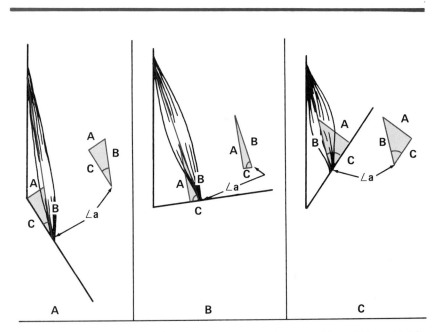

Figure 3-5. Effect of the angle of pull of a muscle upon the external force (A) provided for equal amounts of internal muscular force (B). Side (C) in each case represents wasted internal force.

which is held the same through 3.5A, 3.5B, 3.5C, to the net force available to do the work (side A) and to the wasted force (side C). It is easily seen that there is an optimal value of the angle of pull that is closely approximated by the condition in 3.5B. When the muscle pulls at right angles to the bone it is moving, sides A and B will coincide, and all of the muscle's force becomes available to do useful work. At angles of pull greater or less than the optimal value, the wasted force, side C, becomes larger, and the externally available force, side A, becomes smaller for any given value of muscular effort (side B).

For example, the most difficult points in a chin-up seem to be at the very bottom and top of the exercise which are represented by 3.5A and 3.5C respectively. If a subject is able to start the chin, he can probably get past the midpoint where the angle of pull is favorable, but he will have difficulty in stretching his neck to get over the bar at the top.

Length of Muscle. At any given time during contraction, the length of the muscle determines how much internal force or tension it can generate. It has been demonstrated that in an isolated muscle fiber the ten-

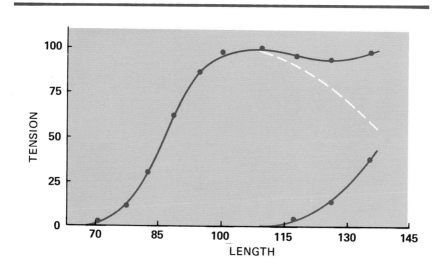

Figure 3-6. Relation between length and tension. One-hundred is rest length and maximum tension. Monotonic increasing curve at lower right represents effect of passive stretch on tension. Upper solid curve is obtained from system as a whole. Broken line represents behavior of contractile elements when passive stretch curve is subtracted from upper curve. (From Zierler, Kenneth L.: Mechanism of muscle contraction and its energetics. In Mountcastle, Vernon B., editor: Medical physiology, ed. 13, St. Louis, The C.V. Mosby Co. [in press].)

sion developed in a tetanus is maximum at the maximum resting length, and decreases with greater and with lesser lengths (15). The same general conditions have been observed in intact skeletal muscle (1).

Thus the principle for physical education is "Put the muscle on stretch to obtain the greatest force of which the muscle is capable." However, it is important to realize that the stretch factor that provides the greatest internal forces may be working at odds with the angle of pull (described above), which determines how much of the internal muscle force will be externally available for useful work. Thus the intelligent analyst of athletic activity must consider the interaction of both factors to achieve the best results.

Velocity of Muscle Shortening. This factor affects the external force available. It has been found that as the speed of shortening increases, the force decreases, in exponential fashion (5). This would indicate that force falls off disproportionately as the speed of contraction increases, and this in turn would dictate an optimum speed for a needed amount of force.

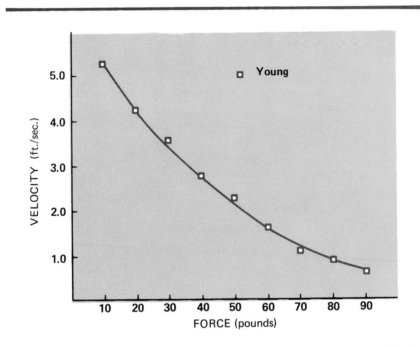

Figure 3-7. Force-velocity relationship in healthy young men. (From Damon, E.L. *An Experimental Investigation of the Relationship of Age to Various Parameters of Muscle Strength,* Doctoral dissertation, Physical Education U.S.C. 1971.)

A. V. Hill (7) believes the optimum speeds for muscular efficiency and power are approximately the same: twenty to thirty percent of the maximum speed at which the muscle can shorten under zero load. Further research is needed to determine how these figures could be applied to power events, such as the shot put.

Improvement of Force and Work Delivery by Dynamic Stretching of Muscle. Cavagna, Dusman, and Margaria (3) have recently provided us with some new concepts in muscle physiology which have direct application to improving athletic performance in certain events. Having found that the efficiency of running was considerably better (forty percent) than that usually calculated for simple ergometer work (twenty-five percent), they looked for the source of this increased efficiency in the possible storage of energy in elastic tissues during negative work which could be released to aid the subsequent positive contraction. Thus in running, as the extended leg strikes the ground, the quadriceps is forced into lengthening to accept the weight of the body and in so doing accumulates elastic energy which is immediately used to augment the following positive work of striding. They found that the maximal positive work (W') done by a muscle shortening immediately after being stretched, is greater than the work (W) done when shortening from a state of isometric contraction, and further found that the improvement represented by the ratio W'/W increases with the speed of stretching and shortening and also with the length of the muscle. Not only is this true for the work produced but the same principle holds true for the force production.

Thus for such events as the discus or the shot put the ultimate results will be better the farther and more rapidly that the preparatory windup is made. This also requires optimal development of flexibility, of course, to achieve.

MUSCLE TONUS

It has probably been customary since time immemorial for one urchin to assess the status of another's musculature by squeezing the biceps, construing a certain degree of hardness as a condition much to be desired and as reflecting a goodly amount of strength. In a sense, this has been an evaluation of what we term muscle tonus in physiology, and palpation of muscles for assessment of tonus may occasionally be used by physicians.

There seems to be agreement that the firmness of a muscle to palpation reflects, to some extent at least, its physiological condition. However, exactly how firmness is brought about is the subject of much research, and we are only beginning to see glimmers of light.

The classic experiments of Sherrington on stretch reflexes (16) resulted in the theory that muscle tonus was the result of a partial tetanus of muscle tissue in which there is a *constant* state of activity by a small portion of the muscle fibers. This constant state of activity was thought to be the result of *myotatic* (stretch reflexes) that originated in the muscle spindles and reflexly innervated the alpha motor neurons (chapter four). Forbes (6) speculated that this muscle tonus was brought about not by constant contraction of the same fibers but by a *rotation of duty* among many different motor units. Thus it was considered that the skeletal muscles were never in a state of complete rest.

By these concepts, postural tonus was the result of a constant feedback mechanism in which a postural muscle was stretched due to slight swaying, and thus muscle spindles were deformed, bringing about afferent impulses to the spinal cord that reflexly innervated the motor units of the stretched muscle to contract. The resulting contraction checked the sway, and balance was restored.

However, with the advent of electromyographic equipment of ultra-high sensitivity pioneered by Jacobson (8) with the help of Bell Telephone Laboratories, it was found that skeletal muscles in relaxed subjects (supine or sitting) could be electrically silent for minutes at a time. Since it was well known that any muscular contraction, no matter how small, is accompanied by muscle action potentials, this required modification of the traditional concept of muscle tonus. The findings of electrical silence in relaxed, resting muscles in man have been corroborated by many other laboratories (although not always with the same rigorous level of sensitivity). Thus Jacobson (8, p. 229), as early as 1938, suggested redefining muscle tonus in skeletal muscles as ". . . meaning a state of slight contraction, more or less constant, or irregular, often present, but *sometimes absent* in health.

In the light of recent research, the most acceptable definition of general muscle tonus is that of Basmajian (2, p. 41):

. . . the general tone of a muscle is determined both by the passive elasticity or turgor of muscular (and fibrous) tissues and by the active (though not continuous) contraction of muscle in response to the reaction of the nervous system to stimuli. Thus, at complete rest, a muscle has not lost its tone even though there is no neuromuscular activity in it.

Resting Muscle Tonus. Over a period of many years, since electromyographic recording of MAPs has become a common laboratory procedure, many investigators have reported electrical silence in relaxed, resting muscles. However, it is an obvious truism that to demonstrate the absence of a physiological phenomenon it is necessary to use equipment that has the capacity to render observable any and all phenomena under consideration. Obviously, the use of a magnifying glass to observe bacteria might result in a false conclusion that no such organisms exist. It must always be considered a more hazardous conclusion to show the absence of an event than its presence.

Seen in this light, most evidence has not been conclusive because of deficiencies in equipment. Investigators have at times been satisfied that electrical silence existed when their sensitivity did not allow detection of anything under fifty microvolts. Furthermore, the use of needle electrodes to find electrical silence is akin to sampling the opinion of only a few persons to predict the outcome of a national election. Obviously, the smaller the sampling the greater the potential error in the conclusion.

Nevertheless, electrical silence has been demonstrated by a few investigators such as Jacobson, whose work is unimpeachable. The conclusion that muscles can indeed be entirely inactive rests upon their work. The author has found that, without special training, ten of twenty-nine physical education students could achieve complete relaxation (electrical silence) in the right quadriceps femoris muscle for a period of two minutes. Under similar conditions, only four of the twenty-nine could achieve electrical silence in the right elbow flexors. Jacobson has demonstrated that the ability to relax voluntarily can be improved by training.

Nothing that has been said should be construed as denying the activity of the neuromuscular system as a participant in general muscle tonus. Electrical silence is achieved only by relaxed subjects, under the best laboratory conditions. How often, how long at a time, or in how many muscles this may occur in everyday activity is quite another question. The best we can say at the present time is that it is possible for some persons to achieve in selected muscles complete relaxation on some occasions and under certain conditions. It is felt that the definition for general muscle tonus stated by Basmajian, and referred to earlier, is the best summation of the present state of our knowledge.

Postural Muscle Tonus. There is little agreement upon the mechanisms of postural tonus, and, more specifically, upon the presence or absence of neuromuscular activity in the extensor muscles involved in maintaining the erect posture in man.

In a comprehensive review of the work done in this area, Ralston (13) and Ralston and Libet (14) concluded that during easy standing there is no electrical activity, even in such postural muscles as the erector spinae, unless the subject sways sufficiently. Kelton and Wright (10) reported long periods of silence during easy standing in all of thirty-eight muscles studied, except only in the tibialis anterior and soleus, and only intermittent activity in them. Their study included such postural muscles as quadriceps femoris, erector spinae in which they apparently found no electrical activity.

On the other hand, Jacobson (9), who used higher sensitivity and integration procedures, was unable to find periods of electrical silence in the anterior tibialis and calf muscle.

Kelton and Wright (10) present evidence that gross movement of a magnitude and velocity much greater than that occurring in the sway of erect posture is needed to bring about *simple* stretch reflexes. This may be so, but in any event corroboration with more sensitive equipment is needed. They postulate maintenance of erect posture by mechanical arrangement of body segments around the gravital line, in such fashion that any support needed is furnished passively by connective tissues.

It seems rather difficult to accept the hypothesis of "hanging on the ligaments" as it were, in anything that approaches normal erect posture. Therefore, the author reinvestigated this question with highly sensitive equipment (4). Table 3.1 shows the results for the postural muscles of the lower leg—the gastro-soleus group and the anterior tibialis. Hghly significant differences were found in muscular activity between resting and easy standing (standing in a very relaxed fashion). Every subject showed a marked increase in both muscles when he changed from the resting (seated position) to the standing position. Furthermore, no convincing evidence of electrical silence was found, even for brief periods, in either muscle in any subject. This agrees completely with the work of Jacobson (9), the only other investigator whose equipment achieved the same sensitivity. It would seem that those who found electrical silence in these muscles did so because of deficiencies in equipment.

Table 3.2 shows the results of a similar experiment in the author's laboratory on the erector spinae muscle. Although other investigators had been unable to find evidence of electrical activity in this muscle, significant differences were again found in all subjects for this muscle when comparing the standing posture with lying prone. The differences between sitting and lying prone were not significant, although even here there were bursts of activity (when sitting) in all subjects.

Occasional but very brief periods of electrical silence were found in some of the eight subjects of Table 3.2. For this reason, an outstanding athlete (four gold medals in Olympic diving) was selected for more intensive study. In repeated, alternating periods of prone rest and easy standing, even this subject was unable to approach electrical silence in

normal posture. Very short periods of electrical silence could be identified
if the subject adopted a position of extreme hyperextension of the spinal

TABLE 3.1

Postural **versus** Resting Tonus in Gastro-soleus and
Anterior Tibialis Muscles
(Mean Microvoltages of 1-minute Integrals
Corrected for Electrical Noise)

Subject	Gastrosoleus		Anterior Tibialis	
	Resting	Easy Standing	Resting	Easy Standing
M. A.	1.02	4.17	0.82	3.72
D. B.	1.38	2.12	0.68	3.27
S. C.	0.0	10.06	0.0	2.24
G. D.	0.0	7.16	0.47	3.57
T. G.	0.32	1.53	0.38	3.44
A. F.	0.0	2.74	0.0	14.70
Y. I.	0.0	2.62	0.50	10.88
L. G.	0.0	3.84	0.0	2.47
S. S.	0.0	12.98	0.0	3.02
C. W.	2.04	7.20	1.12	11.05
Mean	0.48	5.44	0.40	5.84

TABLE 3.2

Postural **versus** Resting Tonus in Erector Spinae Muscle Group
(Mean Microvoltages of 1-minute Integrals
Corrected for Electrical Noise)

Subject	Prone	Sitting	Easy Standing
D. B.	0.0	6.93	8.01
J. D.	5.08	5.19	8.18
A. K.	6.56	14.95	18.55
Y. I.	4.51	10.95	17.55
G. J.	6.66	6.29	8.58
R. S.	5.38	13.85	14.05
B. W.	5.54	5.89	8.00
J. L.	5.32	5.21	7.74
Mean	5.58	8.65	11.32

column, but this was a very abnormal posture and it resulted in palpable tension of the abdominal wall.

The quadriceps femoris and hamstring muscle groups were also investigated. These turned out to be the easiest muscles for most subjects to relax completely. Again, significant differences were found between the electrical output of the resting muscle compared with normal easy standing. The difference was less than one microvolt, however, and would have been completely obscured with equipment that had a basic noise level above 0.3 microvolts which apparently was the case with investigators who have reported electrical silence in these muscles.

In consequence of these experiments (4), it would seem that the traditional concepts of postural tonus are still tenable, and that the more recent research that purports to find electrical silence in postural muscles rests on insufficient evidence from equipment of insufficient sensitivity to justify the conclusions.

Effects of Exercise upon Resting Muscle Tonus.   It has long been thought that one of the benefits of exercise is the improvement of muscle tonus. It has also been observed that the lack of exercise from casting a fractured leg or forced bed rest, results in a degree of flaccidity. Although these statements are probably true, they seem to be unsupported by experimental evidence at this time.

Physiology of Muscle Tonus.   The most logical explanation of muscle tonus, based upon the research cited above, would seem to rest upon a *passive component* and an *active component*.

Passive Component.   The passive component needs little further discussion. It is composed of the elasticity of muscle and connective tissues, plus the tissue turgor, which may be defined as the pressure with which body fluids tend to distend their surrounding tissues. This factor is present regardless of the state of innervation.

Active Component.   The active component rests upon the discussion of the gamma loop discussed in chapter four and is hypothetical in large part. The most logical explanation that encompasses all experimental results is as follows.

1. Muscle tonus rests on a reflex basis.
2. The afferent limb of the reflex arises in the receptor of the muscle spindle and enters the spinal cord, where it synapses directly with the alpha ventral horn cells.
3. A constant facilitation effect is brought about by impulses from subcortical nuclei, reticular substance and vestibular and cerebellar pathways.
4. Firing of the alpha ventral horn cells innervates a small proportion of the motor units in all muscles concerned with posture probably

(although not demonstrably), in rotating fashion, as postulated by Forbes (6).

5. In muscles other than the postural muscles, and if the subject is sufficiently relaxed, complete inactivity may exist at least for short periods of time.

SUMMARY

1. The *myogram* illustrates the contraction of a whole muscle (muscle twitch) when it is artificially innervated by a single stimulus. Its response consists of a *latent period* of 0.001 to 0.01 second, a *contraction phase* of approximately 0.04 second, and a *relaxation phase* of approximately 0.05 seconds.

2. If, during the above *muscle twitch,* a second stimulus occurs, a *summation of contractions* will occur that results in greater tension than either twitch separately.

3. A *tetanus* or *tetanic contraction* results from repeated stimulation of muscle when the intervals between stimuli are too short to allow complete relaxation to occur. If *no* relaxation occurs between stimuli, it is a complete tetanus and the tension developed may be three to four times that of a single twitch.

4. Low muscle temperatures result in slow contraction and relaxation phases, and this effect is relatively much greater in the relaxation phase. High temperatures have a converse effect; and these two facts have important implications for warm-up and the prevention of muscular distress.

5. The *all or none law* states that a muscle fiber (or motor unit) contracts either maximally, or not at all, in response to a single stimulus.

6. *Gradation of response* in muscle tissue is brought about by two methods: (1) innervation of varying numbers of motor units and (2) variation of the frequency of stimulation.

7. The *site of local muscular fatigue* seems to be peripheral, and probably involves either the contractile mechanism itself or the coupling of the muscle action potential to the contractile mechanism—or both.

8. The *external muscular force* available for useful work is the resultant of three component factors: (1) the angle of pull of the muscle, (2) the length of the muscle, (3) the velocity of shortening.

9. Resting muscle tonus is the result of *active* and *passive components.* The active component is due to neuromuscular activity, and is not always present, whereas the passive component is due to tissue pressure and the elastic quality of muscle and connective tissue, and is continuous during the life of the organism.

10. Postural muscle tonus has been shown to have both components in all muscles that are involved in maintaining the erect posture. Investigations that have failed to show the active component probably suffered from deficiencies in equipment.

REFERENCES

1. Banus, M. G., and Zetlin, A. M. 1938. The relation of isometric tension to length in skeletal muscle. *Journal of Cellular and Comparative Physiology* 12:403-20.
2. Basmajian, J. V. 1962. *Muscles alive.* Baltimore: Williams & Wilkins Co.
3. Cavagna, G. A.; Dusman, B.; and Margaria, R. 1968. Positive work done by a previously stretched muscle. *Journal of Applied Physiology* 24:21-32.
4. deVries, H. A. 1965. Muscle tonus in postural muscles. *American Journal of Physical Medicine* 44:275-91.
5. Fenn, W. O., and Marsh, B. S. 1935. Muscular force at different speeds of shortening. *Journal of Physiology* 85:277-97.
6. Forbes, A. 1922. Spinal reflexes. *Physiological Reviews* 2:401.
7. Hill, A. V. 1956. The design of muscles. *British Medical Bulletin* 12:165-66.
8. Jacobson, E. 1938. *Progressive relaxation.* Chicago: The University of Chicago Press.
9. Jacobson, E. 1943. Innervation and tonus of striated muscle in man. *Journal of Nervous and Mental Disease* 97:197-203.
10. Kelton, I. W., and Wright, R. D. 1949. The mechanism of easy standing by man. *Australian Journal of Experimental Biology and Medical Science* 27:505-15.
11. Merton, P. A. 1956. Problems of muscular fatigue. *British Medical Bulletin* 12:219-21.
12. Petajan, J. H., and Eagan, C. J. 1968. Effect of temperature and physical fitness on the triceps surae reflex. *Journal of Applied Physiology* 25:16-20.
13. Ralston, H. J. 1957. Recent advances in neuromuscular physiology. *American Journal of Physical Medicine* 36:94-120.
14. Ralston, H. J., and Libet, B. 1953. The question of tonus in skeletal muscle. *American Journal of Physical Medicine* 32:85-92.
15. Ramsey, R. W., and Street, S. 1940. The isometric length-tension diagram of isolated skeletal muscle fibers of the frog. *Journal of Cellular and Comparative Physiology* 15:11-33.
16. Sherrington, C. S. 1923. *Integrative action of the nervous system.* New Haven: Yale University Press.
17. Tuttle, W. W. 1941. The effects of decreased temperature on activity of intact muscles. *Journal of Laboratory and Clinical Medicine* 26:1913-15.
18. Tuttle, W. W. 1943. The physiologic effects of heat and cold on muscle. *Athletic Journal* 24:45.
19. Wilkie, D. R. 1956. The mechanical properties of muscle. *British Bulletin* 12:177-82.

4 The Nervous System and Coordination of Muscular Activity

The human individual has at his disposal several hundred muscles, each of which may include a thousand or more motor units. Since each of these motor units can be innervated independently, the possibilities for movement are almost unlimited, and the degree to which an individual can organize and integrate his potential movement possibilities into meaningful, efficient patterns determines—to a very large extent—how well he will succeed in the skills of physical education and athletics. Although the nervous system also serves the more important functions of maintaining homeostasis of the internal environment and adjustment to the external environment, the interests of the physical educator and coach center upon the movement aspects, which apply most directly to their profession. For this reason, the discussion in this chapter will provide a background for a better understanding of the principles involved in (A) learning physical education and athletic skills, (B) achieving maximum human performance, and (C) understanding the limitations imposed by the nervous system. Since the student is assumed to have had a basic physiology course, the general organization of the nervous system is covered in somewhat cursory fashion.

THE NEURON AND THE MOTOR UNIT

The *neuron*, a single nerve cell, forms the basic structural unit of the nervous system; it is specialized for its function by having a high degree of irritability and conductivity. There are billions of neurons in the nervous system, and usually several neurons are interconnected by *synapses* to form pathways for conduction of nervous impulses. The neurons that conduct sensory impulses from the periphery to the central nervous system are called *sensory* or *afferent* neurons; the neurons that conduct impulses from the central nervous system to the muscles and other effectors are called *motor* or *efferent* neurons. Although neurons are microscopic in width, one cell may extend in length from the cerebral cortex almost to the caudal end of the spinal column, or an equal distance from the spinal cord to a muscle in the foot, a distance of approximately three feet.

The typical motor neuron (fig. 4.1) has two types of processes from its cell body: (1) *dendrites* which receive impulses and conduct them to the cell body and (2) an *axon* which conducts the impulses away from the cell and accounts for the great length of some neurons. The cell body of the motor neuron, which innervates skeletal muscle, lies in the gray matter in the ventral horn of the spinal cord, and its axon joins many other axons from other motor neurons (also many sensory axons) to form a spinal nerve. This spinal nerve is thick enough to be seen and handled grossly in dissection.

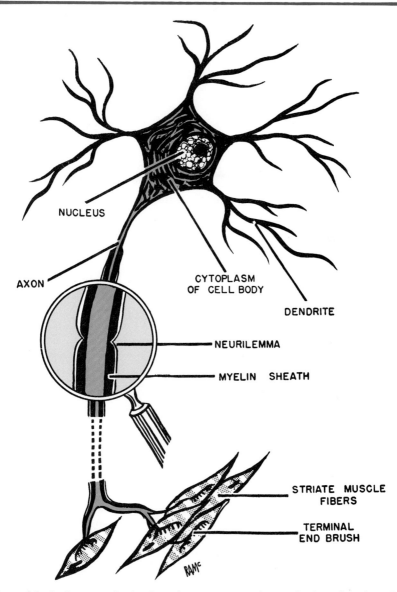

NUCLEUS

AXON

CYTOPLASM
OF CELL BODY

DENDRITE

NEURILEMMA

MYELIN SHEATH

STRIATE MUSCLE
FIBERS

TERMINAL
END BRUSH

Figure 4-1. A diagrammatic drawing of a neuron. At the top is the cell body and its numerous branchings, the dendrites. They make up the soma of the neuron. The axon, of which there is only one, extends downward. The point at which the axon leaves the soma is the axon hillock. Axons, and sometimes dendrites, may be covered with a myelin sheath, and, outside the nervous system, with a neurilemma. (From *Physiological Psychology* by Morgan and Stellar. Copyright 1950. Used by permission of McGraw-Hill Book Company.)

The motor nerve, after entering the muscle through the epimysium, branches and rebranches until one axon enters a fasciculus. The axon then branches into many twigs, each of which innervates one muscle fiber. Thus the cell body in the ventral horn, plus the axon and all its twigs together with the many muscle fibers innervated by the twigs form one *motor unit.*

THE REFLEX ARC AND INVOLUNTARY MOVEMENT

A great deal of muscular activity is accomplished by reflex control. A *reflex* is most simply defined as an involuntary motor response to a given stimulus. An illustration is the automatic, unthinking response to touching a hot surface. In its simplest form, a reflex consists of a discharge from a sensory nerve ending, called a *receptor* or *sensory endorgan,* whose impulses are propagated over the sensory nerve fiber to a *synapse,* or junction, in the spinal cord with a motor neuron. When the motor neuron is stimulated to discharge, impulses are propagated over its axon to the *effector* (muscle or gland), bringing about the reflex response. The sensory pathway is *afferent* and the motor pathway is *efferent.*

This simple reflex arc (fig. 4.2) occurs only in the *myotatic* or stretch reflex, and, since there is only one synapse in the cord, it is called a

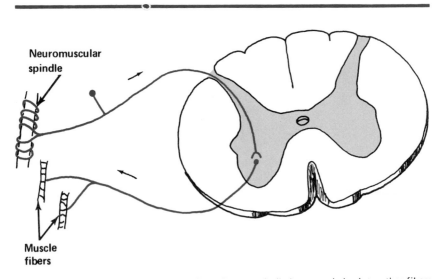

Neuromuscular spindle

Muscle fibers

Figure 4-2. Diagram of a two-neuron reflex—from a spindle in a muscle back to other fibers of the same muscle. Arrows indicate direction of conduction. (From Gardner. *Fundamentals of Neurology,* 1958. Courtesy of W.B. Saunders Company, Philadelphia.)

monosynaptic reflex. Other reflexes, such as the *flexion reflex* (involved in removing the hand from a hot surface), involve at least three neurons and two synapses, and these are called *disynaptic reflexes* for three or *multisynaptic* for four or more neuron arcs (fig. 4.3). The short neuron that serves to connect the sensory and motor neurons in this case is called an *internuncial* or *association* neuron.

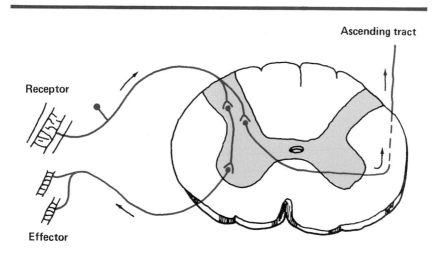

Figure 4-3. Diagram illustrating how impulses from a cutaneous receptor reach an effector (skeletal muscle) by a three-neuron arc at the level of entrance. (From Gardner. *Fundamentals of Neurology,* 1958. Courtesy of W.B. Saunders Company, Philadelphia.)

The preceding discussion is an oversimplification of what actually occurs. For example, in the case of the flexion reflex, in order that it might proceed with dispatch, the antagonistic extensor muscle group must be prevented from acting. This inhibition of the antagonists is accomplished by kinesthetic impulses from the muscle spindles of the flexor muscle and these synapse not only with the flexor motor neuron directly but also, indirectly, with the motor neurons of extensor muscles of the same joint. This process is called *reciprocal inhibition.*

Applying this same flexion reflex to the foot (in stepping on a sharp object), we find that not only does the reflex result in withdrawal of the foot with its concomitant reciprocal inhibition of the extensor muscle of the same leg, but it may also result in the extension of the contralateral (opposite) leg to support the body during the flexion reflex. This action of the contralateral limb is called the *crossed extensor reflex;* it is the result of *facilitation* that is also brought about by action of the afferent neuron from the muscle spindles but upon the motor neuron of the extensor muscles of the opposite limb.

This is still not a complete account of even these simple reflexes, and the interested reader is referred to a text in neurology for further discussion. At this point, it is well to realize that even the simplest reflex involves organization and integration of responses into meaningful movement patterns.

Knowledge of the reflex mechanism of the stretch reflex will greatly facilitate the student's understanding of the scientific principles involved in recent research in flexibility which is discussed in Part 3.

INTERSEGMENTAL AND SUPRASEGMENTAL REFLEXES

Reflexes are not necessarily limited to causing action at the same spinal cord level as the incoming afferent stimulus. For example, in the scratch reflex of the dog, the stimulus (or flea bite) may occur at a level where the afferent part of the reflex arc enters the cord in the upper thoracic area, and the response is brought about by the hind leg muscles, whose efferents leave the cord at the sacral level. The association neuron travels down the dog's spinal cord a considerable distance before synapsing with the motor neuron, which forms the efferent pathway to bring about the scratching response. This is illustrated in figure 4.4 which also shows the possibilities for contralateral responses as well as upward or downward conduction pathways in the spinal cord. Reflexes, that involve more than one spinal segment (or level) are called *intersegmental reflexes.*

So far we have considered only spinal reflexes. When attention is directed to postural mechanisms it is seen that, although these are indeed reflex in that they do not require conscious volitional control, they are abolished in the absence of the centers and pathways of the brain. For example, in a faint, or in anesthesia, postural reflexes fail. The spinal or segmental portion of the reflexes involved in posture may still be elicited with the proper stimulus.

Thus it is apparent that higher brain centers are necessary for postural reflexes, and for this reason we refer to this group of reflexes as *suprasegmental reflexes.* The stretch or myotatic reflex, described above, forms the basic component of the postural reflexes, but it depends upon facilitation from higher centers in order that incoming sensory impulses may achieve threshold value, and thus bring about total postural responses. Furthermore, higher brain centers seem to be necessary to coordinate and control these mechanisms.

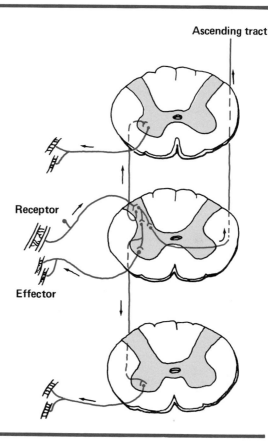

Figure 4-4. Diagram of the connections by which impulses from a receptor reach motor neurons at different cord levels. (From Gardner. *Fundamentals of Neurology,* 1958. Courtesy of W.B. Saunders Company, Philadelphia.)

Ascending tract

Receptor

Effector

OVERVIEW OF THE NERVOUS SYSTEM

The nervous system may be divided in two principal ways. First, we may think of it as divided structurally into *central* and *peripheral* components. The central component consists of the brain and spinal cord, and the peripheral component consists of all the ganglia (groups of nerve cells not in the spinal cord) and nerve fibers (the axons described above). Second, it is divided functionally into the *somatic* and *autonomic* systems, and both systems have central as well as peripheral components. The autonomic system controls the internal environment, and innervates the smooth muscles of the gastrointestinal tract, the blood vessels, etc., as well as the endocrine glands.

The autonomic system has two divisions: (1) the *sympathetic division,* whose central outflow is from the thoracic and lumbar regions of the spinal cord, and (2) the *parasympathetic division,* which originates in the cranial nerves and in the sacral region of the spinal cord. In a very general way, these two divisions of the autonomic system are antagonistic, and balance each other. The sympathetic has to do with "fight or flight" adjustments of the organism to a dangerous situation, to the stress of sport, etc. The parasympathetic, on the other hand, is related in a general way to vegetative functions, such as digestion.

The *somatic system* consists of the central and the peripheral components of the nervous system that have to do with peripheral reception of nervous impulses, conduction to the spinal cord or brain, organization of motor patterns, and conduction back to the skeletal muscles to bring about the desired movements. The remainder of this chapter will deal with the somatic system.

PROPRIOCEPTION AND KINESTHESIS

For the effective coordination of motor patterns to take place in the brain and spinal cord, a constant supply of sensory information must be available to feed back the results of movement as it progresses. This feedback of sensory information about movement and body position is termed *proprioception.* The receptors for proprioception are of two types: vestibular and kinesthetic.

The *vestibular receptors* are found in the nonauditory labyrinths of the inner ear. Each of these two labyrinths, one on each side in the temporal bone of the skull, consists of a small chamber, the *vestibule,* which communicates with three small canals known as *semicircular canals* (fig. 4.5). Within the semicircular canals is a fluid called *endolymph.*

The inertia of the endolymph which results in its remaining stationary at the first part of a movement of the body and also its continued movement when the body has returned to a resting position, causes disturbance of a sensory receptor organ, the *crista.* This disturbance is transmitted to the brain by way of the vestibular branch of the eighth cranial nerve. Thus the sensory information from the cristae of the semicircular canals provides the data regarding movement, and, more specifically rotational acceleration or deceleration of movement as in twisting or tumbling. Movement in itself is not recognized; for example, moving at almost the speed of sound in an airliner produces no sensation, unless a change of direction or velocity occurs.

Along with the semicircular canals, the *utricle* and *saccule* of the vestibule complete the vestibular system. Apparently, the saccule has little if any function in equilibrium or position sense; it seems to be involved in sensory perception of vibration only. The utricle, however

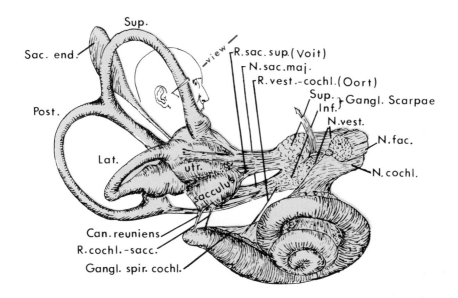

Figure 4-5. Drawing showing structural relations of innervation of the human labyrinth (by Max Brodel). (From *The Anatomical Record* 59:403-18, 1934.)

is the sense organ that provides the data necessary for positional sense. The *otolith organ* in the utricle responds to linear acceleration and to tilting, and thus seems to be the source of data that informs us of our posture in space.

Although no sensation of movement is engendered in a passenger in an airliner (in smooth air), the *orientation* of the body in space is clearly recognized, even with the eyes closed; for instance, in standing upright or lying down. This recognition of spatial orientation is the result of interpretation of sensory information received from the otolith organ in the utricle.

The kinesthetic sense and its receptors are of even greater interest. At least five types of receptors serve the muscle sense, or *kinesthesis*: (1) the muscle spindle[1] (2) the Golgi tendon organ, (3) the pacinian corpuscle, (4) Ruffini Receptors, and (5) free nerve endings. It has long been known that these receptors provide the individual with muscle sense. The individual can tell what his limbs or body segments are doing, at any given time, without having to look. For instance, the nor-

1. Spindle afferents, although extremely important in their sensory input to reflex behavior, do not contribute to subjective sensations.

mal individual has no difficulty making accurately controlled movements, such as bringing his finger from arm's length to touch the end of his nose, even when blindfolded. Furthermore, he can usually make reasonably accurate guesses as to the weight of an object by lifting it (see fig. 4.6).

This muscle sense or kinesthesis, as it is properly called, is important in providing sensory information for skilled movement; however, recent research indicates that this system, particularly the muscle spindle and its attendant nerve supply, may be even more important in functioning as *autogenetic governors of motor-nerve* activity (7). The muscle spindles have their own motor-nerve system, which is important enough to constitute about one-third of the total efferent fibers that enter skeletal muscle (18).

Therefore, let us consider the muscle spindle first, and in some detail (fig. 4.7, p. 68). The spindle is large enough to be visible to the naked eye, and it is fusiform—as the name implies. That muscle spindles are widely distributed throughout muscle tissue is clearly illustrated by the large number of efferent fibers that serve them. However, the distribution is quite different from muscle to muscle. In general, the muscles used for complex movements (such as finger muscles) are abundantly supplied, with up to thirty spindles per gram of muscle while muscles involved in only very gross movements such as latissimus dorsi may have only one to two per gram. In some of the cranial muscles no spindles were found (2).

Each spindle consists of a connective tissue sheath four to ten millimeters long that contains from five to nine *intrafusal muscle fibers* (IF) in mammalian tissue. These IF fibers are quite different from the typical fibers (extrafusal or EF) of muscle described in chapter one which are involved in bringing about gross muscle contraction. Spindle structure

---

Figure 4-6. Schema of the innervation of mammalian skeletal muscle based on a study of cat hindlimb muscles. Those nerve fibres shown on the right of the diagram are exclusively concerned with muscle innervation; those on the left also take part in the innervation of other tissues. Roman numerals refer to the groups of myelinated (I, II, III) and unmyelinated (IV) sensory fibres: Greek letters refer to motor fibres. The spindle pole is cut short to about half its length, the extracapsular portion being omitted. b.v., blood vessel; c., capsule; epi., elimysium; ex.m.f., extrafusal muscle fibres; n.b.m.f., nuclear-bag muscle fibre; n.c.m.f., nuclear-chain muscle fibre; n.s., nodal sprout; m.e.p., motor end-plate; P, primary ending; p_1, p_2, two types of intrafusal end-plates; peri., perimysium; pf.c., paciniform corpuscle; S, secondary ending; tr., trail ending; vsm., vasomotor fibres. (From Barker (1973) in *Handbook of Sensory Physiology,* Vol. III, pt. 2. Courtesy of Springer-Verlag: Berlin, Heidelberg, New York.)

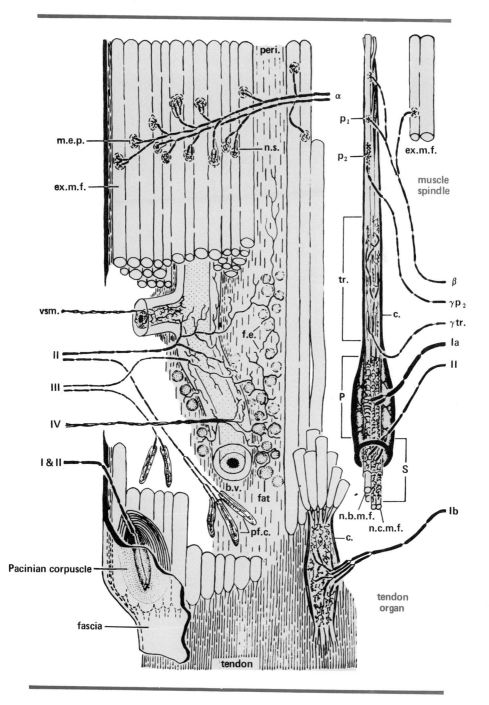

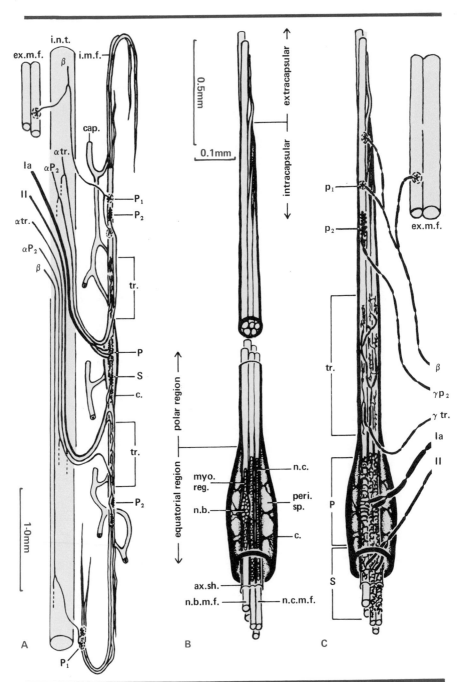

Figure 4-7. Schematic diagrams illustrating the structure and innervation of the mammalian muscle spindle as found in cat hindlimb muscles. *A* shows the general proportions of the receptor; the ends of the poles are curled round so as to fit into the figure. *B* shows the morphology of the equatorial region and about half of one pole, and the same figure is used in *C* with the addition of the sensory and motor innervation. ax.sh., axial sheath; c., capsule; cap., capillary; ex.m.f., extrafusal muscle fibres; i.m.f., intrafusal muscle fibres; i.m.t., intramuscular nerve trunk; myo.reg., myotube region; n.b., nuclear bag; n.c., nuclear chain; n.b.m.f., nuclear-bag muscle fibre; n.c.m.f., nuclear-chain muscle fibre; P, primary ending; p_1, p_2, two types of intrafusal motor end-plates; peri.sp., periaxial space; S, secondary ending; tr., trail ending. Sensory nerve fibres indicated by Roman numerals, motor fibres by Greek letters. (From Barker (1973) in *Handbook of Sensory Physiology,* Vol. III, pt. 2. Courtesy of Springer-Verlag: Berlin, Heidelberg, New York.)

is shown in figure 4.6 and 4.7. It is important to note that the spindles are always oriented parallel to the EF fibers. There are two types of IF fibers:

1. Usually there are two *nuclear bag* fibers which are thicker and longer and in which as many as a dozen crowed nuclei occupy the middle section of the fiber.
2. From three to seven *nuclear chain* fibers so named because their nuclei, although also in the midsection, are fewer in number and are arranged in single file because the fiber is thinner as well as shorter.

At each end of the IF fiber are the motor poles which are the contractile elements composed of striated myofibrils.

The sensory end-organs within the spindles are of two types, the *annulo-spiral endings* (also called primary ending) and the *flower spray ending* (also called secondary ending). The large annulo spiral type Ia afferent nerve axon (only one per spindle) sends individual twigs to wrap around the middle of each nuclear bag fiber and other less well developed spiral terminals to most of the nuclear chain fibers. The flower spray endings are so named because they arborize in spray-like formation from a smaller afferent nerve fiber (type II) and wrap themselves around nuclear chain fibers almost exclusively. There may be one or two flower spray endings per spindle and they attach not at the nuclear area but at one or both sides of it in the transition zone between the motor pole and the nuclear area.

Both of these endings are deformed by stretching of the intrafusal fibers. Since these intrafusal fibers lie lengthwise, parallel with the skeletal (extrafusal) fibers, an externally applied stretch results in stretching the intrafusal as well as the extrafusal fibers. The consequent deformation of the annulo spiral ending evokes an afferent discharge in its large, type Ia sensory nerve (fast-conducting); simultaneously, the flower spray ending discharges into its type II sensory nerve (slower conducting). This afferent discharge from the spindle results in a motor response: contraction of the muscle that was stretched. This response, called a *stretch* or *myotatic reflex,* is typified by the tendon jerk elicited by the physician when he strikes the patellar tendon.

The annulo spiral ending responds to both phasic and static stretching whereas the flower spray ending responds to static stretch but is relatively insensitive to phasic stretch (4).

The Golgi tendon organ (fig. 4.6, p. 67), a somewhat simpler end-organ, is found in the musculotendinous junction, and throughout the perimysial connective tissues. It should be noted that this ending is in series with the skeletal muscle fibers, and therefore is deformed by tension in the tendon whether by passive stretching or by active shortening of the muscle. It therefore discharges under both conditions, whereas the spindle discharges only when stretched. The spindle ceases to fire when contraction begins because it is in parallel with the extrafusal muscle fibers, and is thus unloaded as soon as the extrafusal fibers shorten in contraction (see figure 4.8).

A further difference in function between the spindle and the tendon organ is that the spindle facilitates—indeed, may cause—contraction, whereas the tendon organ seems to be a protective device, inhibitory not only to its muscle of origin but to the entire functional muscle group as well (24). The stretch reflex that originates in the muscle spindles is the basis for unconscious muscular adjustments of posture where a slight stretching of the extensor muscles at the knee, for instance, is immediately corrected by reflex shortening to prevent collapse. The tendon reflex that prevents overstressing of the tissues is called the *inverse myotatic reflex.* Granit (7) points out that "the muscle machine is working under self-regulation from autogenetic governors, first aiding it to contract, then damping the discharge from its motoneurons."

The pacinian corpuscle is a large encapsulated end-organ, made up of several layers of fibrous tissue in which nerve endings ramify. These receptors, although widely distributed throughout the body, do not lie within the muscle tissue proper. They are found concentrated in the region of the joints and in the sheaths of tendons and muscles, and consequently are pressed upon when muscles contract. They are excited by the deformation of deep pressure, and may be more important than the spindles and tendon organs in detecting passive movement or position of a body segment in space.

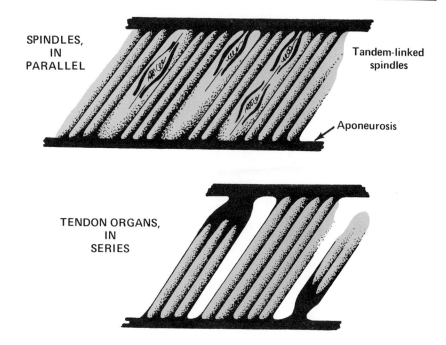

SPINDLES,
IN
PARALLEL

Tandem-linked
spindles

Aponeurosis

TENDON ORGANS,
IN
SERIES

Figure 4-8. The principle of "in series" and "in parallel" arrangement of muscle receptors with reference to extrafusal (non-spindle) muscle fibers. Spindles lie between muscle fibers, either with both poles ending in interfascicular connective tissue, with one pole attached to a tendon, or in some short muscles with both poles inserting into muscle tendons or aponeuroses. In muscles with long extrafusal fascicles, several spindles may be linked in tandem by one or more long intrafusal fibers that pass from one capsule to another. This histological distinction of series and parallel arrangements has a physiological counterpart in response characteristics of the afferent during contractions. (From Eldred, E. *Am. J. Phy. Med.* 46:83, 1967. Courtesy of the Williams and Wilkins Company, Baltimore, Md.)

Ruffini receptors are scattered throughout the collagenous fibers of joint capsules and are differentially activated by joint movement. Consequently, they are probably most important in sensing joint position and motion. As can be seen in figure 4.9 (p. 72) each individual receptor ending monitors a well-defined and restricted range of the total movement. The sensing of the complete movement is thus the result of integration by the nervous system of the bits and pieces of information provided by the many Ruffini receptors.

Unmyelinated, free nerve endings are thought to be widely distributed through muscles, tendons, joints, fascia, and ligaments, but the only

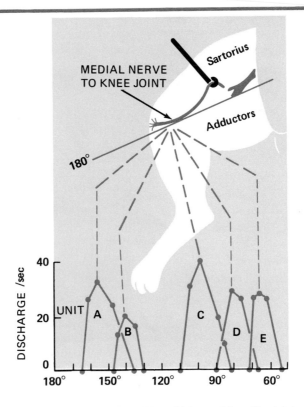

Figure 4-9. "Range fractionation" in signalling of joint position. Five joint receptor units were isolated from the medial nerve to the knee joint of the cat. Each unit discharged only over a restricted range of knee positions and had a maximum at one fairly sharply defined point. The discharge was constant at a stable position of the joint, but became elevated during movements within the response range for that unit. (From Eldred, E. and adapted from S. Skoglund. *Am. J. Phy. Med.* 46:69, 1967. Courtesy of the Williams and Wilkins Company, Baltimore.)

definite histological information seems to indicate their distribution to these tissues is not direct but indirect—by serving the blood vessels that supply these tissues. Their function as kinesthetic receptors is also largely unknown.

In sumary, proprioception involves sensing five aspects of muscle status:

1. *Active contraction,* by the tendon organ discharge
2. *Passive stretch,* by spindle discharge only since tendon-organ threshold is high
3. *Tension,* by tendon-organ discharge

4. *Position*, by discharge of Ruffini receptors
5. *Pressure sensation* from Pacinian corpuscles

Kinesthesis rests largely on the last two elements of proprioception.

THE ALPHA AND GAMMA SYSTEMS FOR MUSCULAR CONTROL

Recent evidence has shown that approximately a third of all the efferent nerve fibers that enter a muscle have no connection with skeletal, extrafusal muscle fibers (18); rather, these nerve fibers have been demonstrated to innervate the intrafusal fibers of the muscle spindles (described on page 66). The importance of this has been suggested, and it is of practical significance to understanding muscular control. The smaller motor-nerve fibers that make up this one-third of the total efferent nerve fibers are called *gamma efferent fibers*, in contrast to *alpha efferent fibers* which are larger, and are the motor-nerve fibers for the extrafusal or skeletal muscle fibers.

In figure 4.10 the myonosynaptic response to stretch can be traced as follows:

1. Stretching the main muscle fibers of the quadriceps results in stretching the muscle spindle and its intrafusal fibers.
2. The annulospiral nerve ending in the intrafusal fibers is distorted and causes propagation of nervous impulses to the cord via the large Ia spindle afferent.
3. The large spindle afferent synapses directly with the large alpha efferent which brings about muscular contraction (stretch reflex) of the quadriceps.

It will also be noted in figure 4.10 that the flower spray receptor activates its smaller, slower conducting type II afferent which goes through an internuncial neuron to end in an inhibitory synapse with the alpha motor neuron pool. Activation of the flower spray ending also brings about a facilitating effect on the alpha motor neuron going to the antagonistic flexor muscle shown as the hamstring group in the diagram. Typically, the flower spray ending, if it is in an extensor muscle, facilitates contraction of the antagonistic flexors and inhibits its own extensor muscle. When this ending lies in a flexor, it helps to bring about the stretch reflex or shortening of the flexor. Threshold for stimulation of the flower spray ending is much higher so the action is usually controlled by the annulospiral ending until stretch is of considerable magnitude.

As the extrafusal fibers contract, the intrafusal fibers in the spindle go slack (see fig. 4.11); thus the deformation of the annulospiral ending

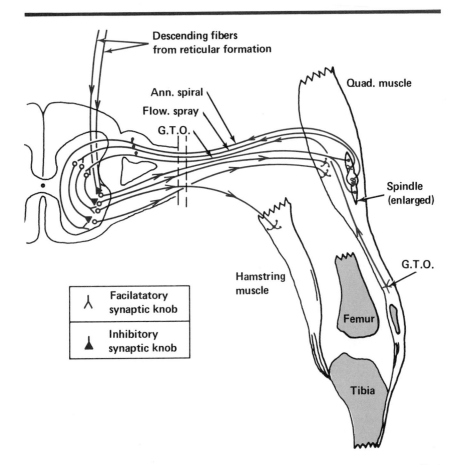

Figure 4-10. The myotatic and inverse myotatic reflexes as "autogenetic governors" of movement at the knee joint. Note that supraspinal influence, both facilitatory and inhibitory is brought to bear on the gamma efferent neuron thus setting the bias of the spindle.

is relieved, and consequently the innervation of the large spindle afferent ceases, and the stretch reflex is over. In voluntary movement, however, the situation is somewhat more complex. As the extrafusal fibers contract, the intrafusal fibers are innervated by their motor nerves, the gamma efferents, which causes a shortening of the intrafusal fibers and a consequent resetting of the spindle length, as it were, so that they are again (and constantly) sensitive to any stretching of spindles. Thus a system is set up in which the innervation of the intrafusal fibers sensitizes the spindle, and the spindle firing causes more contraction of the

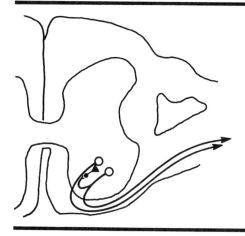

Figure 4-11. The Renshaw internuncial neuron or Renshaw cell is the short interneuron with the inhibitory synaptic knob which is activated by a recurrent collateral from an alpha motor nerve.

extrafusal fibers. This is an alternative method for initiating movement and provides the feedback information as to *length* of the muscle.

One other system (fig. 4.11) should also be noted. When the alpha efferent neuron fires, a recurrent axon collateral is also innervated, which synapses with an internuncial neuron in the cord called a *Renshaw cell* which has the property of synapsing with and inhibiting other motoneurons. This system constitutes what is termed a *feedback loop*. In other words, the fact that the alpha neuron is initiating contraction in the main muscle is *fed back* and is used to inhibit other muscle fibers from making the contraction too strong. This is negative feedback, in that action tends to limit itself from getting out of control. The process by which a physiological (or mechanical) mechanism controls itself by feeding back information that reflexly governs the action is called a *servomechanism*.

Another factor enters into the reflex control of muscular movement. It will be recalled from our discussion of kinesthetic receptors that the Golgi tendon endings are also sensitive to stretch. The response, however, is inhibitory in nature; and good evidence is available that these endings inhibit not only the muscle from which the afferent impulse arises but the entire functional muscle group (24). The tendon endings have a higher threshold to stretch than the spindles, and consequently do not fire until considerably more force is expended. However, they are very sensitive to tension brought about by active contraction of the muscle fibers with which they are in series. Even one-tenth gram of force results in impulse propagation from the Golgi Tendon Organ (GTO). Consequently, the GTO is thought to be important in providing feed back information with respect to tension produced by the muscle. It must also be considered important as a peripheral source of inhibition to protect the muscle against too great an overload.

As has been pointed out by investigators in this area such as Granit (8), Holmgren and Merton (17) and Mountcastle (25), muscles seem to be controlled by a system of *autogenetic governors*. Muscular activity seemingly may be initiated by either the alpha or gamma efferents, and a constant feedback of information by the muscle spindles and tendon organs provides the central nervous system with the data needed to control the movement as it progresses. The spindles are, in the words of Granit, "the private measuring instruments of the muscle's servomechanisms. They do not record length so much as differences in length between the extrafusal muscle fibers and intrafusal fibers of the spindles. The tendon organs apply the brakes to muscular contraction to prevent the development of too great a tensile force, which could result in injury to muscle and or tendon.

As has been pointed out in earlier discussions, the motoneurons are affected by impulses that impinge upon them from the higher centers of the brain and brain stem. In the light of the evidence presently available (5, 8, 9), it would seem that after the cerebral cortex has decided upon the movement to be made, the cerebellum arranges the pathway by the straight route of the large fiber alpha efferents or through the small fiber gamma efferent system. The work of Granit and Kaada (8) indicates that the gamma efferent system is tonically activated from central regions, such as the diencephalic reticular system, the motocortex, and the anterior lobe of the cerebellum. This tonic activity of the gamma efferents results in a degree of tonus in the muscle spindles, which in turn tonically innervates the large spindle afferents for postural reflexes, resulting in postural tonus of the extensor muscle groups throughout the body.

Furthermore, the stretch reflex has some very interesting qualities for muscle stretching in developing flexibility or warming-up athletes. There is very good evidence that the stretch reflex has two components, one of which is the result of phasic (jerky) stretching and the other the result of static (maintained) stretch (18, 22, 25). The phasic response seems to be faster and stronger, and typified by synchronous discharges of the spindles, whereas the static response is slower and weaker, and typified by a synchronous discharge of the spindles.

From the practical standpoint, then, we may say that the *amount* and *rate* of response of a stretch reflex are proportional to the *amount* and *rate* of stretching. In other words, the use of bouncing or jerky movements in stretching will cause the muscle to contract with a vigor proportional to that of the bouncing and jerking. It is rather obvious that this is not desirable either in warming-up cold muscles for athletic participation or in work that is designed to improve flexibility.

There is also a difference between the stretch reflexes of the flexor and extensor muscles. The phasic component of the reflex is well developed in both, but the static stretch component is well defined only in the extensors, where it is needed for the sustained muscular activity of maintaining posture.

It would seem intelligent for the physical educator and coach to apply known principles. If it be desired to loosen up, lengthen, or relax muscle tissue, the use of a sustained pull on the muscle would tend to eliminate the phasic component of the stretch reflex, and the pull should be of sufficient force to reach the threshold of the tendon organs or flower spray endings; this will then initiate the inverse myotatic reflex, which will inhibit the muscle under stretch and thus further aid in stretching the muscle.

Other areas where these reflex patterns have application come to mind. It seems reasonable to believe for example, that the upper limits of muscle strength and power must be set by the level of inhibition brought about centrally by the Renshaw cell and peripherally by the Golgi tendon organ and the flower spray endings. Learning to disinhibit may be an important part of strength training!

In the light of the preceding discussion it is easy to see how muscle cramp can be brought about by making a maximally vigorous contraction of a muscle in a shortened position. You may demonstrate this to your satisfaction by making a maximal contraction of the fully flexed biceps. What happens is that in the shortened position, no tension can be placed on the tendon organ (see the length tension diagram in chapter three p. 47). So we have maximum innervation with minimal inhibition and the result in a large percentage of trials is cramping. Fortunately, you can apply your new found knowledge to also relieve the cramp by simply forcing the muscle into its longest position thereby creating tension in the tendon and the Golgi tendon organ with resulting inhibition which relieves the cramp.

HIGHER NERVE CENTERS AND MUSCULAR CONTROL

So far the discussion of muscular control has centered about the involuntary reflex systems; now we will consider the voluntary control of muscular activity by the brain. It will be convenient to consider this in three parts: (A) the *pyramidal system*, (B) the *extrapyramidal system*, and (C) the *proprioceptive-cerebellar system*. Although much is known about the function of the brain in controlling muscular activity, a much greater portion awaits further research. Furthermore, a complete discussion of what is known of the motor functions of the brain is beyond the scope of this text and unnecessary for its purposes. Therefore, the discussion is somewhat brief and is confined to those aspects that are of interest to the physical educator.

The Pyramidal System.   The cerebral cortex has been mapped out in fair detail, over a period of time, by two methods: (1) by relating clinically observed motor defects with the lesions seen in surgery and autopsies, and (2) by electrical stimulation of the cortex of experimental animals and observation of the resulting motor effects. This research has resulted in cytoarchitectural maps of the human cortex. The most commonly used map is that of Brodmann, and our areas of interest are shown in figure 4.12.

The pyramidal system originates in large nerve cells, shaped like pyramids, that lie mainly in area four of the cortex. It had once been thought

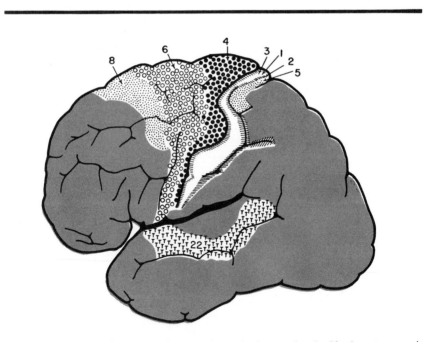

Figure 4-12. Diagram of the areas of the human cerebral cortex involved in the extrapyramidal system. In the frontal lobe are areas 4, 6, and 8. In the postcentral region are areas 3, 1, 2, and 5. Down in the temporal lobe, area 22 is concerned in the extrapyramidal pathways. (From *Physiological Psychology* by Morgan and Stellar. Copyright 1950. Used by permission of McGraw-Hill Book Company.)

that the giant Betz cells were the entire source of the pyramidal tracts, but recent research has indicated they are only about two percent of the total motoneurons of the pyramidal system. The axons from the moto-neuron cell bodies in area four form large descending motor pathways, called *pyramidal tracts,* that go directly (in most cases) to synapses with the motor neurons in the ventral horn of the spinal cord with which we have already dealt. The neurons whose cell bodies are in the brain are commonly called *upper motor neurons,* and those in the spinal cord are called *lower motor neurons.* Seventy to eighty-five percent of the nerve fibers of the pyramidal tract cross from one side to the other; some at the level of the medulla, others at the level of the lower motoneuron.

Area four of the cortex is also referred to as the *motor cortex,* or be-cause of its location, as the *precentral gyrus.* The mapping of the motor cortex clearly demonstrates a neat, orderly arrangement of stimulable areas. It is of interest that the area of cortex devoted to a given body part is not proportional to the amount of tissue served but rather to the complexity of the movement potential of the body part. It has been shown that the hands and the muscles of vocalization involve a dispro-portionate share of motoneurons.

It should be pointed out that the motor cortex is oriented by *move-ment,* not by *muscle.* That is, stimulation of the motor cortex results not in a muscle twitch of one muscle but in a smooth, synergistic movement of a group of muscles.

The Extrapyramidal System. The extrapyramidal system has its origin mainly in area six according to Brodmann's nomenclature. This area is rostral to area four, the motor area, and is sometimes called the *pre-motor cortex.* Good evidence, however, indicates that some of the fibers descending in the extrapyramidal tracts also originate with cell bodies in other areas, notably areas eight and five and also in areas three, one and two which are usually considered the sensory areas for somesthetic impulses.

The descending tracts that are composed of the axons from the neurons of the premotor cortex are considerably more complex. These fibers do not go directly to synapses with the lower motoneurons, but by way of relay stations, which are called *motor nuclei.* The most important nuclei are: (A) *corpus striatum,* (B) *substantia nigra,* and (C) *red nu-cleus.* Some fibers also go by way of the pons to the cerebellum.

For the physical educator, the most important differences between the pyramidal and extrapyramidal systems are the functional differences. Whereas electrical stimulation of area four produces *specific movements,* stimulation of area six produces only large, general *movement patterns.* Consequently, it is believed that learning a new skill in which conscious attention must be devoted to the movements (as in learning a new dance step, where every movement is contemplated) involves area four. As skill progresses (the dancer no longer concentrates on his feet but rather on very general patterns of movement, so that he can interpret the music better), the origin of the movement is thought to shift to area six. However, area four still participates as a relay station, with fibers connecting area six to area four.

The Proprioceptive-cerebellar System. We have already dealt with some of the sensory functions of this system, namely, the proprioceptive system concerned with kinesthesis and vestibular function. In general, the pathway of vestibular proprioception leads to the cerebellum, either directly or by way of the vestibular nucleus in the medulla. Of the fibers that conduct kinesthetic information, some go to the thalamus and cortex to provide sensory knowledge of movement at the conscious level. Others go to the cerebellum. The confluence of sensory data on position, balance, and movement upon the cerebellum is indicative of the importance of this organ to movement.

The cerebellum rivals the cerebral cortex in complexity, but unfortunately, it is not so well understood. Removal of the cerebellum of experimental animals results in a loss of function that has three distinct components: (A) impairment of volitional movements, (B) disturbances of posture, and (C) impaired balance control. Consequently, its functions may be deduced. Without entering into anatomical detail we may say that the cerebellum receives constant sensory information from receptors in muscles, joints, tendons, and skin; and also from visual, auditory, and vestibular end-organs.

Despite all this sensory reception, however, no conscious sensation is aroused in the cerebellum; this function is served by the sensory cortex of the cerebral hemispheres. The cerebellum is intimately connected with the motor centers, from the motor cortex all the way to the spinal cord, and may be considered to modify muscular activity from the beginning to the end of a movement pattern.

POSTURE, BALANCE, AND VOLUNTARY MOVEMENT

It is now appropriate to consider how all of the foregoing discussion relates to a better understanding of human muscular activity which is the purpose of this text.

Posture. Human upright posture is mainly brought about through suprasegmental reflexes. The major part of these suprasegmental reflexes is the basic stretch, or myotatic reflex which has been described; let us therefore direct our attention to the postural mechanism that occurs about the knee joint. If the joint starts to collapse (flex) immediately as the muscle spindles of the quadriceps are stretched, an impulse is generated that is propagated over large afferents to the cord where synapse is made with a motoneuron which innervates fibers in the quadriceps to contract and thus reextend the joint into its proper position. This reflex, however, occurs only in the presence of facilitation by the vestibular nucleus in the medulla, whose fibers in the cord tend to maintain a state of excitation of the motoneurons innervating the muscles, so that a relatively small afferent impulse can reach threshold value. Furthermore, postural reflexes also depend upon effects of the extrapyramidal system and the autogenetic governor system (described earlier) to bring about smoothly coordinated contraction of the proper strength.

Balance. This aspect of muscular activity is best discussed by reference to the *righting reflex,* which illustrates the underlying principles rather well. If one drops a cat from a small height in supine position (upside down), observations can be made of the sequential events that invariably lead to its righting and landing upon all four feet. The first reaction is a turning of the head toward the floor in the attempt to normalize the sensations coming from the otolith organs which inform him he is not oriented in space as he would wish to be. This turning of the head innervates muscle spindles, tendon receptors, and other nerve endings in the neck muscles, that initiate kinesthetic impulses that reflexly bring about the execution of a half twist usually long before the cat hits the ground.

As the cat turns right side up, its visual receptors bring the necessary sensory data to the cerebellum for organization of muscle activity in the extensors, to bring about a gradual acceptance of the force involved in landing. As the cat lands, the force that flexes the legs invokes the stretch reflex in the extensors and if the cat was an unwilling subject the muscles of propulsion will already be underway. These principles apply equally well in diving, trampolining, and all other activities in which balance is a factor.

Voluntary Movement. Let us now take a very simple voluntary movement and analyze the neural activity involved in bringing it about. Assume the right arm is at the side-horizontal position and the desired movement is to bring the right index fingertip to the end of the nose. Since this is not a usual movement, it will probably originate in the arm area of area four of the motor cortex and proceed by way of the pyramidal tracts to synapse with the lower motoneuron in the cord and out to the appropriate muscles by way of the brachial plexus. At the same time, kinesthetic impulses traverse the afferent pathways to the cerebellum and bring about the proper control and coordination so that the shoulder muscles are activated to support the arm as it is moved through horizontal flexion adduction.

Furthermore, the same kinesthetic impulses act reflexly at the segmental level to relax the antagonists through reciprocal inhibition, and the gamma efferent system is busy all the while innervating the muscle spindles so that constant measurements of the progress of the movement can be fed back. As the movement accelerates, more and more motor units are innervated and the rate of impulse transmission to each motor unit increases, with each motor unit participating at the proper time in the sequential development of the movement (1). Finally, the movement has to be decelerated in reverse fashion.

This may seem rather complex, but this discussion is really a superficial treatment of a relatively simple movement. Highly skilled movements made every day in the gymnasium may be infinitely more complex, and may defy detailed analysis.

PRACTICAL CONSIDERATIONS

Much of the discussion in this chapter has been technical; however, an understanding of the foregoing material can be of value in very practical situations in physical education and coaching. Some of these situations will now be considered.

Effects of Hypnosis and Emotional Excitement upon Performance. It is well known that emotional excitement can greatly increase muscular strength and endurance. Every coach and athlete is aware of the improvement of performance in the game situation, compared with that under practice conditions. Upon occasion, however, a coach may also see examples of a decrement in performance due to overexcitability of a young, inexperienced athlete.

Explanations of these phenomena rest upon a knowledge of the neural factors involved (as well as humoral factors, to be discussed later). Gellhorn (6) explains improved performance during emotional excitement in terms of an excitation of the hypothalamus that accompanies excitement. He cites studies that have shown that hypothalamic stimulation (which by itself does not elicit muscular movement) increased the intensity of a cortically induced movement, and also increased the complexity of the induced activity. Furthermore, many muscles that were not activated by cortical stimulation alone became active, and even activity in other extremities was noted. Gellhorn attributes these effects to summation processes that take place at two sites:

1. In the spinal cord, as the result of the interaction of the subthreshold

extrapyramidal discharges from the hypothalamus and of the efferent discharges from the motor cortex.

2. In the motor cortex itself, due to the intensification of pyramidal discharges as the result of hypothalamic-cortical discharges (5).

This discussion serves to explain both the commonly seen improvement and the less common decrease in athletic performance, sometimes referred to as *tying up,* due to emotional excitement. The rationale for improved performance is obvious from the above; and an explanation for tying up, though less obvious, is also at hand. Nervous overflow to other muscles, and even to other extremities, could well be expected to result in innervation of synergistic muscles; and in some cases, antagonistic muscles may be innervated in a portion of the desired athletic movement. When the latter occurs, a performance decrement results.

Thus, to summarize the effect of emotional excitement upon muscular performance, we may say that under normal conditions only a portion of the available motor units are activated, but that this number can be augmented by activity of the hypothalamus due to emotional excitement. If the activity of the hypothalamus and humoral factors, such as an increased level of adrenaline in the muscle tissue results in an activation of other muscles, some of which are antagonists, tying up and a decrement in performance may result.

Although great feats of strength and endurance have been claimed as the result of hypnotic trance states, demonstrations by competent investigators under controlled laboratory conditions have been less spectacular. Johnson and Kramer were unable to demonstrate significant changes in the strength or power of ten athletes under hypnotic conditions, although muscular endurance was enormously improved for one professional athlete.

Roush (1951), in a study noted for its large number of subjects (twenty) and rigid criteria of the state of trance, found significant improvements in grip strength, arm strength, and muscular endurance, but Johnson's (1961) summary of the available research points out that the use of hypnosis to improve muscular strength or endurance is unreliable, even though great improvements have been found in a few individuals. It is also his opinion that the beneficial effects, when found, are the result of the neurophysiological mechanisms described in regard to emotional excitement. In any event, hypnosis is certainly not a practice to be indulged in by coaches and physical educators, unless it is supervised or directed by medical or other qualified personnel.

The Cross-Education Effect. Before the turn of the century, psychologists demonstrated that training one limb resulted in significant improvements not only in the exercised limb but in the symmetrical, un-exercised limb as well. This phenomenon, the *cross-education effect,* was found to apply both to the learning of skills and to the improvement of strength.

Cross-education has recently been thoroughly investigated for its use-fulness in physical education and rehabilitation by Hellebrandt and her co-workers (10, 11, 12) and by Walters (28). Their work demon-strated the cross-education effect in relation to the gross motor activities of physical education. As a result of training one limb, they found that significant improvements in strength, endurance, and skill occurred not only in the trained limb but also in the contralateral (opposite), un-trained limb. To produce a well-defined effect, it was necessary to go into an overload training condition; in fact, it seems that the nondomi-nant arm could be trained as well by cross-education with an overload condition as by direct practice with an underload. Furthermore, the nondominant arm sometimes gained as much in skill by cross-education as it did in direct practice; but this was not true for the dominant arm.

The rationale for this cross-education effect has not yet been clearly elucidated; however, from what is known of the motor pathways from the cortex, logical deductions can be made. As was pointed out in the description of the pyramidal system, seventy to eighty-five percent of the descending nerve fibers cross from one side to the other in their descent to synapse in the cord. Some of the remainder seem to descend ipsilaterally, and it is known that ipsilateral effects are obtainable by stimulation of the posterior premotor area of the cortex. Thus it seems likely that the cross-education effect is brought about by an overflow of nervous energy from neurons in the motor cortex which innervate the crossed pyramidal fibers, to a smaller number of neurons that supply the uncrossed fibers. Sufficient overflow apparently occurs only under the conditions of strong volition that are involved in overloading. It should be pointed out that the untrained limb was frequently observed to pro-duce isometric contractions during the training of its symmetrical partner. So that technically, it was not unexercised.

The implications of this work for the maintenance of muscle tone and prevention of atrophy in immobilized muscles is obvious. From the fore-going rationale, it will also be obvious that intact motor innervation is necessary for achievement of the cross-education effect.

The Dynamogenic Effect of Cocontractions. Hellebrandt and Houtz (12), after observing isometric contractions in the "unexercised" limb during the cross-education experiments postulated that the concurrent contraction of homologous (corresponding) parts (e.g., right and left arms) might function in augmenting the work output of a tiring or a weakened muscle. Their experiments, as well as the earlier experiments of Karpovich (21), demonstrated that this is indeed the case. When a limb was fatigued ergographically by rhythmic, contractions bringing the other, unfatigued limb into synchronous movement resulted in a marked improvement of the work output of the fatigued limb. This phenomenon has much practical significance for corrective physical education, and may prove of value in athletics as well.

Reaction Time and Movement Time. Of great interest and importance to all concerned with physical education and athletics is the speed with which an individual can react in a game situation. For example, this factor partly determines how successful a basketball player can be on defense. When the offensive player makes his move (commits himself to a course of action), the difference between a slow and a fast reaction by the defensive player (possibly 0.10 second) can result in the offensive player's getting a lead of several additional feet simply because the defense man must react to the offensive move. In swimming races a difference in reaction to the pistol shot can result in several feet gained or lost. On such slim margins hang the fruits of victory in closely fought contests.

Reaction time is defined, for purposes of physical education, as the interval between presentation of the stimulus and the first sign of response. The measurement is easily made by electric circuitry, which applies current to an electric timer (chronoscope) at the presentation of the stimulus and cuts the current when the subject removes his hand from a push-button switch. The stimulus may be visual, audible, or tactile.

Movement time is defined as the interval between the start and the finish of a given movement. The movement may be terminated if it ends in striking an object; or it may be nonterminated if the chronoscope is stopped by interruption of a light beam or similar device that allows follow-through.

An interesting question here is that of the specificity versus the generality of these measures. In other words, if an individual has a fast reaction time for removing his hand from a switch in response to a stimulus, can we expect him to be equally fast with his leg on the same or the opposite side? Well-controlled studies by Henry and Rogers (15), Clark and Glines (3), and Lotter (23) seem to indicate a relatively high degree of specificity by limb and movement. Thus an individual may be quick in reacting with an arm but slow when reacting with the legs.

Another question that has occupied the attention of investigators in recent years is whether movement time can be predicted from reaction time. The research (3, 14, 15, 16, 23) fails to demonstrate a relationship between reaction and movement times, although one investigator (26) found a correlation of $r = 0.56$ which had to be reduced to $r = 0.31$ when corrected for the contribution of the aging factor. There is fairly good agreement on the effects of age upon reaction time; fastest reactions being found in the college-age group, and slower reactions in both younger and older groups.

In regard to sex, adequate data for the college-age group indicate that reaction and movement times are slower in women by approximately fourteen and thirty percent, respectively (13, 15).

Motor Set Versus Sensory Set. *Set* has been defined as the direction of the subject's attention preliminary to an anticipated movement. Thus *motor set* is obtained by directing the subject's attention to the move-ment response as in thinking of the starting movement in track. *Sensory set* is the direction of attention to the stimulus, as in concentrating upon the gunshot for the start.

It has been the accepted procedure in athletics to use the motor set on the assumption that it results in faster reaction; however, as a con-sequence of the *memory drum theory*, Henry (15) hypothesized that attempts to institute conscious control of movement will interfere with the programming, thus increasing reaction time and resulting in a slower start. His experiment on college-age men and women indicated that both sexes react approximately 2.6 percent slower and move 2.1 percent slower when using the motor set, compared with the sensory set. It should be pointed out, however, that he found twenty percent of his subjects had a natural preference for the motor set and that these subjects performed better with the motor set.

Although this phase of performance research cannot yet be consid-ered closed, the evidence weighs in favor of the sensory set, contrary to widespread opinion.

SUMMARY

1. The basic structural unit of the nervous system is the nerve cell, the *neuron*. The cell body has two types of processes: *dendrites* which bring impulses to the cell body and the *axon* which conducts nerve impulses away.

2. The *reflex arc*, in its simplest form, is a discharge from a sensory receptor that is transmitted by an *afferent* pathway to a synapse in the spinal cord with a motor neuron, which conducts the *efferent* impulse to an *effector* organ (muscle or gland).

3. Reflexes may occur entirely at one level of the spinal cord (*segmental reflexes*), or they may traverse upward or downward in the cord (*intersegmental reflexes*), or they may be influenced by higher brain centers (*suprasegmental reflexes*).

4. The nervous system may be divided in two ways: (A) structurally, into *central* and *peripheral* components, and (B) functionally, into *somatic* and *autonomic* systems.

5. Coordination of movement depends upon feedback information of what the muscles are doing. This feedback is called *proprioception,* and consists of two types of information: (A) *kinesthetic,* from receptors in the muscles, tendons, and joints, and (B) vestibular, from receptors of the nonauditory labyrinths of the inner ear.

6. Muscular control is mediated directly through the large *alpha motor nerve fibers* and indirectly through the smaller *gamma nerve fibers.* The alpha motor nerve fibers and their skeletal muscles, together with the gamma motor nerve fibers and their intrafusal fibers, form an interlocking servomechanism in which each reacts to the other's actions, thus bringing about very fine control of movement.

7. The *pyramidal system* is comprised of area four of the motor cortex, and the nerve fibers emanating therefrom, which descend through the pyramidal tracts to synapse directly or indirectly with the lower motoneuron in the cord. This system is involved mainly in conscious, specific, volitional movement.

8. The *extrapyramidal system* originates mainly in area six of the *premotor cortex.* Its descending fibers go to the cord indirectly, by way of various relay stations called *nuclei.* It is involved in general, diffuse motor patterns.

9. The *proprioceptive-cerebellar system,* though it arouses no conscious sensory sensation, is the clearing house for sensory data necessary for the coordination of movement patterns, which is mainly accomplished here.

10. *Upright posture* is maintained largely through the operation of *stretch reflexes,* also called *myotatic reflexes.* These reflexes make the minute adjustments in extensor tone that is necessary when extensor muscles start to slacken.

11. *Emotional excitement* or *hypnotic suggestion* can lead to an augmentation of the number of motor units participating in a given motor activity and thus improve performance. Both, however, can lead to a decrement in performance under certain conditions; e.g., by *tying up* an overly emotional or inexperienced athlete due to overexcitement.

12. The *cross-educational effect* is well-established in respect to strength, endurance, and skill. It requires intact motor innervation and overload conditions of the trained limb for its best manifestation. The *dynamogenic effect of muscular cocontractions* in augmenting the work output of fatiguing muscles has also been established, and the rationale is probably similar for both phenomena.

13. *Reaction time* and *movement time* appear to be unrelated, and neither is a general quality; i.e., quick eye-hand reactions are not necessarily evidence that other reactions in the same individual will be similarly fast.

14. Tests of a hypothesized *memory drum theory* of neuromotor reaction have produced evidence that tends to overthrow older opinions of motor versus sensory set. Evidence indicates that, for most people, a sensory set results in quicker reactions.

REFERENCES

1. Bigland, B., and Lippold, O. C. J. 1954. Motor unit activity in the voluntary contraction of human muscle. *Journal of Physiology* 125:322-35.
2. Bourne, G. A. 1960. *The structure and function of muscle*, vol. 1. New York: Academic Press.
3. Clarke, H. H., and Glines, D. 1962. Relationships of reaction, movement and completion times to motor strength, anthropometric and maturity measures of 13-year-old boys. *Research Quarterly* 33:194-201.
4. Eldred, E. 1967. Peripheral receptors: their excitation and relation to reflex patterns. *American Journal of Physical Medicine* 46:69-87.
5. Eldred, E.; Granit, R.; Holmgren, B.; and Merton, P. A. 1954. Proprioceptive control of muscular contraction and the cerebellum. *Journal of Physiology* 123:46-7.
6. Gellhorn, E. 1960. The physiology of the supraspinal mechanisms. In *Science and Medicine of Exercise and Sports*, ed. W. R. Johnson, p. 737. New York: Harper & Row.
7. Granit, R. 1950. Reflex self-regulation of muscle contraction and autogenetic inhibition. *Journal of Neurophysiology* 13:351-72.
8. Granit, R., and Kaada, B. R. 1952. The influence of stimulation of central nervous structures in muscle spindles in the cat. *Acta Physiologica Scandinavica* 27: 130-60.
9. Hammond, P. H.; Merton, P. A.; and Sutton, G. G. 1956. Nervous gradation of muscular contraction. *British Medical Bulletin* 12:214-18.
10. Hellebrandt, F. A. 1951. Cross education: ipsilateral and contralateral effects of unimanual training. *Journal of Applied Physiology* 4:136-44.
11. Hellebrandt, F. A.; Parrish, A. M.; and Houtz, S. J. 1947. Cross education: the influence of unilateral exercise on the contralateral limb. *Archives of Physical Medicine* 28:76-84.

12. Hellebrandt, F. A.; Houtz, S. J.; and Kirkorian, A. M. 1950. Influence of bimanual exercise on unilateral work capacity. *Journal of Applied Physiology* 2:446-52.
13. Henry, F. M. 1960. Influence of motor and sensory sets on reaction latency and speed of discrete movements. *Research Quarterly* 31:459-68.
14. ———. 1961. Stimulus complexity, movement complexity, age, and sex in relation to reaction latency and speed in limb movements. *Research Quarterly* 32:353-66.
15. Henry, F. M., and Rogers, D. E. 1960. Increased response latency for complicated movements and "memory drum" theory of neuromotor reaction. *Research Quarterly* 31:448-58.
16. Henry, F. M.; Lotter, W. S.; and Smith, L. E. 1962. Factorial structure of individual differences in limb speed, reaction and strength. *Research Quarterly* 33:70-84.
17. Holmgren, B., and Merton, P. A. 1954. Local feedback control of motoneurons. *Journal of Physiology* 123:47-8.
18. Hunt, C. C. 1952. The effect of stretch receptors from muscle on the discharge of motoneurons. *Journal of Physiology* 117:359-79.
19. Johnson, W. R. 1961. Hypnosis and muscular performance. *Journal of Sport Medicine and Physical Fitness* 1:71-9.
20. Johnson, W. R., and Kramer, G. F. 1961. Effects of stereotyped non-hypnotic, hypnotic, and post-hypnotic suggestions upon strength, power and endurance. *Research Quarterly* 32:522-29.
21. Karpovich, P. V. 1937. Physiological and psychological dynamogenic factors in exercise. *Arbeitsphysiologie* 9:626.
22. Katz, B. 1950. Depolarization of sensory terminals and the initiation of impulses in the muscle spindle. *Journal of Physiology* 111:261-82.
23. Lotter, W. S. 1960. Interrelationships among reaction times and speeds of movement in different limbs. *Research Quarterly* 31:147-55.................
24. McCouch, G. P.; Deering, I. D.; and Stewart, W. B. 1950. Inhibition of knee jerk from tendon spindles of crureus. *Journal of Neurophysiology* 13:343-50.
25. Mountcastle, V. B. 1961. Reflex activity of the spinal cord. In *Medical Physiology*, ed. Philip Bard. St. Louis: C. V. Mosby Company.
26. Pierson, W. R. 1959. The relationship of movement time and reaction time from childhood to senility. *Research Quarterly* 30:227-31.
27. Roush, E. S. 1951. Strength and endurance in the waking and hypnotic states. *Journal of Applied Physiology* 3:404-10.
28. Walters, C. E. 1955. The effect of overload on bilateral transfer of motor skill. *Physical Therapy Review* 35:567-69.

5 The Heart and Exercise

It is the function of the heart and the circulatory system to provide the flow of blood necessary to maintain homeostasis of the various tissues of the body. *Homeostasis* can be defined as the sum total of regulatory functions that maintain a constant environment for the cells of the tissues. The *internal environment,* i.e., the tissue fluid, must be held relatively constant in regard to nutrients and metabolites, oxygen and carbon dioxide, temperature and hormonal content. The blood must transport nutrients from the digestive tract, wastes to the kidney, etc. The greatest concern in the physiology of exercise lies, however, with the transport of oxygen and carbon dioxide. This is so because during exercise the supply of oxygen to the tissues is the most urgent of the factors mentioned; oxygen cannot be stored, in any real sense, and its supply or lack of it is usually the critical factor in any endurance exercise. The removal of carbon dioxide is intimately related with the blood's carriage of oxygen (as will be seen in a later discussion).

In other words, in the study of exercise physiology we are primarily interested in the heart as an organ of the *cardiorespiratory system,* in which it serves as the pump to provide the energy for the proper pressure and flow of blood to the active muscle tissues.

REVIEW OF THE CARDIAC CYCLE

The salient anatomical features of the heart may be reviewed by considering figure 5.1. Blood flows into the right atrium from the systemic circulation by way of the superior and inferior vena cava. The thin-walled atrium acts as a combination storage basin and pump primer for blood flow through the tricuspid valve into the right ventricle which provides most of the energy for blood flow through the pulmonary valve and artery into the pulmonary circuit, then through the lungs and back through the pulmonary veins into the left atrium. Blood flow proceeds from the left atrium, through the mitral valve, and into the left ventricle. Contraction of the left ventricle provides the energy for blood flow through the aortic valve, then through the aorta and through the systemic arterial system to the capillary beds of the various tissues.

From the capillaries, the blood flow is returned through veins, of ever-increasing size, to the great veins: the superior and the inferior vena cava. Thus the circulatory system comprises two loops, each with its own pump. The right heart and the pulmonary circuit form one loop, and the left heart and the systemic circuit form the other.

Origin and Transmission of the Heartbeat. The muscle tissue of the heart possesses *autorhythmicity*. It requires no innervation or stimuli from without to produce its regular contractions. Under normal conditions,

HEAD and UPPER EXTREMITY

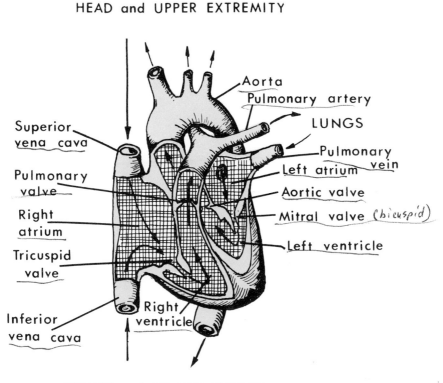

TRUNK and LOWER EXTREMITY

Figure 5-1. Details of the functional parts of the heart. (From Guyton, A.C. *Function of the Human Body,* 1959. Courtesy of W.B. Saunders Company, Philadelphia.)

the wave of excitation originates at the *sino-auricular node;* however, all cardiac tissue has the property of autorhythmicity. If, under abnormal conditions, the rate of emission from the SA node should slow unduly, any area of the myocardium that has a faster inherent rate may assume the role of pacemaker. This is what occurs in abnormal heart rhythms.

Figure 5.2 illustrates the transmission of the wave of excitation from the SA node by way of the syncytium of muscle fibers in the auricle to the auriculoventricular or AV node, thence into the Purkinje system which conducts the impulse throughout the ventricular myocardium.

Pressure Relationships of the Cardiac Cycle. Relating the events of the cardiac cycle to each other and placing them in time is best done by

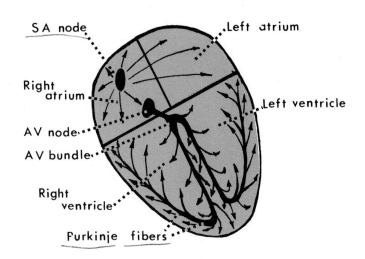

Figure 5-2. Transmission of the cardiac impulse from the SA node into the atria, then into the AV node, and finally through the Purkinje system to all parts of the ventricles. (From Guyton, A.C. *Function of the Human Body,* 1959. Courtesy of W.B. Saunders Company, Philadelphia.)

considering the *pressure relationships* that are basic to valve action in the heart. It is important to realize from the outset that all valve action is brought about by pressure differentials on the two sides of any given cardiac valve.

The pressure changes in figure 5.3 are recorded along with the events of the electrocardiogram, phonocardiogram (recording of heart sounds), and the heart volume curve. The vertical lines intersect these tracings to indicate events that occur simultaneously. The pressure curves depict the changes in the left heart, but the occurrences in the right heart are similar —though at a considerably lower pressure level.

Table 5.1, p. 96, represents the events of an average cardiac cycle, under resting conditions, with a rate of seventy-four beats per minute. Under conditions of exercise, which necessitate higher heart rates, the relative durations of the phases of systole and diastole are altered somewhat. The most notable change and the change most important to the physiology of exercise is that the period of *diastasis* is the first to be shortened, and it may be eliminated completely as the heart rate increases. Because diastasis is the period during which the entire myocardium is at rest, a decrease in resting time at higher heart rates results in losses of efficiency.

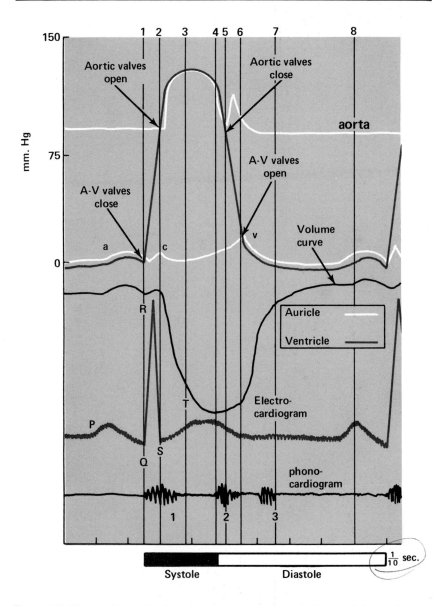

Figure 5-3. The cardiac cycle. Superimposed curves of ventricular, auricular, and aortic pressures, together with a ventricular volume curve, an electrocardiogram and a phonocardiogram. (From Best and Taylor. *The Physiological Basis of Medical Practice*, 3rd ed., 1943. Courtesy of the Williams and Wilkins Company, Baltimore.)

TABLE 5.1
Cardiac Cycle

Line	Nomenclature	Pressure Events	Valve Action	Average Duration
		SYSTOLE		
1		Ventricular pressure overcomes auricular pressure	AV valves close	
1-2	Period of isometric contraction (presphygmic)	Ventricular pressure increases	AV valves closed, aortic valve closed	0.05 sec.
2		Ventricular pressure overcomes aortic pressure	Aortic valve opens	
2-3	Period of maximal ejection	Ventricular pressure continues to increase	Aortic valve open, AV valves closed	0.12
3-4	Period of reduced ejection	Ventricular pressure decreases	Aortic valve open, AV valves closed	0.14
			Systole Total	0.31 sec.
		DIASTOLE		
4-5	Protodiastolic phase	Ventricular pressure drops		0.04 sec.
5		Ventricular pressure falls below aortic pressure	Aortic valve closes	
5-6	Isometric relaxation phase (postsphygmic)	Ventricular pressure continues to drop rapidly	Aortic valve closed, AV valves closed	0.08
6		Ventricular pressure falls below auricular pressure	AV valves open	
6-7	Period of rapid filling	Ventricular pressure falls to zero	Aortic valve closed, AV valves open	0.09
7-8	Diastasis—period of slower filling	Auricular and ventricular pressure both low	Aortic valve closed, AV valves open	0.19
8-1	Auricular systole	Increase in both auricular & ventricular pressure due to auricular contraction	Aortic valve closed, AV valves open	0.10

Diastole Total   0.50 sec.
Total Cardiac Cycle   0.81 sec.
Heart Rate 74

THE CARDIAC OUTPUT

The cardiac output is the volume of blood ejected by the heart per unit of time, and is usually expressed in liters per minute. At rest, in the average sized man, it is approximately five liters per minute, and it can be increased to forty-two liters per minute in a well-trained athlete. The amount of this increase in cardiac output is one of the most important limiting factors in athletic performance. The output of the heart is determined by two factors: the heart rate and the stroke volume (the amount of blood ejected with each beat). Consequently, the cardiac output equals the heart rate times the stroke volume.

Measurement of Cardiac Output. The most direct method is based upon the *Fick principle*. If we know how much O_2 an individual is consuming per unit time and if we also know the concentration of O_2 in the arterial and mixed venous blood, then we can calculate the cardiac output (CO) as follows:

$$CO \text{ in L/min} = \frac{O_2 \text{ consumption in ml/min}}{\text{A-V difference in } O_2 \text{ in ml/L of blood}}$$

For example, in a resting subject we find an O_2 consumption of 250 ml/min. His arterial O_2 concentration is 20 vol. % and his mixed venous concentration is 15 vol. %. First we convert the vol. % which means the volume in ml carried by 100 ml of blood, to ml per liter (1,000 ml). Thus each liter of arterial blood carries 200 ml of O_2 while the mixed venous blood only returns 150 ml to the heart and the lungs. Therefore we calculate the cardiac output:

$$CO \text{ (L/min)} = \frac{O_2 \text{ consumption (ml)}}{\text{A-V diff. in } O_2 \text{ (ml/L)}} = \frac{250}{50} = 5 \text{ L}$$

What we are really saying is that if we know the O_2 consumption has been at a rate of 250 ml/min and that the delivery of O_2 by the blood is such that it requires 1.0 L blood to deliver 50 ml then 250 ml would require the service of 5L of blood to deliver the 250 ml we know have been consumed. This is simple and direct, but unfortunately the calculation requires the value of O_2 in *mixed* venous blood which can only be gotten by catheterization of the right heart to get a measure of truly mixed venous blood. This procedure involves inserting a tube into an arm vein and feeding it through the vein into the auricle. Although this is a standard hospital procedure for evaluation of cardiac patients, it is not often used in exercise physiology.

Noninvasive techniques have been developed which involve the rebreathing of CO_2 and the estimation of mixed venous CO_2 from the rate at which CO_2 approaches a plateau. (The Fick principle is used just as above but substituting CO_2 values for O_2 values.) This method is attractive in that no trauma is involved for the subject and it is feasible in the well-equipped physiology of exercise laboratory. It is reasonably accurate and reproducible under exercise conditions (6), but the author has found the reproducibilty under resting conditions to be poor (4).

Control of Heart Rate. The rate of the heartbeat is determined by the frequency of impulse generation at the SA node. The activity of the SA node, in turn, is controlled by other factors, most important of which seems to be the effect of autonomic innervation upon the SA node. The autonomic nervous system supplies both parasympathetic and sympathetic fibers to the SA node. Parasympathetic fibers are supplied by the *vagus nerve,* and sympathetic fibers by the *accelerator nerve.* In both cases the innervation arises in the cardioregulatory centers of the medulla.

It has long been known that severing the vagus fibers to the SA node results in an immediate quickening of the heart rate, and thus we know that these fibers are inhibitory, and also that they exhibit *tone;* that is, they are chronically active. Further, the accelerator fibers also are constantly active, in the other direction; they have an accelerating effect called *accelerator tone.* Thus the heart rate is precisely adjusted by a balance of activity of the two divisions of the autonomic system.

For the adjustment of the heart rate to be meaningful and to serve the changing needs of the organism, it must reflect the demands of changing metabolic activity. To understand how this servomechanism works, we must know the origin of the afferent impulses that form the sensory side of the cardioregulatory reflexes, whose center lies in the medulla. These afferent nervous impulses come from a number of sources, and are *pressor* (increasing the activity) or *depressor* (decrease the activity). The sources of pressor afferent stimulation are:

1. *Proprioceptive impulses* from the working muscles and joints
2. Impulses arising in the chemoreceptors of the *carotid body* and the *aortic body*
3. Impulses arising in the *cerebral cortex*

The sources of depressor afferent stimuli are mainly from the *stretch receptors* of the *carotid sinus* and the *aortic arch.*

The effects of the autonomic nervous system in controlling the heart rate in an exercise bout may be summarized in three phases.

1. The anticipatory rise in heart rate, frequently seen before exercise begins, is undoubtedly the result of reflexes that arise in the cerebral cortex, due to anxiety, excitement, etc.

2. As exercise begins, stimuli from the working muscles influence the cardioregulatory centers (mainly, they inhibit the cardio-inhibitory center), which results in a release from vagal inhibition, and consequently produces an increased heart rate.

3. As exercise continues beyond thirty or forty seconds, increases in heart rate—if the exercise is demanding—are mainly brought about by increases of tone in the accelerator nerve, and this through stimulation of the chemoreceptors in the carotid and aortic bodies by decreasing pH and increasing concentrations of carbon dioxide.

On the other hand, the frequency of the impulses in the pressure receptors of the carotid sinus and the aortic arch rises with increasing blood pressure, and exerts a mitigating influence to prevent too high a rise in blood pressure. The receptors also function in bringing about an increase in heart rate (and blood pressure) when their discharge slows because of decreasing blood pressure as occurs, for example, in a change of posture from lying to standing.

In addition to the nervous control of the heart rate, at least two other factors are of considerable importance. An increase in adrenal activity also plays a large part in the increased heart rate of the third phase (described above). Both the nervous and the hormonal effects are superimposed, as it were, on the basic effects of body temperature on the heart rate. Increased body temperature results in increases in heart rate, and vice versa, in accordance with the reaction of all metabolic processes to temperature.

Control of Stroke Volume. Until quite recently, the stroke volume of the heart had been considered a simple and direct function of the end diastolic volume of the ventricle, a conclusion based on the classic work of Frank and Starling. Starling's law of the heart stated that the mechanical energy set free on passage from the resting to the contracted state depends on the length of the muscle fibers at the end of diastole; and this is in agreement with the length-tension law of skeletal muscle discussed in chapter two. Now that there is equipment to take X-ray motion pictures and X-ray kymograms, there is evidence that the end diastolic volume of the heart is not larger in exercise than at rest, and may even be smaller (8). Furthermore, whether the results of the Frank and Starling experiments on thoracotomized (open chest) dogs can be extrapolated to normal intact dogs—let alone to intact man—is open to question (9). Because the classic work had been done on heart-lung preparations in dogs, these limitations were serious challenges to its validity, and further research has shed more light on the mechanisms that control the stroke volume of the heart (2, 12, 15, 17, 18, 27).

First of all, there is no reason to challenge Starling's law as a determinant of stroke volume in a heart-lung preparation. Second, there is every reason to believe that a physiological law that can be as elegantly displayed as Starling's law of the heart must have some use for the intact organism. However, the weight of accumulating evidence indicates that although end diastolic volume may be a determining factor under certain conditions (postural changes and gravital changes), several other factors are probably more important in the adjustments of stroke volume to the demands of exercise.

It would seem that the stroke volume of the heart is controlled by a physiological interplay of at least four factors:

1. Effective filling pressure
2. Distensibility of the ventricle in diastole
3. Contractility
4. The systemic arterial blood pressure

The first and second items are, in a sense, expressions of Starling's law; and the third item needs elaboration. The *contractility* of the heart means its ability to produce force per unit of time or, in other words, power. Randall (17) has summarized the evidence that demonstrates increased contractility as the result of sympathetic stimulation. Under sympathetic stimulation, systolic pressures rise much faster, and reach higher levels, because of the development of augmented myocardial fiber tension. This means that, in addition to the obvious advantage of a more forceful beat, there is greater time for diastolic filling because systole is completed more rapidly within each cardiac cycle, resulting in even more advantage to the succeeding cycle due to the complete filling.

The importance of the fourth factor, systemic arterial blood pressure, is rather obvious in that the magnitude of this pressure is the resistance against which the blood must be ejected into the aorta. As this resistance grows higher, the stroke volume must inevitably grow smaller for any given force of contraction.

To summarize Starling's law of the heart, while entirely valid in the experimentally controlled heart, is not nearly so important in the normal physiological control of stroke volume as was once believed. Furthermore, the law should probably be amended, as suggested by Rushmer (19) ". . . . the energy released during contraction is related to the initial length of the muscle fibers *under equal states of responsiveness.*"

Starling's law probably functions quite importantly when the venous return is altered due to changes in posture, etc., without concomitant changes in innervation or humoral content of the blood. During exercise, then, the most important changes in ventricular performance for providing the needed increase in cardiac output are (A) an accelerated heart rate and (B) an increased contractility due to increased sympathetic stimulation of the ventricular myocardium which results in a more complete emptying of the heart during systole.

Importance of the Venous Return. With the accumulating evidence against a greater end diastolic volume during exercise, there may be a tendency to neglect the importance of the necessity for an increased venous return during exercise. It is an obvious truism that the heart cannot eject more blood than it receives. Therefore, although the increase in venous return can no longer be considered the determining factor in increasing cardiac output, it is nevertheless a very important limiting factor where venous return may be curtailed in exercise. For example, in hot and humid environments. Furthermore, it is undoubtedly the major factor in increasing cardiac output when an erect man lies down; venous return is indeed temporarily increased due to the smaller effect of the force of gravity upon the circulatory system. The reduction of cardiac output in the change from the supine position to the standing position must be explained on a similar basis, and will be discussed at greater length in chapter six.

CORONARY CIRCULATION AND EFFICIENCY OF THE HEART

It has been pointed out that cardiac output is usually the limiting factor in determining the level at which work output can be maintained. This is so because skeletal muscle tissues depend upon a constant supply of oxygen from the blood to maintain their metabolic needs. As a consequence, the supply of blood to the heart muscle might be supposed to be the determinant of the upper limits of cardiac output, and thus, indirectly, the determinant of the maximum exercise load to be sustained by the skeletal muscles.

This, as it turns out, seems to be very sound reasoning. Arterial blood usually contains approximately 19 ml of oxygen per 100 ml of blood. In mixed venous blood, this may be reduced to 12 to 14 ml per 100 ml of blood at rest, thus leaving some room for greater utilization in exercise. In the coronary veins under resting conditions, however, the oxygen content has already been reduced to 4 to 6 ml per 100 ml of blood. Thus the oxygen extraction from blood in the coronary vessels is relatively high even at rest, and consequently leaves little coronary venous oxygen reserve for the demands of exercise loads. For these reasons, the maximum sustained cardiac output is limited by two factors: the volume of the coronary blood flow and the efficiency of the heart muscle in performing its work.

Coronary Circulation.   Let us discuss first the control of the coronary blood flow and its adjustment to the demands of exercise. It is obvious that the blood flow through the heart is dependent upon two factors: (1) the difference in pressure (pressure gradient) between the entering arterial blood and the venous outflow, and (2) the resistance to the flow, which in turn depends upon the state of vasoconstriction or vasodilatation of the coronary vessels. The first factor, the pressure gradient, is determined largely by aortic pressure since the coronary arteries derive from the aortic sinus. The resistance to flow is probably the more important factor of the two. Decreased oxygen tension has been shown to have a very strong dilatory effect upon the coronary vessels.

During exercise several factors tend to increase myocardial O_2 requirements and therefore would operate to decrease coronary vascular resistance and thus increase coronary blood flow:

1. Heart rate
2. Arterial pressure
3. Cardiac output
4. Left ventricular work
5. Myocardial contractility

Experiments on dogs have shown that about one-third of the increment in coronary flow and three-fourths of the decrease in coronary resistance during severe exercise can be accounted for by the tachycardia unaffected by any of the other factors (26).

It seems, then, that increased coronary flow during exercise is brought about by at least two factors: (1) the increased arterial blood pressure provides a greater pressure gradient for driving blood through the myocardium; (2) as the myocardial tissue increases its oxygen consumption, the lowering levels of oxygen result in dilatation of the coronary vessels.

Efficiency of the Heart.   Before we enter this discussion it will be well to define some of the necessary terms. *Efficiency*, in general, is the ratio of work production to energy input; thus in this case:

$$\text{Efficiency} = \frac{\text{Work of the heart}}{\text{Energy input (in terms of } O_2 \text{ consumption)}}$$

The *work of the heart* can be measured, as can any work done by fluid pressure:

$$\text{Work} = \text{Pressure} \times \text{Volume moved}$$

It should be noted here that pressure and volume moved (or flow rate) are independent of each other; that is, an increase in pressure may be associated with an increase or a decrease or no change at all in flow rate.

A simple law of physics, the law of La Place, can also help our understanding of the cardiac function:

Tension (in the cylinder wall) = Pressure × Radius of cylinder

This formula tells us that the tension in the muscle fibers of the myocardium must be proportionately greater as the pressure rises. In other words, the tension required of the heart to move a given volume of blood increases as the arterial blood pressure rises. The formula also tells us that to move the same quantity of blood under equal pressures, the large heart (of greater radius) must exert greater tension than the small heart. Because the energy requirements of the heart are determined largely by the tension demanded of it, this means that a small heart is more efficient in working against pressure, other things being equal.

The work of Sarnoff and his associates (21, 22) illustrates the conformance of practice to theory in this regard. Ingeniously devised experiments allowed measurement of the oxygen utilization of the myocardium of dogs when aortic pressure was increased and cardiac output and heart rate were held constant. In these *pressure runs* it was found that a 175 percent work increase was accompanied by a 178 percent increase in oxygen consumption. On the other hand, in *flow runs* where the work output was increased 696 percent through increasing the cardiac output while holding aortic pressure and heart rate constant—an oxygen consumption increase of only fifty-three percent was noted. Even this fifty-three percent seemed to be accounted for by an inadvertent increase in aortic pressure. Thus a striking difference in cardiac efficiency is seen when the work output of the heart is increased by pressure-load increases compared with volume-load increases.

Another very important observation in this series of experiments was that if the amount of work done by the heart was held constant by holding the cardiac output and the mean aortic pressure constant while increasing the heart rate, the oxygen consumption of the myocardium increased. Consequently, we may say that *high heart rates are less efficient than low rates*, other things being equal.

The researchers concluded that the principal, if not the sole, determinant of myocardial oxygen utilization is the *Tension-Time Index* (mean systolic aortic pressure × duration of systole).

Recent work has shown that a reasonably valid estimate of the myocardial O_2 consumption (equivalent to work load stress on the heart muscle) can be made even from the heart rate-blood pressure product using systolic pressure measured with a cuff (13, 14). This is important in any conditioning or testing program involving middle-aged or older adults since the work of the heart is not always proportional to the work of the total body. Data from the authors laboratory will be presented in chapter seventeen to illustrate this point.

Some practical conclusions can be drawn from the above discussion that have large implications for exercise physiology. For any given set of conditions (A) the heart of a subject with abnormally high blood pressure must work much harder than that of the normal subject; (B) the slower the heart rate for any given work load, the more efficiently is the cardiac work performed.

FACTORS AFFECTING THE HEART RATE

The heart rate at rest varies widely from individual to individual, and also within the same individual from one observation to another under similar circumstances; therefore, it is almost meaningless to speak of a *normal* heart rate. We may, however, say that the *average* heart rate is seventy-eight beats per minute without implying that a rate of forty (observed in highly trained endurance athletes) or 100 is necessarily *abnormal*. Although heart rate during the stress of exercise or during the recovery period after exercise is a very valuable source of information for the exercise physiologist, the resting rate is affected by so many variables that it has very little meaning for the prediction of physical performance. Some of the factors that affect the resting rate will now be discussed.

Age. The heart rate at birth is approximately 130 beats per minute, and it slows down with each succeeding year until adolescence. The average rate in a resting adult male is approximately seventy-eight in the standing position. The maximal attainable heart rate decreases with increasing age in the adult.

Sex. The resting heart rate in adult females averages five to ten beats faster than adult males under any given set of conditions.

Size. In the animal world in general, it seems to be a general biological rule that the heart rate varies inversely with the size of the species. For example, the canary has a rate of approximately 1,000, whereas that of an elephant is in the neighborhood of twenty-five beats per minute. However, no consistent relationship between size and heart rate in adult humans has been demonstrated.

Posture. Posture has a very definite effect upon the heart rate. Although the results of different investigators show variances, the typical response to the change from the recumbent to the standing position seems to be an increase of ten to twelve beats per minute. It was at one time thought that this change in heart rate due to posture was related to physical fitness, and consequently it has appeared as a test item in some tests of physical fitness; however, its value in this regard is open to serious doubt.

Ingestion of Food. The resting heart rate is higher while digestive processes are in progress than in the post-absorptive state. This is also true in exercise; a given exercise load elicits a greater heart rate after a meal, and this is one of many reasons that militate against heavy exercise immediately after a meal.

Emotion. Emotional stress brings about a cardiovascular response that is quite similar to the response to exercise. An increase in heart rate is the most notable factor, and it occurs in all but the most experienced athletes as an anticipatory reaction. Dill (5) found a mean increase of nineteen beats per minute in the resting rate of teen-age boys waiting to be tested in his laboratory. The effect of emotional excitement is most easily observed at rest, but it also occurs during exercise, where it tends to result in an excessive cardiovascular response (1). Under these conditions the response to a standard exercise load may be considerably greater, with the heart rate being elevated by the summation of the stimuli from exercise and from the emotional situation. The recovery period may also be unduly prolonged.

Body Temperature. With increases in body temperature above normal, the heart rate increases. Conversely, with decreases in temperature the rate slows, until a temperature of about 26° C. is reached, at which temperature abnormal electrocardiograms are obtained that show danger of heart failure.

Environmental Factors. Ambient temperature is one of the most important factors affecting the heart rate and the total cardiovascular response to exercise. In moderate exercise, an increase of from ten to forty beats per minute may occur, depending upon the magnitude of the temperature rise. At rest, small increases in heart rate are seen as temperature increases. However, humidity and air movement also are factors. For any given temperature and work load, the rise in heart rate will be greater if the humidity is high and the air is motionless.

Effects of Smoking. It has been found that smoking even one cigarette significantly increases the resting heart rate, in either the sitting or the standing position (23).

THE HEART RATE DURING AND AFTER EXERCISE

The ready availability of the pulse rate as a measure of what transpires internally has resulted in the accumulation of much interesting data that relate various exercise conditions and heart rate. We have pointed out that cardiac output is a determinant in deciding the exercise load that may be tolerated, and that the cardiac output is the resultant of two components: heart rate and stroke volume. Since heart rate is easily obtained, it is indeed fortunate that research has shown the heart rate is the more important variable in the response to the demands of exercise. The greater importance of heart rate is due to at least three reasons.

1. Stroke volume probably increases very little with an increase in metabolism until a level approximately eight times the resting level is reached (20).
2. Heart rate is proportional to the work load imposed.
3. Heart rate is proportional to the oxygen consumption during an exercise.

All three of these factors are true only during the steady state, however, when the work is done aerobically.

It is obvious from preceding discussions that the slower the heart rate in response to a given exercise work load the more efficient is the myocardium—and again for at least three reasons.

1. The oxygen consumption of the heart increases with increasing heart rate, even though the work load is held constant (21).
2. As the heart rate increases, the filling time decreases.
3. Diastasis, the only resting period for the myocardium, is disproportionately shortened in faster rates, and may disappear entirely at high rates.

All things considered, the rate of the heart beat furnishes data that quite accurately reflect the degree of stress created by an exercise work load; conversely, it provides insight into the adequacy of physiological responses to the exercise.

The Typical Heart Rate Response to Exercise. As exercise begins, the pulse rate elevates very rapidly. If the exercise is light or moderate, a plateau (leveling off) is seen in thirty to sixty seconds, and this pulse rate is relatively constant until cessation of the exercise. This rate is proportional to the work load of the exercise in any individual. If the work load is heavy (ten or more times the resting metabolic rate), the rate increases until exhaustion supervenes (fig. 5.4). For the first two to three minutes after the end of the exercise, the heart rate decreases almost as rapidly as it increased. After this initial decrease, further decline in the heart rate occurs more slowly at a rate that is roughly related to the intensity and duration of the work.

isometric Response of the Heart Rate to Differences in Exercise

Static Versus Dynamic Exercise. In exercises that involve a held position, or a straining of the musculature against a heavy load—as in weight

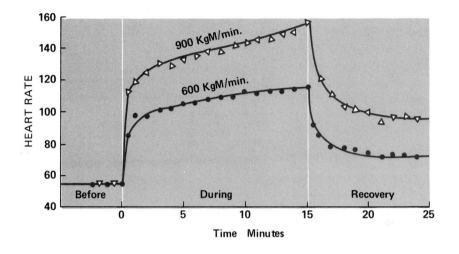

Figure 5-4. Heart rate changes in a moderately conditioned, middle-age subject at work loads of 600 and 900 Kgm/min on a bicycle ergometer.

lifting—only a very slight increase in heart rate is observed. At the other end of the continuum are exercises that involve rapid and vigorous alternating contractions, such as running, cycling, etc., in which a large increase in heart rate occurs. This difference can be explained on two bases.

1. Venous return may be decreased in the straining exercise due to the increased intrathoracic pressure (chapter six), and it may be increased in dynamic exercise due to the pumping action of the muscles.
2. The heart rate is proportional to the work load per unit of time, and slow, straining exercises seldom create a work load sufficient to bring about large responses in heart rate.

Intensity of the Exercise. Intensity is the number of foot-pounds of work per minute expended in an exercise. Since *work = force × distance,* in a simple exercise such as bench-stepping, the work load and thus the intensity may be increased by increasing the height of the bench, by increasing the rate of stepping, or by increasing both. Both factors would of course increase the distance per unit of time, and the force could be increased by having the subject carry a weight on his back. Any and all of these factors increase the intensity of the exercise, which is the most important factor in determining the heart rate during exercises.

Duration of the Exercise. If a moderate work load is maintained over a considerable period of time, a secondary increase in heart rate can be observed after the plateau has been attained and held. This can best be explained in terms of fatigue of the skeletal musculature, resulting in the recruitment of larger numbers of motor units, which results in a greater metabolic demand for the same level of exercise work load and thus an increase in the heart rate. This secondary increase is usually progressive, and continues until exhaustion ends the exercise (4).

Rest Periods in Discontinuous Exercise. Our discussion has so far centered about work or exercise that is done continuously. However, because of the advent of interval training methods in track, swimming, and many other sports, a discussion of the importance of rest periods and of their interaction with work load in influencing the stressfulness of the exercise or workout is in order.

It is of interest that although both resting and exercise heart rate decrease, the physiology involved is quite different. Experiments involving autonomic blockade (7) suggest that the lowered resting rate is due to enhanced parasympathetic influence, but the decreased exercise rate is due to a decreased sympathetic drive.

For a light work load, a rest period of constant size can result in a return of the heart rate to the prework level after many work sessions; but if the intensity of the work session is increased beyond a certain point, recovery is no longer completed in each successive rest period unless the length of the rest periods is also progressively increased. On the other hand, if the rest interval is held constant and the intensity is increased, a progressively ascending heart rate will be observed during the work or exercise (3), and exhaustion will result if the work is carried on too long. A coach will of course end a workout after sufficient fatigue has occurred in bringing about the desired training effect, and before exhaustion ensues.

In industry, on the other hand, where a six- to eight-hour day is involved, the rest periods must be adequate to prevent a progressive heart rate increase, or the intensity of the work must be decreased. In general, then, the stress of a day's work, or of an interval of a training and conditioning program, is the result of an interaction of two components: (1) total work done and (2) total amount of rest periods. The final recovery of the heart rate will be the resultant of these two components.

Heart Rate as a Measure of Stress. It is frequently desirable to evaluate the degree of stress imposed upon an individual's cardiovascular system by work loads in athletics and in industry. This is particularly important where the total load is increased by unfavorable environmental conditions, such as high ambient temperatures (see Chapter 16). Again, observation of the heart rate response to the work load provides the easiest and quickest evaluation.

Brouha (3) suggests the concept of *cardiac cost* as a means of comparing different work loads. The cardiac cost during exercise is expressed as follows:

Cardiac cost = Total heart beats during exercise minus resting rate for the same period of time

Recovery cost = Heart beats between end of exercise and return to resting minus resting rate for the recovery period

Total cardiac cost = Cardiac cost during exercise plus cardiac cost during recovery

The use of this concept provides reasonably valid information on the total stress an individual's cardiovascular system is subjected to under conditions in which the stress of exercise is complicated by the summation of the exercise stress and the stress imposed by the environment.

EFFECTS OF ATHLETIC TRAINING ON THE HEART

Heart Rate. As training progresses, the heart rate for any given work load decreases, as is illustrated in figure 5.5. We may also say that, other things being equal, the physically fit or athletically trained individual has a lower heart rate for any given exercise work load. Furthermore, at the maximum heart rate which is similar for the trained and the untrained states the trained individual will be able to produce a greater work load.

Stroke Volume. A preponderance of evidence indicates that the increased maximum cardiac output in athletes is due largely to an increase in stroke volume. This is not to say that the immediate adjustment to exercise, which was discussed earlier, is the result of an increased stroke volume; rather, the stroke volume increase seems to be a long-term effect of training, and is also manifest in the slower resting rate of the endurance-trained athlete. This greater stroke volume is the result of the greater contractility and consequent greater systolic emptying of the ventricle in the heart of the trained athlete (2).

Heart Size. The effect of exercise upon the heart in animals is well established. Many investigators have found increases in the weight of the heart in different species as the result of heavy, endurance exercise. There is a temptation to extrapolate these data to man; but there is very little direct evidence, or agreement, on the effects of exercise upon heart size in man.

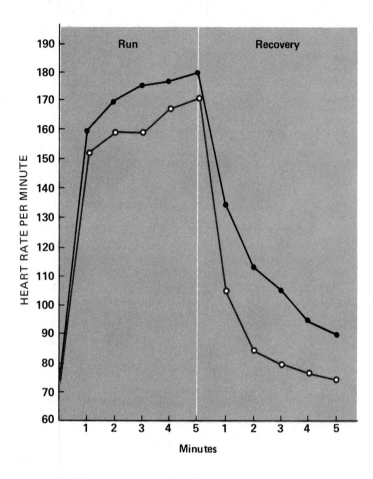

Figure 5-5. Effect of training on the heart rate of an oarsman doing a standard amount of exercise. Solid dots represent "out of training" values; open circles represent "in training" values. (From Brouha. *Work and the Heart,* ch. 21, Rosenbaum and Belknap, eds., 1959. Courtesy of Harper & Row, Publishers, New York.)

Some investigators have found increases in heart size that they attribute to (A) physiological hypertrophy of the musculature, (B) greater diastolic size due to the greater filling of the slower heart rate, or (C) greater end systolic size at rest and a smaller size as exercise commences. Still other investigators have found that the heart size of athletes is within the normal range.

The important fact to be noted is that a change in heart size would be a normal physiological reaction, in all respects similar to the physiological hypertrophy of skeletal muscle as a result of training. It is certainly not to be confused with the pathological increase of heart size that occurs as a compensatory mechanism for heart disease and that imposes greater loads upon the myocardium twenty-four hours a day for many years. There is no evidence that strenuous exercise can injure a normal heart.

Training in Childhood and Old Age. The training of prepubescent children in swimming and other strenuous sports is becoming widespread. With the advent of many age-group programs, children as young as six are competing in several organized sports, and questions are frequently raised of possibly deleterious effects upon the growing child's heart. Karpovich (10) recalculated the data of an older investigation that purported to show that the aorta and pulmonary arteries did not keep up with the heart in the growth rate of children; the recalculated data showed a parallel growth rate, and no contraindication for vigorous exercise. Although there seems to be no evidence of injury to the cardiovascular system of children through strenuous exercise, competitive athletics for small children must also be evaluated on other bases, such as psychological effects and possible bone and joint injuries, which—however—are beyond the scope of this text.

The effects of exercise upon the heart of older persons will be discussed in chapter seventeen.

THE INTENSITY THRESHOLD FOR A TRAINING EFFECT ON THE HEART

A question of interest in the training of athletes is how much work is required to achieve the physiological changes that are reflected by a lowered heart rate in the trained athlete, and pilot studies have been done in this area by Karvonen (11). Untrained medical students were used as subjects, and treadmill running was instituted for a daily, half-hour period for four weeks. The speed of the treadmill was adjusted according to the pulse rate of the subjects, so that each subject ran at a specific, predetermined pulse rate. As exercise tolerance improved, and the heart rate slowed for a given work load, the speed of the treadmill was increased to keep the heart rate at the original level.

Karvonen concluded that to improve the exercise tolerance of the heart the intensity of the workout must exceed a critical threshold value. This was expressed as attaining a heart rate sixty percent of the way between the resting and the maximal rate. For a subject with a resting rate of seventy and a maximum of 200, the critical threshold would be 70 + 0.60 × (200 − 70) or 148 beats per minute. This concept is important for anyone who wishes to apply scientific methods to athletic training. Further experimental data along these lines are needed.

THE CARDIAC RESERVE CAPACITY

Vigorous physical exercise provides the greatest challenge to the cardiovascular system. In the normal individual, only the increased metabolic demand of strenuous work loads can raise the output of the heart to its maximum values. Let us now consider the mechanisms available to the heart in its adjustment to supply the oxygen needs of exercised muscle tissue. It is convenient to think of these mechanisms, in total, as the *cardiac reserve.*

The first and probably the most important factor is the *reserve of heart rate.* In exercise, the rate can increase from its resting value of seventy to eighty beats per minute to a rate of 170 to 180 beats per minute. Although the heart rate can exceed these values, cardiac output will not be improved above approximately 180 because stroke volume will decrease as a result of the decreased diastolic filling times. Thus the cardiac output can be increased two to two and one-half times by increases in heart rate.

The second factor is the *stroke volume reserve.* As was mentioned before, this factor probably comes into play only at a very high level of exertion. However, at very high levels of oxygen consumption the heart has two means by which stroke volume may be increased:
1. By reducing the blood volume remaining at the end of systole, a more complete ejection as the result of greater contractility
2. By increasing the diastolic filling as the result of a greater effective filling pressure and possibly a more distensible ventricle

The third factor is the possibility for *increased oxygen utilization* by the active muscle tissues. At rest, the arterial oxygen level supplied to the muscles is approximately 19 ml per 100 ml of blood and the venous blood may have 13 to 14 ml per 100 ml of blood with a consequent utilization of 5 to 6 ml per 100 ml of blood supplied. However, when the muscle is exercising strenuously, 16 to 17 ml of oxygen per 100 ml of blood may be extracted, which results in a much larger arteriovenous oxygen difference—mainly at the expense of a lowered venous oxygen content in the blood flow from the active muscles.

The question of where the ultimate limits to performance are set is not yet completely resolved but theoretical considerations of the *Oxygen Conductance Equation* as elucidated by R. J. Shephard (24, 25) strongly suggest that aerobic work capacity in normal young men at sea level is set by the capacity for increases of cardiac output. The best controlled experimental evidence supports this theoretical position (16).

HEART MURMURS

A heart murmur is the sound created by turbulent blood flow. The degree of turbulence necessary to create vibrations that can be heard is determined in the cardiovascular system by the velocity of blood flow, and by the amount of eddy currents caused by obstructions, restrictions, etc. Because the flow within the vascular system is normally streamlined (or laminar) and not turbulent, ordinarily no murmurs are heard; however, the velocity of flow in the roots of the aorta and in the pulmonary artery is sufficient to create murmurs during the rapid ejection phase of systole (20). These normal sounds, when they are heard or recorded, are termed *functional murmurs,* and have no pathological significance.

On the other hand, cardiac valves are frequently damaged by disease; and the murmurs caused by regurgitation of blood through an insufficient valve, or by the increased velocity due to a damaged valve (which creates a restriction in the orifice), are valuable diagnostic signs to the physician. The physical educator should at least understand the significance of these murmurs.

The significance of murmurs that result from valvular insufficiency is that in pumping a given volume of blood flow to the tissues to meet metabolic demands the heart must, in a sense, pump the blood that regurgitated twice. This results in a greater-than-normal *volume load* on the heart, and it responds by increasing its stroke volume through an increase in size (and probably by hypertrophy). In doing this, however, a portion of the cardiac reserve is lost because greater tension is required in the myocardial wall to maintain a given blood pressure in the systemic arteries, according to the law of La Place. Because our discussion of the tension-time index indicated a rise in oxygen consumption with tension, it is apparent that the heart is now less efficient. This lessened efficiency may be so slight in some cases as to be a limiting factor only in very strenuous exercise, but in other cases it may severely limit the exercise tolerance.

In a murmur that is due to a valvular restriction, the result is of course an increased *pressure load,* and the heart responds by hypertrophy of the ventricular walls. Again, there is increased tension in the wall of the myocardium, of even greater magnitude, and the consequent lessening in efficiency. Obviously, participation of individuals with heart murmurs in strenuous exercise or athletics should be under the control of a physician. Present-day physicians and cardiologists recognize the advantages that accrue from exercise programs commensurate to the needs of the individual and his limitations. Both professions would be immeasurably helped in their efforts to attain a corrective physical education program if the physical educator and the physician were able to communicate, in quantitative terms, on exercise work loads. These terms might be kilogram meters per minute of work, liters of oxygen per minute, or the number of times the work load demand is greater than the resting metabolic demand. We will discuss this further in chapter nine.

SUMMARY

1. The heart and the vascular system maintain *homeostasis* of the various tissues of the body. Most important to the physical educator is an understanding of oxygen and carbon dioxide transport to and from the skeletal muscles.
2. Although the nervous impulse that stimulates the heart to beat originates within the myocardium, the rate is controlled to a large extent by a balance of the effects of the parasympathetic and sympathetic divisions of the autonomic system, acting through the *vagus* and *accelerator nerves,* respectively.
3. All cardiac valve action is the result of differences in pressure on the two sides of each valve. The cardiac cycle can best be understood in light of the pressure changes that occur in the heart.
4. One of the most important factors that limits human physical performance is the ability to increase cardiac output. Cardiac output = Heart rate × Stroke volume. Consequently, the cardiac output can be increased by an increase in rate, or stroke volume, or both.
5. The rise in heart rate with exercise seems to occur in three phases: (1) a pre-exercise, anticipatory rise due to cortical activity, (2) an early rise due largely to inhibition of vagal activity, and (3) a later rise that is probably the result of a combination of accelerator nerve activity and increased adrenal activity.
6. Starling's law undoubtedly operates under all conditions, but it is the principal determinant of stroke volume only in changes of posture and other manifestations of gravitational changes. Under conditions of exercise, stroke volume is more likely determined by an interplay of the following factors: (1) effective filling pressure, (2) the distensibility of the ventricle in diastole, (3) contractility, and (4) the systemic arterial blood pressure.
7. Coronary blood flow is the limiting factor in cardiac output responses, and thus it indirectly sets the upper limit of exercise tolerance. Prob-

ably the most important factors that effect the increased coronary flow necessary for exercise conditions are: (1) increased arterial blood pressure and (2) lowering levels of oxygen in the myocardium to bring about vasodilatation of the coronary vessels.

8. Many factors affect the resting heart rate, and in many cases, the rate during exercise. All of the following factors must be considered in observing the effects of exercise upon heart rate: (1) age, (2) sex, (3) size, (4) posture, (5) ingestion of food, (6) emotion, (7) body temperature, (8) environmental factors, and (9) smoking.

9. The heart rate responds to light or moderate exercise loads with a rapid increase to a plateau, at which the rate is proportional, in any individual, to the work load and to the oxygen consumption. In very heavy exercise, the rate continues to increase without leveling off, until exhaustion ends the work bout. After exercise ends, the return to normal is very rapid for the first two to three minutes, then slows considerably to a rate of decrease that is roughly related to the intensity and duration of the exercise.

10. The heart rate responds differently to different types of exercise. In general, dynamic muscular activity brings about a much greater increase in heart rate than static, straining types of exercise. Increases in heart rate vary directly with the intensity and duration of the exercise, and inversely with the amount of rest periods in a long, continued work bout.

11. *Cardiac cost* has been proposed as a method for evaluating the stress imposed upon the cardiovascular system by a combination of exercise and environmental stress. Total cardiac cost includes the increase in heart rate during the work bout and the increase during recovery.

12. Athletic training brings about a complex of changes in heart rate, stroke volume, and other factors, all of which together interact to bring about a more effective and efficient adjustment of the organism to the increased metabolic demands of exercise. There seems to be no evidence that indicates a normal heart is harmed by the stress of exercise.

13. Evidence indicates a threshold of exercise intensity below which no *training effect* is observed. This threshold is estimated to be sixty percent of the heart's potential for rate increase.

14. The *cardiac reserve* for conditions of strenuous exercise is the result of three factors: (1) increase in heart rate, (2) increase in stroke volume, (3) increased oxygen utilization of the active muscle tissues.

15. Heart *murmurs* are heart sounds that are brought about by increased turbulence in the blood flow through the heart or large vessels. This

increased turbulence can be the result of increased velocity or of increased eddy currents in the blood flow. In some cases the velocity reaches the critical value without the existence of an abnormality, and the murmur is said to be *functional*. Heart murmurs are usually brought about by a valvular insufficiency that allows regurgitation of blood through a small opening at high velocity, or by restriction of a valvular orifice as a result of disease. Exercise or athletic participation under these conditions should be evaluated and controlled by the individual's physician.

REFERENCES

1. Antel, J., and Cumming, G. R. 1969. Effect of emotional stimulation on exercise heart rate. *Research Quarterly* 40:6-10.
2. Asmussen, E., and Nielsen, M. 1955. Cardiac output during muscular work and it regulation. *Physiological Reviews* 35:778-800.
3. Brouha, L. A. 1959. Effect of work on the heart. In *Work and the Heart*, eds. F. F. Rosenbaum and E. L. Belknap. New York: Paul B. Hoeber, Inc.
4. deVries, H. A. 1970. Physiological effects of an exercise training regimen upon men aged 52-88. *Journal of Gerontology* 25:325-36.
5. Dill, D. B. 1959. Regulation of the heart rate. In *Work and the Heart*, eds. F. F. Rosenbaum and E. L. Belknap. New York: Paul B. Hoeber, Inc.
6. Ferguson, R. J.; Faulkner, J. A.; Julius, S.; and Conway, J. 1968. Comparison of cardiac output determined by CO_2 rebreathing and dye dilution methods. *Journal of Applied Physiology* 25:450-54.
7. Frick, M. H.; Elovainio, R. O.; and Somer, T. 1967. The mechanism of bradycardia evoked by physical training. *Cardiologia* 51:46-54.
8. Gauer, O. H. 1955. Volume changes of the left ventricle during blood pooling and exercise in the intact animal: their effects on left ventricular performance. *Physiological Reviews* 35:143-155.
9. Gregg, D. E.; Sabiston, D. C.; and Thielen, E. O. 1955. Performance of the heart: changes in left ventricular end-diastolic pressure and stroke work during infusion and following exercise. *Physiological Reviews* 35: 130-36.
10. Karpovich, P. V. 1937. Textbook fallacies regarding a child's heart. *Research Quarterly* 8:33.
11. Karvonen, M. J. 1959. Effects of vigorous exercise on the heart. In *Work and the Heart*, eds. F. F. Rosenbaum and E. L. Belknap. New York: Paul B. Hoeber, Inc.
12. Katz, L. N. 1955. Analysis of the several factors regulating the performance of the heart. *Physiological Reviews* 35:91-106.
13. Kemp, G. L.; Ellestad, M. H.; Beland, A. J.; and Allen, W. H. 1969. The maximal tread mill stress test for the evaluation of medical and surgical treatment of coronary insufficiency. *Journal of Thoracic and Cardiovascular Surgery* 57:708-13.

14. Kitamura, K.; Jorgensen, C. R.; Gobel, F. L.; Taylor, H. L.; and Wang, Y. 1972. Hemodynamic correlates of myocardial oxygen consumption during upright exercise. *Journal of Applied Physiology* 32:516-22.
15. McC. Brooks, C. 1962. The laws of the isolated heart. In *Cardiovascular Functions*, ed. A. A. Luisada. New York: McGraw-Hill Book Co. Inc.
16. Ouellet, Y.; Poh, S. C.; and Becklake, M. R. 1969. Circulatory factors limiting maximal aerobic exercise capacity. *Journal of Applied Physiology* 27:874-80.
17. Randall, W. C. 1962. Sympathetic control of the heart-peripheral mechanisms. In *Cardiovascular Functions*, ed. A. A. Luisada. New York: McGraw-Hill Book Co., Inc. 1962.
18. Richards, D. 1955. Discussion of Starling's law of the heart. *Physiological Reviews* 35:156-60.
19. Rushmer, R. F. 1955. Applicability of Starling's law of the heart to intact, unanesthetized animals. *Physiological Reviews* 35:138-42.
20. ———. 1961. *Cardiovascular dynamics*. Philadelphia: W. B. Saunders Co.
21. Sarnoff, S. J.; Braunwald, E.; Welch, G. H.; Stainsley, W. N.; Case, R. B.; and Macruz, R. 1959. Oxygen consumption of the heart, with special reference to the tension-time index. In *Work and the Heart*, eds. F. F. Rosenbaum and E. L. Belknap. New York: Paul B. Hoeber, Inc.
22. Sarnoff, S. J., and Braunwald, E. 1962. Hemodynamic determinants of myocardial oxygen consumption. In *Cardiovascular Functions*, ed. A. A. Luisada. New York: McGraw-Hill Book Co., Inc.
23. Schilpp, R. W. 1951. A mathematical description of the heart rate curve of response to exercise, with some observations on the effects of smoking. *Research Quarterly* 22:439-45.
24. Shephard, R. J. 1967. Physiological determinants of cardiorespiratory fitness. *Journal of Sports Medicine and Physical Fitness* 7:111-34.
25. ———. 1971. The oxygen conductance equation. In *Frontiers of Fitness*, ed. R. J. Shephard, pp. 129-54. Springfield: Charles C. Thomas.
26. Vatner. S. F.; Higgins, C. B.; Franklin, D.; and Braunwald, E. 1972. Role of tachycardia in mediating the coronary hemodynamic response to severe exercise. *Journal of Applied Physiology* 32:380-85.
27. Wiggers, C. J. 1962. Cardiac output, stroke volume, and stroke work. In *Cardiovascular Functions*, ed. A. A. Luisada. New York: McGraw-Hill Book Co., Inc.

6 The Circulatory System and Exercise

From the standpoint of exercise physiology, blood is primarily a tissue of respiration. Its importance lies in its ability to transport the respiratory gasses, oxygen and carbon dioxide, between the respiratory organs and the active tissues. Although blood subserves many other very important general physiological functions, this transport of oxygen and carbon dioxide becomes the limiting factor in physical performance and consequently assumes major importance.

It is tempting to liken the blood flow through the vascular system to the flow of water through a plumbing system; this is a very poor analogy, however, because the pipes in a plumbing system serve only *passively* as conduits for the transport of fluids whereas the blood vessels are *active* participants in the adjustments made by the circulatory system for the demands of exercise. For example, an individual may increase his oxygen intake and his energy output to twenty times the basal rate, and his increase of energy output by the *active muscles* may be as much as fifty times the resting rate, and this difference, of course, is the result of a redistribution of blood (and thus oxygen) by the vascular system through a vasoconstriction in inactive tissues and a vasodilatation of the active muscle tissues.

HEMODYNAMICS: PRINCIPLES GOVERNING BLOOD FLOW

Pressure Gradient.   Blood flows through the vessels of the circulatory system because of differences in pressure. It flows from a point of high pressure to a point of lower pressure, and the difference in pressure between the two points is called a *pressure gradient.* In the systemic circulatory system, the point of highest pressure is within the left ventricle of the heart during systole, and the pressure gradient between this point and the lowest pressure point in the right atrium is the driving force that brings about blood flow through the entire systemic circulation (although this is aided by the muscle pump, to be discussed below). An analogous situation exists in the pulmonary circulation.

Velocity of Blood Flow.   The combination of systemic circulation and pulmonary circulation may be thought of as the two loops of a figure eight (fig. 6.1). The two loops are interconnected in series, each with its own pressure gradient, provided by its side of the cardiac pump. It is apparent that this is in reality a closed, single circuit—although possessed of two pressure gradients in series—and it follows that the *same volume* of blood must pass *each* and *any point* in the system per unit time (if we assume that no retention of blood occurs at any point). This being so, the *velocity of blood flow* past any point obviously depends upon the total cross-sectional area of the vascular bed at that point; where the area is smaller, the velocity must be higher and vice versa (fig. 6.2).

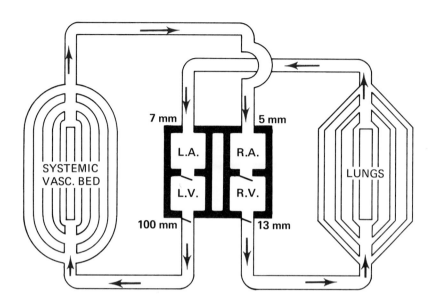

Figure 6-1. Interrelationships of systemic and pulmonary circulations and their pressure gradients.

The aorta has a cross-sectional area of approximately 2.5 to 5.0 square centimeters. As the large arteries bifurcate, the combined area of the branches considerably exceeds the area of the parent vessel. As this branching of the arterial system progresses, the total cross-sectional area of the circulatory system constantly increases, and consequently the velocity of flow decreases proportionately. In the capillary bed, where each vessel is only 10 μ (1/100 of a mm) in diameter, this multiplication has progressed to such an extent that the combined cross-sectional area of all capillaries is about 700 to 800 times the area of the aorta. This means that the flow rate or velocity has decreased in proportion, and the result is a very slow flow of 0.5 to 1.0 mm per second through the capillaries, thus allowing adequate time for the exchange of respiratory gasses, nutrients, etc.

Resistance to Flow. Resistance may be thought of as the sum of the forces opposing blood flow, and may be illustrated by breathing through various sizes and lengths of glass tubing. It is readily seen that exhaling becomes progressively more difficult as the length of the tube is *increased;* it also becomes more difficult as the diameter of the tube is *decreased.* Another factor, the *viscosity* of the fluid, is also important. Other

VOLUME FLOW THROUGH THE SYSTEMIC CIRCULATION

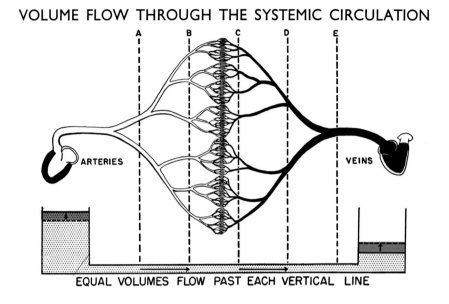

EQUAL VOLUMES FLOW PAST EACH VERTICAL LINE

Figure 6-2. Arborization of the systemic circulatory system is schematically represented with all vessels of the same caliber arranged vertically. This simplified illustration emphasizes the fact that the volume of fluid flowing past each vertical line in a unit of time must be equal to the quantity entering and leaving the system, just as in a single tube. (From Rushmer. *Cardiovascular Dynamics,* 2nd ed., 1961. Courtesy of W.B. Saunders Company, Philadelphia.)

things being equal, the more viscous the fluid the greater the resistance to its flow. For example, the flow of molasses is much slower than the flow of water.

Poiseuille's Law. If we may assume that the walls of the blood vessels are rigid, we can state the relationships discussed above as follows.

$$\text{Volume of blood flow} = \frac{\text{Pressure gradient}}{\text{Resistance}}$$

This can also be stated:

$$\text{Resistance} = \frac{\text{Pressure gradient}}{\text{Volume of blood flow}}$$

$$\text{Pressure gradient} = \text{Volume of blood flow} \times \text{Resistance}$$

A theoretically derived mathematical law, which expresses all these relationships, is frequently used by physiologists. This is Poiseuille's law (see fig. 6.3) an approximation of which (in simplified form) can be stated as follows.

$$\text{Volume of blood flow} = \frac{\text{Pressure} \times (\text{vessel radius})^4}{\text{Vessel length} \times \text{Viscosity}}$$

Hydrostatic Pressure. In diving to the bottom of a swimming pool, an increase in pressure is felt upon the ears. This increased pressure is *hydrostatic pressure*, and it increases with depth. It is also present in any vertical tube that contains a liquid because of the increasing weight of the liquid with increasing height (fig. 6.3). This principle is also applied

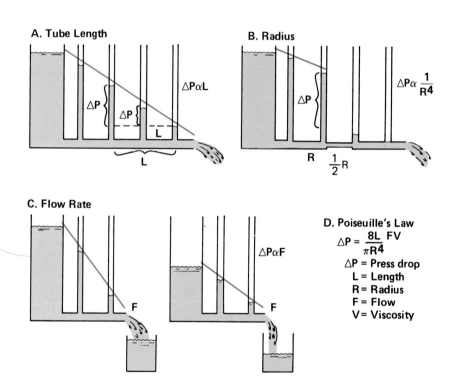

Figure 6-3. A, the drop in pressure (ΔP) during laminar flow of a homogeneous fluid through a rigid tube of constant caliber is directly proportional to the length of the tube. B, under the same conditions, the pressure drop is also inversely proportional to the reciprocal of the radius to the fourth power ($1/R^4$) and directly proportional to the volume flow (F) through

when we *weigh* the atmospheric air by balancing it against a column of mercury to obtain barometric pressure. It is important to remember the effect of hydrostatic pressure in physiology because changes in body position alter the blood pressure in various parts of the body. Thus when blood pressure is taken by a physician, it is taken at the level of the heart. Finding the blood pressure at any other level of the body requires correction for the hydrostatic pressure effect.

For example, in an individual whose mean blood pressure is 90 mm mercury (Hg) at heart level, we should expect to find a decrease of pressure of 30 cm of blood at the ear level. Converting 30 cm of blood to mm of mercury (1 mm Hg = 13.6 mm blood), we would expect a mean blood pressure at the ear of approximately $90 - 22 = 68$ mm mercury. Conversely, at the ankle (in complete rest)—assuming a measurement of 125 cm from ankle to heart level in standing position (and neglecting frictional losses, etc.)—we should expect to find an increased pressure of some $125 \times 10/13.6$, or $90 + 92 = 182$ mm mercury blood pressure at the ankle. These figures correspond rather closely to the pressures found experimentally.

THE MICROCIRCULATION: BLOOD FLOW THROUGH THE CAPILLARY BED

The work of Zweifach (32, 33, 34) and Zweifach and Metz (35) has resulted in a better understanding of the capillary bed and allows much better rationalization of the important circulatory changes that occur in muscle tissue during exercise.

The microcirculation is thought of as a well-organized network in which the arterioles give rise to *metarterioles* (fig. 6.4), which possess a gradually dispersing, thin muscular coat. These metarterioles constitute major thoroughfares, or *preferential channels*, through the tissue, and they remain open even during resting conditions; eventually, they join a collecting venule. The *true capillaries* are endothelial tubes, with no smooth muscle which arise from the metarterioles by way of a *precapillary sphincter* which closes down the true capillaries during resting conditions, and which relaxes during muscle activity to allow the increased circulation demanded by the higher metabolic rate.

There is also a third alternative route for blood flow through the microcirculation, by way of *arterio-venous-anastomoses* (AVA) which form a short and direct connection between (A) small arteries and small veins, (B) arterioles, and venules, (C) metarterioles, and adjacent venules. These AVA have a well-developed muscular coat, and are under sympathetic nervous control. They seem to be most common in the extremities, and they function in bringing about greater losses of heat when

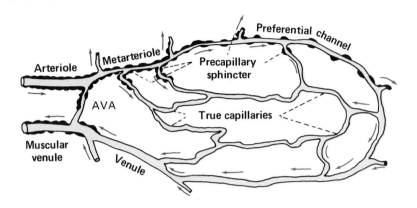

Figure 6-4. A schematic representation of the structural pattern of the capillary bed. The distribution of smooth muscle is indicated in the vessel wall. (From Zweifach. *Basic Mechanisms in Peripheral Vascular Homeostasis,* in 3rd Conference on Factors Regulating Blood Pressure, 1950. Courtesy of Josiah Macy, Jr. Foundation, New York.)

environmental temperature rises or when heat is produced within as during exercise. This loss of heat is brought about because the opening of the AVA causes a greater amount of blood to flow through the venous collection system which is closer to the surface than the arteries and arterioles and thus provides greater heat losses.

We can think of the functions of the peripheral blood vessels as fourfold:

1. Maintenance of blood pressure by the arteries and arterioles
2. Distribution of blood flow to the active tissues by the interaction of metarterioles and the precapillary sphincters in determining how much flow goes through the thoroughfare (preferential) channels and how much through the true capillaries
3. Temperature control, largely by heat loss controlled through the AVA
4. *The return of blood* to the heart, by way of the muscular venules to the small veins, etc.

Various tissues have smaller or larger ranges of metabolic activity. Muscle tissue has the greatest range; from the resting state to forty or fifty times the resting level of energy metabolism. Apparently for this reason, the ratio of true capillaries to thoroughfare channels also varies considerably from tissue to tissue. Zweifach (1961) has estimated the ratio in skeletal muscle as eight or ten to one, whereas in tissues of lesser metabolic activity this ratio may be as low as two or three to one.

CONTROL OF BLOOD DISTRIBUTION

Control of the flow of blood to the various tissues of the systemic circulation is brought about by changes in the diameter of the small arteries and arterioles. The effectiveness of change in the bore of these vessels is seen by referring to Poiseuille's law (p. 122). If the diameter of a small vessel is doubled, the amount of blood flow will not be doubled, but will be increased sixteen times since the flow varies as the fourth power of vessel radius. These changes in diameter are brought about by two mechanisms: *nervous* and *chemical regulation.* Since the main function of the small arteries and arterioles is to control, by their degree of constriction, the resistance to flow, they are properly referred to as the *resistance vessels.* The veins are thin walled but nevertheless also have smooth muscle in their walls and thus can also actively change their diameters. However, changes in their wall tension do not have any great effect upon resistance to flow, but they are very important in altering the *capacity* of the post capillary system. Thus they are important in determining the rate of return flow to the heart, and may be referred to as *capacity vessels.*

Nervous Regulation. So far as we know, all of the nervous regulation of blood flow to the skeletal muscles is brought about by the sympathetic system. However, this system supplies two types of fibers: (1) *adrenergic,* which bring about vasoconstriction, and (2) *cholinergic,* which cause active vasodilatation. The normal state of the resistance blood vessels that supply skeletal muscle tissue is one of vasoconstrictor tone (2). Greater blood supply to an active muscle can be brought about by release of its vasoconstrictor tone or by active vasodilatation. Release of vasoconstrictor tone in the active tissues, with concomitant vasoconstriction in less active tissues—particularly the skin and viscera—seems to be the more important factor. Vasodilatation of resistance vessels appears to function only in emotional reactions or in the expectation of an exercise bout. Further more, active vasodilatation probably does not contribute to the support of an increased metabolic rate since it does not result in an increased flow through the true capillaries but only through the AVA or thoroughfare channels discussed above (5).

Muscular exercise causes a reflex increase in tension of the venous walls in both exercising and nonexercising limbs, which persists throughout the exercise and is proportional to the severity of the work (7). This closing down of the capacitance vessels along with the muscle pump and the abdominal-thoracic pump aids the venous return to the heart.

Chemical Regulation. Greater blood flow to active tissue is also brought about by the chemical results of metabolic activity. Lowered pH, increased CO_2 level, and other local changes in metabolites have such a potent effect upon the microcirculation that these effects can override the more centrally mediated vasoconstrictor stimuli whether bloodborne or neurogenic in origin.

The overall picture in exercise appears to be one in which nervous regulation closes down, to a large extent, the circulation to inactive tissues, and it also opens the precapillary sphincters of the microcirculation so that greater flow is provided through the true capillaries that serve the metabolic needs of the active muscle tissue. Simultaneously, or as soon as metabolic products of the activity accummulate, chemical regulation augments the blood flow by further local vasodilatation.

BLOOD DISTRIBUTION IN REST AND EXERCISE

As we described earlier, the volume of blood flow to a particular tissue depends upon the resistance it offers in relation to the pressure gradient of its blood flow. Thus the resistance to flow is frequently described in *R* units, where:

Resistance to flow
$$R = \frac{\text{Pressure gradient in mm Hg}}{\text{Flow rate in ml/sec}}$$

This is a very convenient method. If we assume an average man at rest has a cardiac output of 5,400 ml/min, then, with the usually accepted average resting mean arterial blood pressure of 90 mm Hg (diastolic + 1/3 pulse pressure), the resistance for the total circulatory system—with essentially zero central venous pressure—becomes:

$$R = \frac{90 - 0}{5,400/60} = \frac{90}{90} = 1$$

This resistance of one *R* unit can be broken down into its component parts, according to the part of the circulatory system that interests us. Thus the resistance of the arterial system can be compared with that of the venous system under resting conditions, as follows:

Flow rate = 90 ml/sec
Central venous pressure = 0.0
Mean arterial pressure = 90 mm Hg
Mean pressure in middle of capillary = 25 mm Hg

Arterial resistance, then, equals: $\dfrac{90 - 25}{90} = 0.72$ R

and venous resistance equals: $\dfrac{25 - 0.0}{90} = 0.28$ R

Total = 1.00 R

Under a moderate exercise load, the same average man will increase his cardiac output some three times, to 16,200 ml per minute. Let us examine some typical figures and determine the resistance changes.

$$\text{Flow rate} = 16{,}200 \text{ ml/min} = 270 \text{ ml/sec}$$
$$\text{Central venous pressure} = 0.0$$
$$\text{Mean arterial pressure} = 120 \text{ mm Hg}$$
$$\text{Mean capillary pressure} = 25 \text{ mm Hg}$$

$$\text{Arterial resistance equals: } \frac{120 - 25}{270} = 0.35 \text{ R}$$

$$\text{and venous resistance equals: } \frac{25 - 0}{270} = 0.09 \text{ R}$$
$$\text{Total} = 0.44 \text{ R}$$

These figures, which are quite realistic, illustrate what happens in the circulatory system during exercise. First, the total peripheral resistance is greatly reduced because the blood pressure gradients do not rise nearly as much as the flow rate. This, of course, is the result of vasodilatation in the active skeletal muscles, which far outweighs the accompanying vasoconstriction in less active tissues. Second, the decrease in resistance is even greater in the venous than in the arterial system. The decrease in the arterial system is the result of vasodilatation of the arterioles, while the decrease in the venous system results from the assistance to blood flow given by the muscle pump. Overall, it is this decreased total peripheral resistance that allows the heart to function at a greatly elevated output without strain.

It is also of interest to know where and to what extent compensatory vasoconstriction occurs to support the increased blood flow to the active muscles in exercise. It has been estimated that the resistance to flow in the muscles is reduced from 3.1 R units to 0.37 R during exercise, while the resistance in the portal arteries increases from 2.6 R to 12.0 R, and the portal venous and liver resistance increases from 1.0 R to 3.0 R (6).

BLOOD PRESSURE

The importance of blood pressure as the driving force for the circulatory system has been emphasized. Now let us consider the practical problem of measurement, and how observed measurements may change under varying conditions.

Measurement of Blood Pressure.   The commonly used indirect method involves a pressure cuff whose pressure is read from a mercury or aneroid manometer. This device is called a *sphygmomanometer*. The sphygmomanometer's cuff is applied to the upper arm, as the subject sits comfortably, so that the cuff is approximately at heart level. The pressure required to occlude the brachial artery is noted by listening to the flow of blood below the cuff, and this is read as *systolic blood pressure. Diastolic blood pressure* is recorded as the pressure at which the sounds resulting from occlusion become muffled, or disappear, as the cuff pressure is reduced. The systolic-diastolic difference is *pulse pressure.*

Blood pressure measurements made by the indirect method during exercise must be viewed with caution. Comparisons between indirect (sphygmomanometer) and direct (catheter) methods showed that systolic pressure was underestimated by mean values of 8 to 15 mm Hg by the indirect method, and overestimated during recovery by 16 to 38 mm Hg (14). Other investigators (22) have found that the indirect method provides satisfactory data on systolic but not diastolic pressure. Some sources of variability in blood pressure follow:

Age. Figure 6.5 illustrates the increase of systolic and diastolic pressures with age. It also shows the more enlightened approach to the problem of *normality,* in which ranges are given instead of single figures. It is of interest that not all cultures show this agewise increment in blood pressure. Henry and Cassel (13) have furnished impressive evidence for a psychosocial effect in which dissonance between the social milieu in later life and expectations based on early experiences brings about the often observed increase in blood pressure with age.

Sex. The blood pressure in women prior to menopause tends to be slightly lower—and after menopause somewhat higher—than men of the same age.

Emotion. The problem of measuring blood pressure is greatly complicated by the fact that the slightest emotional involvement is reflected by significant rises in blood pressure. This fact is used to advantage in the *polygraph* or lie detector because the act of lying creates emotional conflict that is sensed and recorded, along with other physiological variables that react to emotional changes.

Diurnal Variation. Blood pressure tends to rise from a low point during sleep to a high point (15 to 20 mm Hg higher) after the evening meal.

Ingestion of Food. After a large meal, there is normally a considerable rise in systolic, and sometimes a fall in diastolic, pressure.

Posture. In changing from supine to erect posture, the hydrostatic pressure increase requires greater arterial pressure, and the response by the cardiovascular system usually overshoots the mark so that systolic and diastolic pressures usually show an increase of 5 to 10 mm Hg. The pulse pressure usually shows a decrease, due to the relatively greater increase in diastolic pressure.

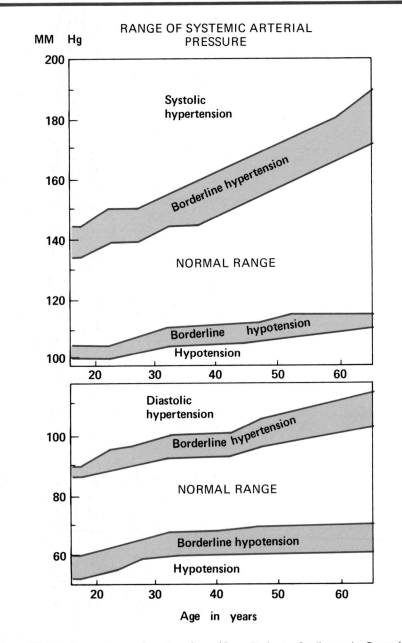

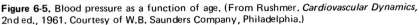

Figure 6-5. Blood pressure as a function of age. (From Rushmer. *Cardiovascular Dynamics,* 2nd ed., 1961. Courtesy of W.B. Saunders Company, Philadelphia.)

Maintenance of Arterial Blood Pressure. The formula: pressure gradient equals volume of blood flow times resistance, shows clearly that blood pressure is maintained by the interaction of two factors, volume of blood flow and resistance. The volume of blood flow is in turn dependent upon (A) heart rate and (B) stroke volume. The resistance is largely determined by the vasoconstrictor tone of the arterioles.

Maintenance of Venous Return to the Heart. The venous blood pressure at the ankle in the standing posture (under conditions of no muscular activity) is roughly equivalent to the hydrostatic pressure 92 mm Hg, if we assume a vertical distance from ankle to right auricle of 125 cm. However, such a pressure, if maintained for any length of time, results in filtration of fluids from the vascular system into the tissue spaces, which results in considerable *edema* (swelling). This happens when a person is forced to stand motionless for a protracted period of time, but it does not occur if the muscles of the leg are active. If the venous pressure is measured in a leg whose muscles are active—as in walking, etc.— the pressure is greatly reduced (to 20 or 25 mm Hg) because of one-way valves in the veins that serve the musculature. Thus the contraction of muscle drives blood toward the heart, and during the relaxation phase these valves prevent a backward flow. This is the first of three major factors that maintain venous return: *the pumping action of contracting muscles.*

A second very important factor is the *abdominothoracic pump.* The descent of the diaphragm in inspiration creates an increase in intraabdominal pressure while simultaneously lowering intrathoracic pressure. This increased pressure gradient, from abdomen to right atrium, aids the venous return. During expiration, the backward flow is prevented by the valves in the veins of the muscles of the legs.

A third factor of importance is the *shortening of the inferior vena cava* during the descent of the diaphragm, which results in its having smaller volume, which in turn aids the flow from abdomen to thorax. The lengthening inferior vena cava during expiration lowers pressure within its walls and allows a better pressure gradient for its filling, preparatory to the next descent of the diaphgram.

ARTERIAL BLOOD PRESSURE DURING EXERCISE

The effects of exercise upon arterial blood pressure can best be described as the end result of the balance struck between the increased blood flow due to the increased cardiac output and the decreased peripheral resistance caused by the vasodilatation of the microcirculation. Consequently, the end result is considerably influenced by the *type* and *intensity* of the exercise and by the physical condition of the subject.

Type of Exercise. In rhythmic exercise that involves moderate to strenuous workloads, the typical response is an elevation of systolic pressure while diastolic pressure usually rises very little if at all, figure 6.6 shows a typical response for a young male. The mean arterial pressure is usually calculated at one-third of the way between diastolic and systolic pressures because of the shape of the arterial pressure wave form. Therefore, the mean pressure is much less affected by exercise.

In static or isometric exercise, where an expiratory effort is made against a closed glottis, the situation is quite different. The intrathoracic pressure is raised from 80 to 200 mm Hg or more, and this increased pressure is transmitted through the thin walls of the great veins; venous return to the right atrium is thus severely decreased, resulting in the following sequence of events.

1. There is a sharp increase in pressure, both systolic and diastolic which reflects the increase in intrathoracic pressure.
2. After a period of several seconds, during which blood in the lungs furnishes the venous return, the decreased venous return brings about a decreased pulse pressure.

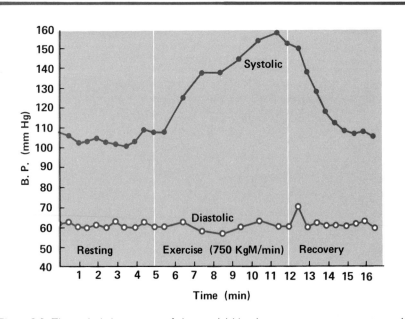

Figure 6-6. The typical time course of the arterial blood pressure response to rest-exercise-recovery in a healthy young man.

3. After release of the straining activity, there is an increase in both mean pressure and pulse pressure due to the improved venous return of blood, which had been blocked.

This sequence of events is called the *Valsalva effect*.

Although exercise physiologists have often cautioned against strength exercises with a large static component because of possibly harmful effects of the increased pressure upon the heart and large blood vessels, the work of Hamilton and others (12) shows that no increased difference in pressure across the walls of the heart and great vessels can exist; as the pressure increases within these walls, it increases proportionately outside them. In fact, the pressure difference decreases.

The vessels of the cerebral circulation are similarly protected in that the increased intrathoracic pressure is also transmitted to the cerebrospinal fluid. The only possible danger, then, is in peripheral vessels; but the peripheral vessels are small in diameter, and the laws of physics tell us they are consequently better able to withstand pressure.

However, it must be recalled from the earlier discussion that the work of the heart is determined to a great extent by the arterial pressure against which it is working. It will also be recalled that during exercise the redistribution of blood flow is accomplished by increased sympathetic adrenergic vasomotor tone in the inactive areas while this tone is overridden in the active muscles by local effects to increase the blood flow to the active muscles.

There is now considerable evidence that the systemic level of arterial blood pressure is set by the perfusion pressure required to get through that muscle tissue which is contracting most strongly (2, 3, 11, 18, 19, 20). That is to say that the level of systemic blood pressure is set not by the total amount of muscle working (level of total body work) but rather by the pressure required to perfuse that muscle which is working hardest even though this may be only one small muscle group (10). Furthermore, the type of exercise is very important. In isometric contraction, the tissue pressure upon the arteries can be very high, thus requiring very high perfusion pressure which in turn requires large increases in systemic pressure to accomplish.

Lind and McNicol (19) performed an experiment in which their subjects walked on a treadmill at three miles per hour against a grade of 22 percent which required an O_2 uptake of 2.8 L/min. In spite of this very heavy work load sustained by the entire body musculature, when they then performed an isometric contraction, while walking, of 50 percent maximum on a handgrip dynamometer for one minute their systolic pressure rose by 45 and diastolic by 40 mm Hg. This illustrates clearly the need to avoid isometric contractions and also high loadings of small muscles in any exercise situation where high cardiac workloads are undesirable as in cardiac rehabilitation exercise or in conditioning programs for older adults.

BLOOD FLOW IN EXERCISING MUSCLES

As soon as exercise begins, the metabolic demands of the active muscle tissue increase (by as much as fiftyfold in all-out activity). Many physiological mechanisms cooperate to supply the demand. In addition to the increased cardiac output and redistribution of blood from inactive to active tissues, changes in blood flow occur within the active tissues. In an interesting experiment—in which India ink was injected into dogs' muscles—Martin and others (1932) showed that in the active gracilis muscle there were 2,010 open capillaries per square millimeter, compared with 1,050 in the same muscle when resting (21).

Concurrently with the increased flow rate through the tissue, the rate of O_2 consumption per cell (muscle fiber) increases rapidly, and this results in a fall in the partial pressure of O_2 within the cell. The partial pressure of O_2 in the tissue fluid bathing the cells, on the other hand, falls very little, and thus a much higher pressure gradient exists to move O_2 from the capillary through the tissue fluid and into the muscle fiber. Better O_2 extraction per volume of circulating blood helps supply the increased metabolic demand. The presence of greater concentrations of CO_2 in the cell further aid the gas exchange (this factor is discussed in chapter eight).

According to the work of Reeves and others (25), it seems that the increased O_2 extraction plays the greater part in making the adjustment to mild exercise (two to three times the resting level), but that in moderate to heavy exercise the increase in cardiac output and the improved flow through tissues is more important.

In general the blood flow through muscle increases in proportion to the metabolic demand and does not appear to be a limiting factor in high level performance (24).

The type of activity is an important factor not only in the circulation through large vessels, but it also affects blood flow within the muscle itself. The classic early work of Barcroft and Millen (1939) on the plantar flexors of the foot demonstrated an increased flow (*hyperemia*) when muscular contractions were 0.1 maximum (or less) but a cessation of flow when the contractions were above 0.3 maximum. More recent work (30, 31) has shown that isometric contraction of the forearm muscles and elbow flexors occludes the blood flow in these muscles also, but requires 0.6 maximal contraction strength. Thus it would seem that muscles held unnecessarily in tension during athletic activity may suffer the effects of ischemia with its accompanying pain and loss of endurance.

As would be expected, training and conditioning have an effect upon the level of blood flow through the muscles involved. Rohter and others (29) demonstrated an increase of almost sixty percent in blood flow through the forearm flexors in swimmers after five weeks of training, compared with controls (fig. 6.7). This work has been confirmed by recent studies by Rochelle et al. (28). It has also been shown that isometric training can increase exercise blood flow, at least when measured with a contraction of not over fifty percent of maximal. (8)

It is tempting to explain this improved blood flow which results from training on the basis of the older and often referred to work which showed increased capillarization to result from training in animals (23). However, this work depended on staining techniques which stained the red

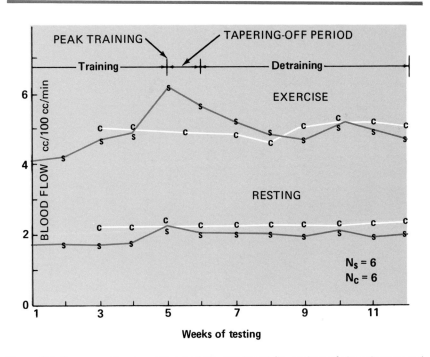

Figure 6-7. Summary of mean resting and exercise blood flow values of six swimmers and six control subjects during a thirteen-week training and detraining program. S = swimmers; C = control. (From Rohter, Rochelle, and Hyman. *Journal of Applied Physiology* 18:798, 1963.)

blood cells and accurate counts can probably not be made in this fashion. More recent work in which the capillary basement membrane itself is stained has shown no increase in the number of capillaries (15). But since the muscle fibers increased in size (human subjects) the training resulted in a more favorable capillary to fiber ratio, 1.5 to 1.0 compared to 1.0 to 1.0 in the untrained. It is possible that this may be related to the improved blood flow found to result from training.

In general, the immediate short-term effects of exercise are an increase of blood flow through muscles that are active in light, rhythmic activity, and a decrease during heavy, sustained contraction which, however, is followed by a period of increased flow, called *reactive hyperemia*. The long-term effect of exercise almost certainly involves an improved perfusion of the active tissues.

BLOOD AND FLUID CHANGES DURING EXERCISE

The total body fluid is composed of four components:

1. Blood plasma ⎫ *extra cellular fluid*
2. Interstitial fluid ⎭
3. Intracellular fluid
4. Miscellaneous components

Only the first three have importance to exercise physiology. Because the capillary wall is freely permeable to most of the substances in the plasma (except the plasma protein), the plasma and interstitial fluid constantly mix, and are very similar in their makeup. Therefore, the two together are referred to as extracellular fluid.

To maintain normal osmotic pressures in intra- and extracellular fluids, water diffuses in the direction needed through the cell membrane. Thus in excessive sweating as in heavy exercise, water that is lost in sweat comes directly from an extracellular component. This raises the concentration of nondiffusible substances of the interstitial fluid which results in transfer of water across the cell membranes of the various tissue cells from intracellular to extracellular components, thus dehydrating the tissues as well. Obviously, ingestion of water causes a reverse reaction, in which tissue hydration is restored toward normal.

Hemoconcentration. Moderate to heavy exercise bouts result in a shift of fluid from the plasma to the interstitial fluid. This, in turn, results in higher hemoglobin and serum protein concentrations, and in a higher proportion of cellular elements in the plasma. If the exercise bouts involve heavy work in a hot environment, dehydration contributes to exaggerate this phenomenon. Weight loss in wrestlers by dehydration has been reported as high as 8.8 pounds, and in marathon runners it may be as high as seven percent of body weight. A dehydration of two percent may cause deterioration of performance in some individuals (1).

Erythrocyte Count. The hemoconcentration discussed above results in a considerable rise in the cell count per cubic millimeter. In the normal male, the count is ordinarily 5.5 million per cubic millimeter (female, 4.8 million per cubic millimeter). These values can be raised by as much as twenty to twenty-five percent in vigorous exercise. Whether this rise is due entirely to hemoconcentration, or in part to release of stored cells, is still unclear. In some animals the spleen releases erythrocytes to the general circulation during exercise, but this does not seem to be the case in man.

BLOOD AND FLUID CHANGES FROM TRAINING

Blood Volume. Evidence indicates that blood volume first falls, then rises, above normal during a four- to nine-week training period in dogs (9). The increased blood volume persisted about four weeks after cessation of training. Kjellberg and others (16) found similar results with men and women: blood volumes were found to be ten to nineteen percent higher after training than before. They also found blood volume was as much as forty-one to forty-four percent higher in an athletically trained group than in a comparable, untrained group.

Changes in the opposite direction occur with prolonged bed rest. Thus it would seem that blood volume varies proportionately with the amount of physical activity. Increased blood volume would be a considerable advantage in heavy exercise because a circulatory demand may exist for purposes of heat dissipation at the same time that active muscle tissues also demand a greatly increased blood volume. Under these conditions, increased blood volume would help assure an adequate venous return to the heart.

Hemoglobin. Increases of *total hemoglobin* have been found in dogs and in man as the result of physical conditioning (9, 16). These increases seem to parallel the increased blood volume, so that no increase in *hemoglobin concentration* (hemoglobin per unit blood volume) seems to occur.

Alkaline Reserve. Alkaline reserve may be defined as the buffering capacity of the blood. Many investigators have shown an increased ability to tolerate acid metabolites (mainly lactic acid) after a period of training. Thus it would seem a likely hypothesis that this increased tolerance might be due to an increase in buffering ability of the blood. Robinson and Harmon (27) have shown, however, that the alkaline reserve did not change during a period of training in which large increases in ability to carry O_2 debt were observed.

Postural Effects on Circulation. Posture during physical activity varies from the usual, upright position to sitting while rowing, to the prone or supine position in swimming, to the head-down position in gymnastics. Changes in posture might be expected to exert effects upon the circulation, and these effects have been demonstrated.

The responses to exercise in supine and sitting (bicycle ergometer) and standing (treadmill) positions have been studied by many investigators. In general, the cardiac output is about 2 L/min greater in supine position than in the upright positions. This is due to the greater stroke volume supine. A higher arteriovenous O_2 difference in the upright position compensates for the lower cardiac output and stroke volume (7).

Tilt-table changes of a subject's position, from standing upright to the head-down position, produced a *vagal rebound phenomenon* (17) in which the subject's heart rates slowed by an average of fifteen beats per minute (fig. 6.8). This can be explained by the fact that in upright posture the peripheral resistance is maintained by sympathetic nervous activity that reflexly maintains a state of vasoconstriction in the arterioles of the lower extremities. When the body is tilted head-downward, the redistribution of blood due to the changed direction of the force of gravity brings about greater stimulation of the carotid sinus and central nervous system receptors which induces vagal efferent stimulation with cardioinhibitory responses. Surprisingly, no relationship was found between the reaction to head-down tilting and physical fitness (measured by endurance in treadmill walking).

The circulatory reserves that can be called upon also seem to vary with body position. As soon as an individual assumes the standing position, his O_2 extraction (as measured by the difference between arterial and venous oxygen levels of the working muscle) has already greatly increased. His circulatory reserve therefore depends largely upon the factors that can increase the flow rate. In the supine position, mild demands of exercise can be satisfied by increased O_2 extraction before any increase in blood flow is demanded.

Cooling Out after Heavy Exercise. It has been the common practice in athletic events that involve large circulatory adjustments—distance running, etc.—to *cool out* at the end of the competitive effort by jogging for a few minutes. This procedure rests upon sound physiological principles, and should be encouraged. If this cooling out is not done, venous return to the heart—which has been largely supported by the muscle pump—drops too abruptly, and blood pooling may occur in the extremities. This, in turn, may result in shock, or at least in hyperventilation, which causes lower levels of CO_2 and muscle cramps.

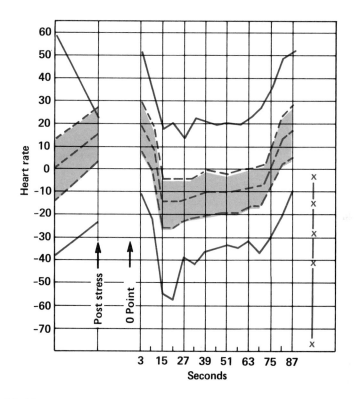

Figure 6-8. The mean change in heart rate from the baseline level for 215 subjects is plotted against time. The O point is a six-second period just prior to the head-down tilt. Heart rate is plotted for each six-second interval thereafter. The increase in heart rate after the sixty-second period is following rotation to the feet-down position. The shaded area is the standard deviation of the mean. The upper and lower graphs represent the extremes, the high and low values for the group. (From Lamb and Roman. *Aerospace Medicine* 32:473, 1961.)

SUMMARY

1. Blood flow is the result of a difference in pressure between two points in the circulation. This difference in pressure is called a *pressure gradient*.

   A. Other things being equal, the velocity of blood flow through any given type of blood vessel varies inversely with the cross-sectional area of the total vessels of that type.

B. A simplification of Poiseuille's law expresses the dynamics of the circulation as follows:

$$\text{Volume of blood flow} = \frac{\text{Pressure} \times (\text{vessel radius})^4}{\text{Vessel length} \times \text{Viscosity}}$$

C. Blood pressure must always be referred to a specific point in the body in order to account for the effects of hydrostatic pressure.

2. There are at least three routes for blood flow through the microcirculation for serving differing physiological conditions: (1) *thoroughfare* or *preferential channels* which serve the metabolic needs of resting tissue; (2) *true capillaries,* which open to serve the needs of an increased metabolic activity; and (3) *arteriovenous anastomoses* which probably serve to dissipate heat.

3. Control of blood distribution is mediated by the sympathetic nervous system and chemical regulation. *Adrenergic fibers* of the sympathetic system bring about vasoconstriction of inactive tissues, and *cholinergic fibers* of the same system cause vasodilatation of the active tissue, which is augmented by chemical activity of the metabolites after exercise is well under way.

4. Approximately seventy-two percent of the resistance of the circulatory system at rest arises in the arterial system (largely in the arterioles) and only twenty-eight percent in the venous system. In exercise, the total resistance may be reduced by at least fifty percent.

5. Blood pressure is subject to the effects of many variables, such as age, sex, emotional state, time of day, nutritional state, and posture.

6. Blood pressure usually shows a rise during exercise in systolic and mean values, but no change or a very small rise in diastolic pressure. The effects vary with the type of exercise.

7. The systemic arterial pressure is set not by the general level of the workload sustained by the total body but rather by the pressure required to perfuse that muscle or muscle group which is working under greatest tension.

8. During exercise, the number of open capillaries is approximately double the number observed during rest.

9. The training and conditioning of athletes has been shown to bring improved blood flow to the active muscles at the peak of training. These changes are reversible, and show a detraining effect within three weeks of the end of training.

10. Exercise which results in heavy sweating causes a loss of intra as well as extracellular fluid which must be replaced during or after the workbout to maintain normal tissue hydration and electrolyte balance.

11. Total blood volume responds to training with significant increases and also declines in individuals confined to the inactivity of bed rest.
12. The response of the circulatory system to exercise varies with posture. Even at rest, changes in posture are reflected by predictable and typical circulatory response patterns.
13. *Cooling out* after heavy exercise is necessary to prevent blood pooling, which may result in muscle cramps, or even shock.

REFERENCES

1. Ahlman, K., and Karvonen, M. J. 1962. Weight reduction by sweating in wrestlers and its effect on physical fitness. *Journal of Sports Medicine and Physical Fitness* 1:58-62.
2. Astrand, P. O.; Ekblom, B.; Messin, R.; Saltin, B.; and Stenberg, J. 1965. Intraarterial blood pressure during exercise with different muscle groups. *Journal of Applied Physiology* 20:253-56.
3. Astrand, I.; Guharay, A.; and Wahren, J. 1968. Circulatory responses to arm exercise with different arm positions. *Journal of Applied Physiology* 25:528-32.
4. Barcroft, H., and Millen, J. L. E. 1939. The blood flow through muscle during sustained contraction. *Journal of Physiology* 97:17-31.
5. Barcroft, H., and Swan, H. J. C. 1953. Sympathetic control of human blood vessels. London: E. Arnold.
6. Bazett, H. C. 1949. A consideration of the venous circulation. In *Factors regulating blood pressure,* eds. B. W. Zweifach and E. Shorr. New York: Josiah Macy, Jr. Foundation.
7. Bevegard, B. S., and Shepherd, J. T. 1967. Regulation of the circulation during exercise in man. *Physiological Reviews* 47:178-213.
8. Byrd, R. J., and Hills, W. L. 1971. Strength, endurance and blood flow responses to isometric training. *Research Quarterly* 42:357-61.
9. Davis, J. E., and Brewer, N. 1935. Effect of physical training on blood volume, hemoglobin, alkali reserve, and osmotic resistance of erythrocytes. *American Journal of Physiology* 113:586-91.
10. deVries, H. A., and Adams, G. M. 1972. Total muscle mass activation v. relative loading of individual muscles as determinants of exercise response in older men. *Medicine and Science in Sports* 4:146-54.
11. Freyschuss, V., and Strandell, T. 1968. Circulatory adaptation to one-and two-leg exercise in supine position. *Journal of Applied Physiology* 25:511-15.
12. Hamilton, W. F.; Woodbury, R. A.; and Harper, Jr., H. T. 1944. Arterial, cerebrospinal and venous pressures in man during cough and strain. *American Journal of Physiology* 141:42-50.
13. Henry, J. P., and Cassel, J. C. 1969. Psychosocial factors in essential hypertension. *American Journal of Epidemiology* 90:171-200.

14. Henschel, A.; De la Vega, F.; and Taylor, H. L. 1954. Simultaneous direct and indirect blood pressure measurements in man at rest and work. *Journal of Applied Physiology* 6:506-12.
15. Hermansen, L., and Wachtlova, M. 1971. Capillary density of skeletal muscle in well trained and untrained men. *Journal of Applied Physiology* 30:860-63.
16. Kjellberg, S. R.; Rudhe, V.; and Sjostrand, T. 1949. Increase of the amount of hemoglobin and blood volume in connection with physical training. *Acta Physiologica'Scandinavica* 19:146-51.
17. Lamb, L. E., and Roman, J. 1961. The head-down tilt and adaptability for aerospace flight. *Aerospace Medicine* 32:473-86.
18. Lind, A. R., and McNicol, G. W. 1967a. Circulatory responses to sustained hand-grip contractions performed during other exercise, both rhythmic and static. *Journal of Physiology* 192:595-607.
19. ———. 1967b. Muscular factors which determine the cardiovascular responses to sustained and rhythmic exercise. *Canadian Medical Association Journal* 96:706-13.
20. ———. 1968. Cardiovascular responses to holding and carrying weights by hand and by shoulder harness. *Journal of Applied Physiology* 25:261-67.
21. Martin, E. G.; Wooley, E. C.; and Miller, M. 1932. Capillary counts in resting and active muscle. *American Journal of Physiology* 100:407-16.
22. Nagle, F. J.; Naughton, J.; and Balke, B. 1966. Comparison of direct and indirect blood pressure with pressure-flow dynamics during exercise. *Journal of Applied Physiology* 21:317-20.
23. Petren, T.; Sjostrand, T.; and Sylven, B. 1936. Der Einfluss des Trainings auf die Häufigkeit der Capillaren in Herzund Skelelmuskulatur. *Arbeitsphysiologie* 9:376-86.
24. Pirnay, F.; Marechal, R.; Radermecker, R.; and Petit, J. M. 1972. Muscle blood flow during submaximum and maximum exercise on a bicycle ergometer. *Journal of Applied Physiology* 32:210-12.
25. Reeves, J. T.; Grover, R. F.; Filley, G. F.; and Blount, S. G. 1961. Circulatory changes in man during mild supine exercise. *Journal of Applied Physiology* 16:279-82.
26. ———. 1961. Cardiac output response to standing and treadmill walking. *Journal of Applied Physiology* 16:283-88.
27. Robinson, S., and Harmon, P. M. 1941. The lactic acid mechanism and certain properties of the blood in relation to training. *American Journal of Physiology* 132:757.
28. Rochelle, R. H.; Stumpner, R. L.; Robinson, S.; Dill, D. B.; and Horvath, S. M. 1971. Peripheral blood flow response to exercise consequent to physical training. *Medicine Science and Sports* 3:122-29.
29. Rohter, F. D.; Rochelle, R. H.; and Hyman, C. 1963. Exercise blood flow changes in the human forearm during physical training. *Journal of Applied Physiology* 18:789-93.

30. Royce, J. 1958. Isometric fatigue curves in human muscle with normal and occluded circulation. *Research Quarterly* 29:204-12.
31. Start, K. B., and Holmes, R. 1963. Local muscle endurance with open and occluded intramuscular circulation. *Journal of Applied Physiology* 18: 804-07.
32. Zweifach, B. W. 1949. Basic mechanisms in peripheral vascular homeostasis. In *Proceedings of Third Conference on Factors Regulating Blood Pressure.* New York: Josiah Macy, Jr. Foundation.
33. ———. 1957. General principles governing the behavior of the microcirculation. *American Journal of Medicine* 23:684-96.
34. ———. 1959. Structural and functional aspects of the microcirculation in the skin. In *The Microcirculation,* eds. S. R. M. Reynolds and B. W. Zweifach, pp. 144-52. Urbana: The University of Illinois Press.
35. Zweifach, B. W., and Metz, D. B. 1955. Selective distribution of blood through the terminal vascular bed of mesenteric structures and skeletal muscle. *Angiology* 6:282-90.

7 The Lungs and External Respiration

Each cell of every tissue in the human body depends upon oxidative reactions to provide the energy for its metabolism. In very simple biological organisms, each cell is in contact with the external environment, and thus derives its supply of oxygen directly. In the human organism, the vast majority of tissues are not in direct contact with the external environment, and for this reason a specialized respiratory system is necessary to provide the oxygen for their metabolic demands.

The respiratory process can be broken down into three component functions:

1. Gas exchange in the lungs, in which the lung capillaries take up oxygen and give up much of their carbon dioxide
2. Gas transport and distribution from the lungs to the various tissues by the blood
3. Gas exchange between the blood and the tissue fluids bathing the ultimate consumers, the cells

The first process is also referred to as *external respiration* or *pulmonary ventilation,* and the third process is referred to as *internal* or *tissue respiration;* the second process, *gas transport,* is the function of the cardiovascular system. This chapter is concerned with external respiration. The respiratory function of the cardiovascular system and internal respiration are discussed in chapter eight.

ANATOMY OF EXTERNAL RESPIRATION

It will be recalled from elementary physiology and anatomy that the flow of air proceeds through the nose (or mouth) into the nasal cavity, where it is warmed, humidified, and agitated by striking the *turbinates.* From the nasopharynx, air is conducted past the *glottis,* where the pharynx separates into the *trachea* for air conduction and the esophagus for the passage of food. The trachea splits into the two chief *bronchi;* one goes to the left lung and the other goes to the right lung (fig. 7.1).

The lungs can be considered a system of branching tubes that perform two major functions: conduction of air and respiration. The conductive portion of the system proceeds from the chief bronchi which branch in the lung root. Subsequent branching of the conductive pathway occurs within the lungs and results in smaller bronchi which in turn branch into smaller tubes called *bronchioles.* Throughout the repeated branchings, each branching results in a larger total cross-sectional area, as was also the case in the circulatory system. The bronchioles eventually branch into the *terminal bronchioles,* the last units of the conductive system which are from 0.5 to 1.0 mm in diameter.

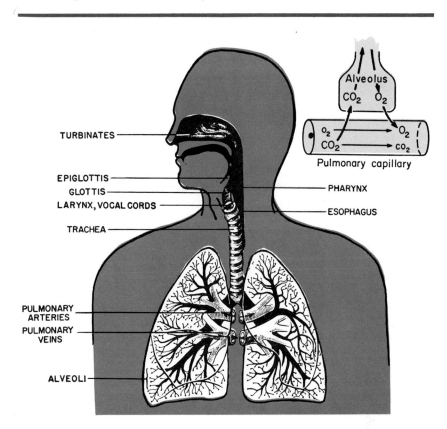

TURBINATES

EPIGLOTTIS

GLOTTIS

LARYNX, VOCAL CORDS

TRACHEA

PULMONARY ARTERIES

PULMONARY VEINS

ALVEOLI

Alveolus

CO_2 O_2

O_2

CO_2

O_2

CO_2

Pulmonary capillary

PHARYNX

ESOPHAGUS

Figure 7-1. The respiratory system, showing the respiratory passages and the function of the alveolus to oxygenate the blood and to remove carbon dioxide. (From Guyton. *Function of the Human Body,* 1959. Courtesy of W.B. Saunders Company, Philadelphia.)

Each terminal bronchiole divides into two *respiratory branchioles*, which in turn may divide once more (or even twice) with these divisions forming *alveolar ducts*. The alveolar ducts may or may not branch, but they eventually terminate in thin-walled sacs called *alveoli* (singular: *alveolus*). These alveoli, with their supporting structures, are highly vascularized. Thus the *lung unit* has been considered to consist of the alveolar duct and its subdivisions (alveoli), together with the blood and lymph vessels and the nerve supply. Within the lung unit, only two very thin endothelial layers separate the air in the system from the blood in the capillaries, thus allowing for very efficient diffusion of gasses. Furthermore, the total cross-sectional area available for diffusion has been estimated to be between 500 and 1,000 square feet.

MECHANICS OF LUNG VENTILATION

The laws governing fluid flow also apply to gasses. It has been pointed out that the flow of blood in the vascular system is brought about through differences in pressure, called a pressure gradient, and the flow of respiratory gas similarly depends upon a pressure gradient between the air in the lungs and the ambient (outside) air. For air to flow into the lungs, the pressure within must be lower than atmospheric pressure. This lowering of pressure in the lungs is brought about by the descent of the diaphragm (contraction of the muscle fibers) and the action of the external and anterior internal intercostal muscles in raising the ribs. Campbell (5) has shown by X-ray technique that the diaphragm descends approximately 1.5 cm in normal, quiet respiration, and as much as 6 to 10 cm during maximal breathing. Thus the volume of the lungs is considerably increased during inspiration largely by virtue of elongation. This increase in volume results in a temporary lowering of pressure within the lungs so that a pressure gradient exists, with the ambient air having the higher pressure and thus moving into the lungs during inspiration.

In the respiratory cycle the inspiration phase is the active phase, and is brought about by the active contraction of the ordinary muscles of respiration: the diaphragm and the intercostals. The expiration phase, under resting conditions, is largely due to the elastic recoil of these muscles and associated structures as they snap back to their resting length. Thus the elastic recoil creates a higher-than-atmospheric pressure within the lung which results in the necessary pressure gradient for moving the air out in expiration.

Ventilation of the alveoli, where the greatest part of the diffusion process occurs, has been attributed to the enlargement of the alveolar ducts in length and in width without a concomitant enlargement of the alveoli themselves. However, recent evidence seems to indicate that the alveoli participate proportionately in the overall enlargement during inspiration, this enlargement being about twofold for the alveolar duct and the alveolus (25). This twofold increase in volume was calculated to result in a seventy percent increase in alveolar area for diffusion.

The description so far holds only for normal resting breathing conditions. During exercise, metabolic demands are greater, and rate and depth of breathing are increased. The increased depth of respiration is brought about by the *accessory muscles* of breathing. In inspiration, greater volume is obtained by activity of the *scaleni* and the *sternocleidomastoid* muscles, through their help in lifting the ribs. In the expiratory phase of heavy exercise, the passive elastic recoil of the ordinary muscles of breathing is greatly aided by the active contraction of the abdominal muscles. The abdominal muscles serve two important mechanical functions: (1) raising the intra-abdominal pressure which results in greater intrathoracic pressure to aid in expiration, and (2) drawing the lower ribs downward and medially. The lateral muscles (obliques and transversi) are more important than the recti abdominis (5).

NOMENCLATURE FOR THE LUNG VOLUMES AND CAPACITIES

Because respiratory physiology had been plagued by an ambiguity of terms, a group of American physiologists agreed in 1950 to standardize terms and definitions (6). The result of this agreement is given in table 7.1 and is illustrated in figure 7.2. Table 7.2 provides illustrative values for the lung volumes in healthy, recumbent subjects.

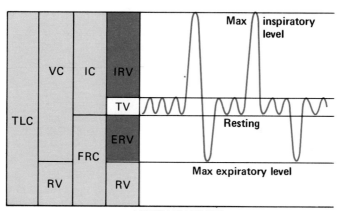

LUNG VOLUMES

Figure 7-2. Lung volumes. (From *The Lung,* 2nd edition, by Julius H. Comroe, Jr., et al., Copyright © 1962, Year Book Medical Publishers, Inc. Used by permission of Year Book Medical Publishers.)

RESPIRATORY CONTROL

The question of how pulmonary ventilation is controlled has been the subject of much physiological research. It is obvious that the rate and depth of respiration must be so controlled as to maintain homeostasis in the face of varying metabolic demands, ranging from rest to the very vigorous exercise of competitive athletics. However, the physiological mechanisms by which this homeostasis is brought about are, as yet, not so obvious.

TABLE 7.1

Lung Volumes and Capacities

A. **Volumes.** There are four primary volumes which do not overlap.
   1. Tidal Volume, or the depth of breathing, is the volume of gas inspired or expired during each respiratory cycle.
   2. Inspiratory Reserve Volume is the maximal amount of gas that can be inspired from the end-inspiratory position.
   3. Expiratory Reserve Volume is the maximal volume of gas that can be expired from the end-expiratory level.
   4. Residual Volume is the volume of gas remaining in the lungs at the end of a maximal expiration.
B. **Capacities.** There are four capacities, each of which includes two or more of the primary volumes.
   1. Total Lung Capacity is the amount of gas contained in the lung at the end of a maximal inspiration.
   2. Vital Capacity is the maximal volume of gas that can be expelled from the lungs by forceful effort following a maximal inspiration.
   3. Inspiratory Capacity is the maximal volume of gas that can be inspired from the resting expiratory level.
   4. Functional Residual Capacity is the volume of gas remaining in the lungs at the resting expiratory level. The resting end-expiratory position is used here as a base line because it varies less than the end-inspiratory position.

From *The Lung*, 2nd edition, by Julius H. Comroe, Jr. et al. Copyright © 1962, Year Book Medical Publishers, Inc. Used by permission of Year Book Medical Publishers.

The nerve cells responsible for the automatic and rhythmic innervation of the muscles of respiration lie in the reticular formation of the medulla. As a group, these nerve cells are referred to as the respiratory center.[1] The best available evidence seems to indicate that this center possesses automatic rhythmicity, which would account for the phases of inspiration and expiration, with expiration being the result of inactivity of the respiratory center.

1. Evidence is accumulating that the respiratory center is probably not as discrete an entity as had been thought. However, for the purposes of this text, the term seems to have utility, and will be retained to eliminate unnecessary discussions of neurological concepts that are as yet not completely elucidated.

Table 7.2

Lung Volumes in Healthy Recumbent Subjects
(Approximate values, in ml)

	Male Aged 20-30 Yr. 1.7 M²	Male Aged 50-60 Yr. 1.7 M²	Female Aged 20-30 Yr. 1.6 M²
Inspired capacity	3600	2600	2400
Expiratory reserve capacity	1200	1000	800
Vital capacity	4800	3600	3200
Residual volume	1200	2400	1000
Functional residual capacity	2400	3400	1800
Total lung capacity	6000	6000	4200
RV/TLC × 100	20%	40%	24%

From *The Lung*, 2nd edition, by Julius H. Comroe, Jr. et al. Copyright © 1962, Year Book Medical Publishers, Inc. Used by permission of Year Book Medical Publishers.

The breathing frequency (f) and depth (tidal volume or *TV*) are adjusted to metabolic demands for oxygen by a complex of factors, some of which act directly upon the nerve cells of the respiratory center (chemosensitive cells of the medulla) and some of which operate reflexly through the aortic and carotid bodies which are sensitive chemoreceptors. The six most important factors are as follows.

Carbon Dioxide and Subsequent pH Changes. In resting man, rises in arterial carbon dioxide tensions have been shown to be a very potent stimulant for the respiratory processes. Lambertsen and others (18) have shown that approximately forty-five percent of this respiratory drive was due to the lowered pH brought about by the increased CO_2. The other fifty-five percent of respiratory drive may be due to extravascular pH changes due to CO_2, or to direct action of the CO_2 itself. The effect of the CO_2 and pH factors seems to be mediated directly through chemosensitive receptors in the medulla.

Oxygen (Anoxia). A low arterial level of oxygen has also been demonstrated to bring about greater ventilatory activity; however, until recently, it was thought the level of O_2 had to drop from a normal arterial partial pressure (PaO_2) of 100 mm Hg to about 60 mm to have any effect. Hornbein and others (14) have shown that very small changes, of 6 to 7 mm Hg, are effective if they are sudden changes, and also that during exercise, responses are elicited to a drop in PaO_2 of 6 to 7 mm Hg. They suggest that this difference in response between the resting and exercise states may be due to increased sympathetic activity during exercise that decreases blood flow to the chemoreceptors of the carotid and aortic bodies where this reflex arises.

Proprioceptive Reflexes from Joints and Muscles. Considerable evidence exists that movement per se, independent of any other change, can have a reasonably large effect in bringing about the increased ventilation that occurs during exercise. This effect has been best demonstrated for the knee joint, but it undoubtedly is also operative at other joints, and arises from receptors in the joints and muscle tissues. Recent work (15) has shown that not only can the afferents from stretch receptors elicit a ventilatory response but even the non medullated C fibers can do so. However, the importance of neurogenic factors in general has been challenged by the work of Beaver and Wasserman (2) who have shown that the rise and fall of ventilation is not generally so precipitous as had been believed; and consequently, the neurogenic factor is no longer necessary to explain a response which was thought to be too rapid for other than a reflex mechanism.

Temperature. As body temperature goes up, the ventilation rate goes up, in direct proportion. Since the body temperature rises from 1 to 5° F. during exercise, this is one of the factors involved. However, it can not be responsible for the early and large ventilatory response to exercise because the temperature rise requires too much time (twenty to thirty minutes for any appreciable increase). It may be noted, in passing, that respiration also drops, in direct proportion to temperatures lower than normal, until death ensues from respiratory failure.

Cerebral Factors. An increase in the ventilation rate is frequently observed in anticipation of exercise before any of the aforementioned factors can have had effect. This increase is attributed to cerebral innervation aroused psychically in the forebrain. Fink supported this concept by demonstrating that the cessation of breathing due to lowered arterial CO_2, which is easily elicited under general anesthesia, was not found in the waking state (more active cerebral state).

Hering Breuer Reflexes. In 1868 Hering and Breuer reported the discovery of stretch receptors in the lungs whose afferent pathway traveled by way of the vagus nerve. These reflexes are named for them, and are twofold; one is the *inhibito-inspiratory* reflex and the other is the *excito-inspiratory* reflex. The inhibito-inspiratory reflex tends to terminate inspiration that is larger than normal by firing inhibitory impulses to the respiratory center. The excito-inspiratory reflex functions only in very deep expiration, or in collapse of the lung.

Control of respiratory activity at rest is undoubtedly brought about by a combination of the above factors in complex interactions that have not yet been completely elucidated. The composite ventilatory response to exercise is best illustrated by figure 7.3. It would seem, on the basis

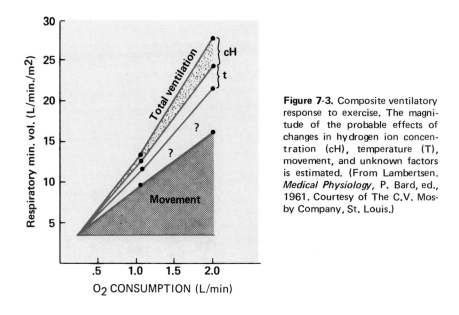

Figure 7-3. Composite ventilatory response to exercise. The magnitude of the probable effects of changes in hydrogen ion concentration (cH), temperature (T), movement, and unknown factors is estimated. (From Lambertsen. *Medical Physiology,* P. Bard, ed., 1961. Courtesy of The C.V. Mosby Company, St. Louis.)

of all available evidence, that the summation of afferent impulses from proprioceptors in moving limbs and muscles is still an important factor in bringing about the increased ventilation of exercise. Changes in hydrogen ion concentration (acidity), reflecting metabolic changes through changes in carbon dioxide concentration, are also important as is the increased body temperature.

Obviously, the muscular movements of breathing are also under voluntary control. Rate and depth can be changed at will, and the breath can be held for varying periods of time.

It is also interesting to note that vibration of the human body, as occurs on trucks, tractors, and high-speed low-flying aircraft, results in hyperventilation (increase over normal ventilation). Exactly how this hyperventilation is brought about is not yet known.

LUNG VENTILATION IN REST AND EXERCISE

Rate Versus Depth.   Lung ventilation rate (minute volume of breathing) is the result of two variable factors: *rate* and *depth,* or tidal volume (TV). There are also two types of resistance to be overcome for the respiratory muscles: the *elastic resistance,* met in stretching the lungs and muscular and connective tissues of the thorax, and *airway resistance,* met by the movement of air in flowing through the small tubes of the lungs. The elastic resistance increases with increasing tidal volume for any given lung ventilation rate because the elastic tissues are stretched farther in deeper breathing. On the other hand, the airway resistance does not increase with rate or with depth if the minute volume of breathing is held constant. On the face of it then, it would seem to be more efficient to breath at a high rate and shallow depth; however, this is not so because of the *anatomical dead space,* which is defined most simply as the volume contained within the conducting portion of the airways of the lung where no gas exchange occurs.

Figure 7.4 illustrates the importance of the anatomical dead space in helping to determine the optimum rate and tidal volume of breathing. It shows that although the minute volume is the same 8,000 ml and the dead space is 150 ml in all three cases, if the tidal volume is small and the rate is high (A), the dead-space air represents 4,800/8,000 of the total minute volume. In (C), where the rate is low and the tidal volume is high, the dead-space air represents only 1,200/8,000 of the total minute volume.

The importance of the dead-space air is perhaps more evident if we consider the extreme case, where the dead-space air is 150 ml, the rate is increased, and the depth decreased, until the tidal volume is also 150 ml. In this case, of course, no real alveolar ventilation can occur because the dead-space air would simply be moved back and forth between conductive airways and the alveoli.

Thus it might be predicted that for each individual, with varying degrees of elastic resistance, airway resistance, and volume of dead space, an optimum rate and depth of breathing exists, and this has proven essentially true. Recent evidence (24) suggests that in near-maximal exercise the rate commonly adopted by the athlete (thirty to thirty-five breaths per minute) is marginally more efficient than either slower or faster rates. This relatively slow breathing pattern probably minimizes the O_2 consumption of the chest muscles and is also most effective in terms of gas exchange. Some typical values of anatomical dead space are given in figure 7.5.

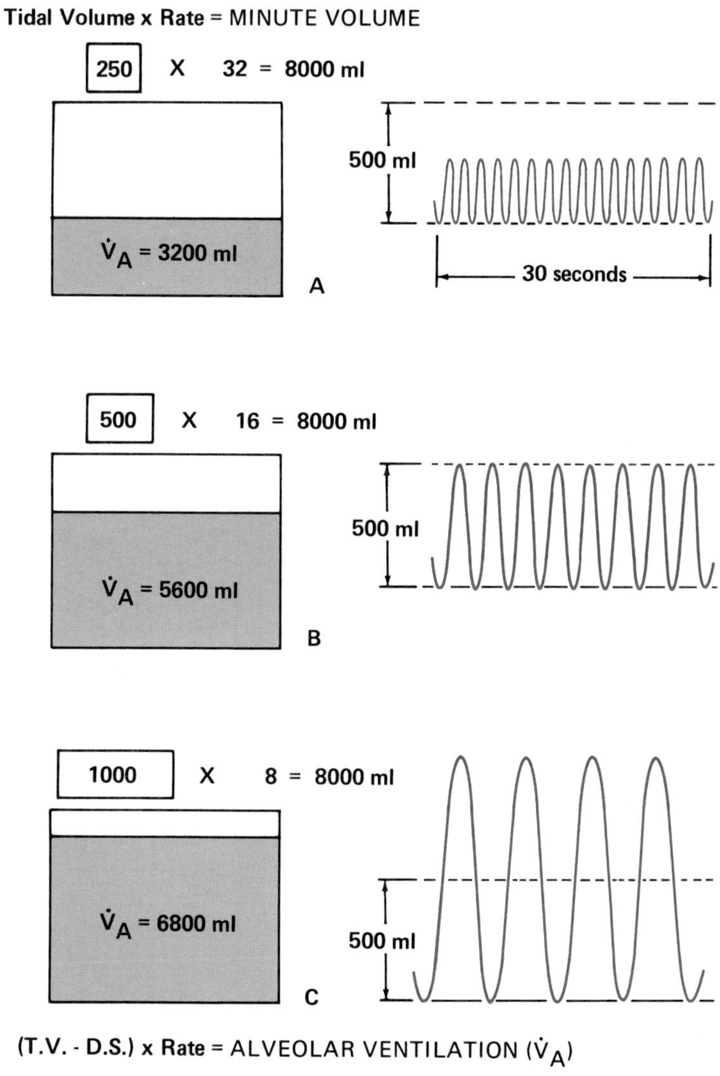

Tidal Volume x Rate = MINUTE VOLUME

250   X   32 = 8000 ml

$\dot{V}_A$ = 3200 ml

500 ml

A

|◄──── 30 seconds ────►|

500   X   16 = 8000 ml

$\dot{V}_A$ = 5600 ml

500 ml

B

1000   X   8 = 8000 ml

$\dot{V}_A$ = 6800 ml

500 ml

C

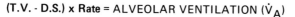

(T.V. - D.S.) x Rate = ALVEOLAR VENTILATION ($\dot{V}_A$)

Figure 7-4. Area of each small block represents tidal volume (250, 500, or 1000 ml). Total area of each large block (shaded + unshaded areas) = *minute* volume of ventilation; in each case it is 8000 ml. Shaded area of each block represents volume of *alveolar* ventilation per minute; this varies in each case since Alveolar Ventilation/min = (Tidal Volume − Dead Space) x Frequency. A dead space of 150 ml is assumed in each case, although actually the dead space would increase somewhat with increasing tidal volume. *Right,* spirographic tracings. (From *The Lung,* 2nd edition, by Julius H. Comroe, Jr., et al., Copyright © 1962, Year Book Medical Publishers, Inc. Used by permission of Year Book Medical Publishers.)

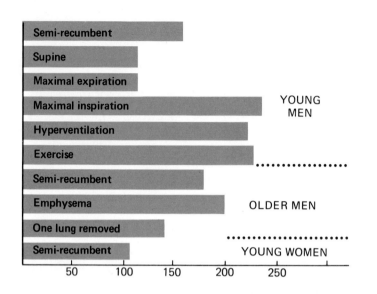

Figure 7-5. Anatomic dead space. (From *The Lung,* 2nd edition, by Julius H. Comroe, Jr., et al., Copyright © 1962, Year Book Medical Publishers, Inc. Used by permission of Year Book Medical Publishers.)

Under resting conditions, the rate of breathing varies from twelve to twenty respirations per minute; during vigorous exercise, it may go as high as fifty to sixty per minute. The tidal volume is roughly 500 ml for an average man, and may increase to approximately 2,500 ml in high-intensity, short-duration (two to three minutes) exercise. The total lung ventilation averages about 7.0 liters per minute for healthy male adults at rest, and may go up to 150 liters per minute or more in heavy exercise.

Factors Affecting Lung Volumes and Lung Ventilation Rate

Age. For adults, the inspiratory capacity, the expiratory reserve capacity, and the vital capacity all become smaller with increasing age, and the residual volume and the functional residual capacity increase (table 7.2). Thus, although the total lung capacity probably does not change, the volumes, which are important for increasing the alveolar exchange during exercise, decrease proportionately with age. These changes are probably brought about by the lessening proportion of elastic components in the tissues with increasing age, and the result is the commonly observed decrease in circulorespiratory capacity.

Anthropometric Measures. For children (six to fourteen years), the work of Lyons and Tanner (20) indicates that all the lung volumes—

except inspiratory capacity—are most highly correlated with height. Total lung capacity was found to correlate 0.898 and 0.975, and vital capacity 0.895 and 0.861—with height—for boys and girls, respectively. Inspiratory capacity correlated best with body surface area: boys 0.881 and girls 0.853.

Posture. Because posture varies in different athletic activities, it is of interest to note its effects upon respiration. The work of Moreno and Lyons (22) showed a decrease in lung ventilation rate in going from the sitting to the supine posture of approximately 0.5 liter per minute in males and 1.0 liter per minute in females. No significant change was found in changing from the sitting to the prone position. The total lung capacity was shown to decrease in both supine and prone positions; and this was also true of vital capacity.

There is reason to believe that these changes in resting volumes are due to the encroachment of a greater volume of blood into the thoracic cavity in the horizontal position, since occlusion of the venous return from the legs results in the return of TLC and VC virtually to the sitting values.

Factors Limiting Depth of Maximal Inspiration.   On the basis of electromyographic evidence (4), it had been thought that the depth of maximal voluntary inspiration was limited by contraction of the abdominal muscles to oppose the further descent of the diaphragm. More recent work (21) indicates that this contraction may be a factor in untrained subjects, but is probably not a factor in trained subjects. The limits for the trained subjects seem to be set by the limits of elastic recoil of the muscles and the associated structures involved in inspiration.

LUNG VENTILATION VERSUS O_2 CONSUMPTION IN EXERCISE

Between the resting state and a moderate level of exercise (approximately 2.0 liters of O_2 consumption), a very constant ratio of ventilation rate to O_2 consumption is maintained. This ratio is usually termed the *ventilation equivalent,* and is defined as the number of liters of air breathed for every 100 ml of oxygen consumed. Thus at rest the ventilation equivalent (VE) is:

$$\frac{7.0 \text{ liters air breathed/minute}}{275 \text{ ml } O_2 \text{ uptake/minute}} \text{ or } \frac{7.0}{2.75 \text{ (hundred ml)}} = 2.54$$

This ratio also indicates that 25.4 liters of air must be respired to achieve

an O_2 uptake of 1 liter: $\dfrac{7.0 \text{ liters}}{.275 \text{ liters}} = 25.4$

This ratio holds until the work load demands more than two liters of O_2 per minute, at which point the ratio grows higher, and this relationship is shown in figure 7.6. The reason for the higher ventilation equivalent at the higher work loads is that the steady state is no longer maintained, and lactic acid accumulates which acts upon the respiratory center through lowering the pH.

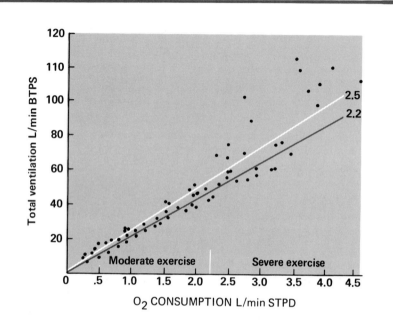

Figure 7-6. Ventilation as a function of O_2 consumption in physical exercise (walking, running, bicycling). The experimental points represent the means of 611 determinations in eighty-six subjects reported by eleven different authors. The straight lines correspond to ventilation equivalents for O_2 of 2.2 and 2.5. (From Gray, J.S. *Pulmonary Ventilation and Its Physiological Regulation,* 1950. Courtesy of Charles C Thomas, Publisher, Springfield, III.)

Oxygen Cost of Breathing. Under resting conditions the muscular work done in breathing is relatively small; probably not much more than one percent of the resting metabolism is devoted to this function. As exercise becomes vigorous, however, the oxygen cost of breathing increases disproportionately. Probably at a point between 150 and 250 liters of ventilation, the cost of moving the air takes all of the additional O_2 provided; however, this range of ventilation is seldom (if ever), achieved in the normal ventilation of even the heaviest work loads. (The experimental values have been achieved through artificially contrived hyperventilation.)

One of the important factors in the physiology of athletic training is the increased efficiency of the breathing mechanics. The ventilation equivalent (discussed above) is smaller in conditioned athletes, meaning that less breathing work is required to maintain a given O_2 supply. It is quite likely that high efficiency of breathing (as measured by the VE) is a very important factor in such feats as the four-minute mile.

RESPIRATORY PHENOMENA

Stitch in the Side. Frequently in the course of making the respiratory adjustment to a heavy exercise load—such as distance running—athletes experience a rather severe, sharp pain on the lower, lateral aspects of the thoracic wall. This pain has been called a *stitch in the side*, but no scientific evidence is available to explain its cause. Because it usually occurs during adjustment to new metabolic demands, it seems reasonable to postulate ischemia of either the diaphragm or intercostal muscles as the cause. Ischemia of any skeletal muscle brings the sensation of pain.

Second Wind. *Second wind*, familiar to most endurance athletes, is typified by the feeling of relief upon making the necessary metabolic adjustments to a heavy, endurance load. Although it is not entirely, and probably not even mainly, a respiratory adjustment, it is treated under respiratory phenomena because the major manifestation to the athlete is the changeover from *dyspnea* (labored breathing, shortness of breath) to *eupnea* (normal breathing).

Again, very little scientific evidence can be brought to bear upon this problem. Close observation seems to indicate a lack of relationship between the time of occurrence and cardiovascular adjustments. Furthermore, the respiratory adjustment is probably only a reflection (an effect rather than a cause) of metabolic adjustment to the exercise load. The most likely explanation of the cause would seem to be one that invokes a change in skeletal muscular efficiency. The work of Tuttle referred to earlier (26), which demonstrated shortening contraction and relaxation phases of muscular contraction with increased temperature, can be used as a basis for rationalization. It will be remembered that contraction and the relaxation phases of contraction are shortened as the muscle temperature increases and that the relaxation phase decreases disproportionately more than the contraction phase. It seems likely that this quicker relaxation of muscles while acting as antagonists in a rapidly reciprocating motion, such as running, etc., would allow the increased efficiency that must be the ultimate cause of the frequently observed effect: second wind. This would likely happen at the time that second wind is usually observed—when muscle temperature has increased enough to bring about sweating, which is often observed concurrently. A recent study by Lefcoe and Yuhasz (19) has shown the intersubject variability in response which makes elucidation of the physiological correlates difficult.

Smoking and Wind.   Although smoking has long been indicted as causing respiratory problems in athletes and has customarily been forbidden for members of athletic teams, the scientific evidence has been meager until recently. Nadel and Comroe (23), in a well-controlled study, demonstrated that fifteen puffs of cigarette smoke in five minutes caused an average decrease in airway conductance of thirty-one percent in thirty-six normal subjects. This finding was highly significant, and was found both in smokers and nonsmokers. Changes occurred as early as one minute after smoking began, and lasted from ten to eighty minutes (mean was equal to thirty-five minutes). These investigators attributed the changes to inhalation of submicronic particles rather than to nicotine or oxides of nitrogen.

In light of the earlier discussion on the cost and efficiency of breathing, it is readily seen that smoking, which can increase airway resistance by thirty-one percent *under resting conditions,* can be a very great detriment under conditions of *maximum ventilation* for an athlete. This scientific evidence—in addition to the evidence cited in chapter five on the effects of smoking on heart action—should reinforce the argument against smoking for athletes (if not the general population).

UNUSUAL RESPIRATORY MANEUVERS

Hypoventilation.   If lung ventilation is decreased, either voluntarily or involuntarily, without a corresponding decrease in metabolic rate, this reduction is called *hypoventilation.* It occurs only in abnormal situations, such as those involving airway obstruction. Because metabolism continues at a faster rate than lung ventilation, CO_2 accumulates and the arterial CO_2 must rise (hypercapnia).

Hyperventilation.   The converse of hypoventilation is *hyperventilation,* in which the lung ventilation rate is greater than is needed for the existing metabolic rate. In this case, CO_2 is *blown off* faster than it is produced, and thus hyperventilation or forced breathing results in decreasing quantities of CO_2 in the circulorespiratory system. This lowering of blood CO_2 is called *hypocapnia.* Hyperventilation and hypocapnia have considerable interest since they occur accidentally—as the result of emotional excitement, particularly in the inexperienced athlete and as an intentional device—to increase breath-holding ability. It should be pointed out here that hyperventilation has no appreciable effect on O_2 values in the blood since blood is virtually saturated with O_2 when it leaves the lungs.

That hyperventilation increases breath-holding time is shown by table 7.3, which illustrates an experiment by the author on sixteen college men and women. One minute of hyperventilation more than doubled the mean breath-holding time. In light of the earlier discussion on the significance of the dead space, it is readily understood why hyperventilation is best performed by increasing the depth rather than the rate of breathing.

There is no doubt that hyperventilation can provide a significant advantage in competitive athletics wherever breath-holding time is a factor in affecting overall performance. In swimming the crawl stroke, for example, turning the head away from the midline to breathe slows the sprint swimmer's time; hyperventilation immediately before an event allows the swimmer to go farther before breathing becomes necessary.

TABLE 7.3

Seconds of Breath-holding with and without Hyperventilation
(Sitting at Rest)

Subject	Without Hyper- ventilation	10 Times in 30 Sec.	20 Times in 60 Sec.	Dizziness at	Other Symptoms
1	35	95	110	20 breaths	none
2	63	83	93	10	cyanosis of fingers
3	80	122	183	20	cyanosis of fingers
4	40	70	152	20	none
5	45	63	105	10	tension in fingers
6	65	125	160	10	cyanosis of fingers
7	45	80	120	20	none
8	63	108	153	20	none
9	90	135	120		none
10	80	180	140		none
11	35	55	80	10	none
12	55	95	120		cyanosis of fingers
13	55	105	145	20	cyanosis of fingers
14	105	150	195	20	tension, headache
15	120	150	160		finger perspiration
16	30	60	75		tension in gastro-cnemius
mean	62.9	104.8	131.9		

Hyperventilation achieved through increasing depth by using both inspiratory and expiratory reserve volumes.

A physical educator or coach will occasionally witness a situation in which an inexperienced individual passes out immediately after completing a sprint run. If the subject's fingernails show cyanosis (blue color) and there is evidence of tetany, such as involuntary flexing of the fingers or toes, the faint may well have been caused by prolonged, unintentional hyperventilation due to the emotional content associated with the run (testing for grading purposes, etc.). In any event, the situation calls for medical attention to determine if more serious factors are involved.

Individual variations in reaction to hyperventilation are illustrated by the symptoms found in table 7.3. If overbreathing is done at a lesser depth, it can be continued for a longer period before symptoms become evident.

Breath-holding. Many athletic events are performed with the breath held, notably swimming and track sprints. The physiology of breath-holding involves respiratory, circulatory, and cardiac changes, all of which are important in the light of recent research. The most obvious changes when the breath is held are the increasing level of CO_2 and the decreasing level of O_2 in the alveolar air. These changes of course reflect the changes in the level of the respiratory gasses in the blood, the result of the continuing metabolism. It will be recalled that O_2 and CO_2 levels are involved in respiratory control, but the rising CO_2 level is more important in determining the length of time the breath can be held.

It has been shown by Craig and his associates (7, 8, 9), that when the partial pressure of CO_2 in the alveolar air exceeds approximately fifty mm Hg, the stimulus to breathe is so strong that the breath can no longer be held. This is called the *break point,* at which breathing recommences. It has, however, become common practice to hyperventilate in preparation for any event that requires breath-holding, and this procedure, since it allows the athlete to start with a lower level of CO_2, also enables him to continue the breath hold longer (see table 7.3 p. 162). As the breath hold continues, lower levels of alveolar O_2 are reached because of the continuing consumption for metabolic needs. When the partial pressure of O_2 in the alveolar air has been reduced from its normal value (approximately 100 mm Hg) to 25 or 30 mm Hg, cerebral function is affected and consciousness is lost. Craig's work (7) indicates this may happen in underwater swimming, at distances of 114 to 185 feet. Thus the combination of hyperventilation and subsequent underwater swimming constitutes a hazardous situation, and may well account for many drownings.

Valsalva Maneuver. This maneuver involves a deep inspiration that is followed by attempted expiration against a closed glottis. Its physiology was described in chapter six.

Diaphragmatic Versus Costal Breathing. There has been considerable recent interest in the relative contribution of the diaphragm and the intercostal muscles to the movement of the tidal volume. Shortening of the diaphragm has been reported to account for one-third (3, 12) to two-thirds of the tidal volume. The discrepancies are probably due to method. In the supine position the diaphragm makes a greater contribution. In general, diaphragmatic breathing is greater in the male and grows more important with age (27). In moderate and heavy exercise tidal volume increases both in inspiratory and expiratory directions. Virtually all of the inspiratory increase is produced by the rib cage and most of the expiratory increase by the abdomen (diaphragm) (12). Physical education and singing instructors have often advised modification of costal breathing (chest) to abdominal breathing (greater use of the diaphragm). Campbell (5) after electromyographic research into the muscular activity of breathing, concluded that the activity pattern of the normal muscles of breathing (diaphragm and intercostals) is probably not changed by any of the breathing exercises advocated even though externally observed movements of the thorax and abdomen may seem different. He feels, however, that the accessory muscles of breathing (abdominals and elevators of ribs) can be trained through breathing exercises but that their activity probably does not become an unconscious habit pattern. Thus a change in the breathing pattern would require constant voluntary control and attention.

It is of practical interest that efficiency of lung ventilation apparently could be improved on theoretical bases (28) by changing the breathing pattern from the normal which approximates a sine wave to that approaching a square wave-involving an end-inspiratory pause. It has been shown in experiments on dogs that such a change in breathing pattern results in an increase in the arterial O_2 pressure of 9.5 percent, decrease in arterial CO_2 of 8.2 percent and 20.3 percent better alveolar ventilation (16). This would appear to be an interesting area for further experimentation by scientifically inclined coaches. To acquire such new breathing patterns would not be a simple matter however.

Artificial Respiration. Whenever respiration ceases because of an accident, such as drowning, shock asphyxiation, etc., artificial respiration must be instituted immediately to save the victim's life by preventing irreversible damage to the respiratory center in the medulla and to the heart which has very little anaerobic capacity.

Until recently, several manual methods had been in vogue, but little research had been done into their effectiveness. The work of Gordon and his associates (11) has established the superiority of the mouth-to-mouth resuscitation method as can be seen from table 7.4. It will be noted that

TABLE 7.4

Mean Pulmonary Ventilation during Artificial Respiration on
8 Apneic Normal Male Adults

Method	Gas Moved per Respiratory Cycle	Cases Not Ventilated
Normal resting tidal volume	540 ml	0
Mouth-to-mouth resuscitation	910	0
Back-pressure arm lift	580	3
Back-pressure hip lift	650	2
Chest pressure arm lift	450	4

From Gordon et al. *Journal of the American Medical Association* 167: 320, 1958.

not only does this method result in moving more air in and out of the lungs but, even more important, airway obstructions are observed by the difficulty in expiring into the victim's airways.

It may be thought that the decreased O_2 and increased CO_2 of the expired air might weigh against the mouth-to-mouth method, but even expired air has approximately sixteen percent O_2. Thus, sixteen percent of 910 ml equals 146 ml of O_2, whereas twenty-one percent (ambient air equals 20.93 percent) by the best of the manual methods provides only twenty-one percent of 650, or 136 ml of O_2 (table 7.4). Furthermore, the increased CO_2 level is also advantageous in providing a greater respiratory drive.

TRAINING EFFECTS ON PULMONARY FUNCTION

The older literature is replete with studies on the effects of training on vital capacity (which is easily measured), but the results show no general agreement. Only recently have data become available on other and probably more important elements of pulmonary function. Bachman and Horvath (1) found significant decreases in functional residual capacity, residual volume and the ratio of residual volume/total lung capacity in swimmers after four months of training. Controls and a similar group of wrestlers showed no significant changes. The swimmers also showed significantly increased vital capacity which was the result of an increased inspiratory capacity. All of these changes would result in better alveolar ventilation and consequently should weigh in favor of improved athletic performance.

SUMMARY

1. The total respiratory process consists of three component functions: (1) gas exchange in the lungs, (2) gas transport to the tissues by the blood, and (3) gas exchange between the blood and the tissue fluids bathing the cells.
2. The lungs consist of two systems: (1) a conductive system, whose smallest components are the *terminal bronchioles*, and (2) a respiratory system, whose function is performed largely by the *alveoli.*
3. Air flow into and out of the lungs depends upon differences of pressure between the ambient air and the air within the lung. This pressure gradient is brought about by the muscular activity of the diaphragm and intercostals in normal resting breathing.
4. Respiration during vigorous exercise brings accessory muscles into play. Inspiration is aided by action of the *sternomastoids* and *scaleni.* Expiration is aided by the abdominal group.
5. Respiratory control is brought about by the interaction of several factors, acting either directly or reflexly upon the respiratory center in the medulla: (1) CO_2 rise and consequent pH depression, (2) anoxia, (3) proprioceptive reflexes from the joints and muscles, (4) body temperature rise, (5) cerebral factors, and (6) Hering-Breuer reflexes.
6. Every individual has an optimal combination of rate and depth of breathing for greatest efficiency. In normal individuals, increases in depth are more effective because of the lessening effect of the anatomical dead space as depth is increased.
7. Posture affects lung volumes and ventilation rates. Other things being equal, better lung ventilation can be obtained in the standing or sitting postures than in the prone or supine positions.
8. Under steady-state conditions, approximately twenty-five liters of air are required to furnish one liter of O_2 to the tissues. The ratio goes even higher during overload conditions.
9. The work of breathing is relatively small at rest. Under vigorous exercise conditions, however, a point is reached at which all the extra

O_2 made available by increased breathing is necessary to supply the needs of the respiratory muscles.

10. Scientific evidence indicts smoking as having a deleterious effect not only upon the circulatory system but also upon the respiratory system.

11. *Hyperventilation* has important physiological advantages in increasing breath-holding time. On the other hand, it also brings about possibly hazardous conditions, of which every physical educator, coach, and athlete should be aware.

12. Recent information proves the physiological advantages of mouth-to-mouth resuscitation over the older manual methods.

REFERENCES

1. Bachman, J. C., and Horvath, S. M. 1968. Pulmonary function changes which accompany athletic conditioning programs. *Research Quarterly* 39: 235-39.

2. Beaver, W. L., and Wasserman, K. 1968. Transients in ventilation at start and end of exercise. *Journal of Applied Physiology* 25:390-99.

3. Bergofsky, E. H. 1964. Relative contributions of the rib cage and the diaphragm to ventilation in man. *Journal of Applied Physiology* 19:698-706.

4. Campbell, E. J. M. 1952. An electromyographic study of the role of the abdominal muscles in breathing. *Journal of Physiology* 117:222-33.

5. ———. 1958. *The respiratory muscles and the mechanics of breathing.* Chicago: The Yearbook Publishers, Inc.

6. Comroe, J. H., Jr.; Forster, K. E. II; Dubois, A. B.; Briscoe, W. A.; and Carlsen, E. 1962. *The lung.* Chicago: The Yearbook Publishers, Inc.

7. Craig, A. B., Jr. 1961. Causes of loss of consciousness during underwater swimming. *Journal of Applied Physiology* 16:583-86.

8. Craig, A. B., Jr.; Halstead, L. S.; Schmidt, G. H.; and Schnier, B. R. 1962. Influences of exercise and oxygen on breath-holding. *Journal of Applied Physiology* 17:225-27.

9. Craig, A. B., Jr., and Babcock, S. A. 1962. Alveolar CO_2 during breath-holding and exercise. *Journal of Applied Physiology* 17:874-76.

10. Fink, B. R. 1961. Influence of cerebral activity in wakefulness on regulation of breathing. *Journal of Applied Physiology* 16:15-20.

11. Gordon, A. S.; Frye, C. W.; Gittelson, L.; Sadove, M.; and Beattie, E. J., Jr. 1958. Mouth-to-mouth versus manual artificial respiration for children and adults. *Journal of the American Medical Association* 167:320.

12. Grimby, G.; Bunn, J.; Mead, J. 1968. Relative contributions of rib cage and abdomen to ventilation during exercise. *Journal of Applied Physiology* 24:159-66.

13. Hornbein, T. F., and Roos, A. 1962. Effect of mild hypoxia on ventilation during exercise. *Journal of Applied Physiology* 17:239-42.

14. Hornbein, T. F.; Roos, A.; and Griffo, Z. J. 1961. Transient effect of sudden mild hypoxia on respiration. *Journal of Applied Physiology* 16:11-14.

15. Kalia, M.; Senapati, J. M.; Parida, B.; and Panda, A. 1972. Reflex increase in ventilation by muscle receptors with non-medullated fibers (C fibers). *Journal of Applied Physiology* 32:189-93.

16. Knelson, J. H.; Howatt, W. F.; and DeMuth, G. R. 1970. Effect of respiratory pattern on alveolar gas exchange. *Journal of Applied Physiology* 29:328-31.

17. Konno, K., and Mead, J. 1967. Measurement of the separate volume changes of rib cage and abdomen during breathing. *Journal of Applied Physiology* 22:407-22.

18. Lambertsen, C. J.; Semple, S. J. G.; Smyth, M. G.; and Gelfand, R. 1961. H^+ and pCO_2 as chemical factors in respiratory and cerebral circulatory control. *Journal of Applied Physiology* 16:473-84.

19. Lefcoe, N. M., and Yuhasz, M. S. 1971. The second wind phenomenon in constant load exercise. *Journal of Sports Medicine and Physical Fitness* 11:135-38.

20. Lyons, H. A., and Tanner, R. W. 1962. Total lung volume and its subdivisions in children: normal standards. *Journal of Applied Physiology* 17:601-4.

21. Mead, J.; Milic-Emili, J.; and Turner, J. M. 1963. Factors limiting depth of a maximal inspiration in human subjects. *Journal of Applied Physiology* 18:295-96.

22. Moreno, F., and Lyons, H. A. 1961. Effect of body posture on lung volumes. *Journal of Applied Physiology* 16:27-29.

23. Nadel, J. A., and Comroe, J. H., Jr. 1961. Acute effects of inhalation of cigaret smoke on airway conductance. *Journal of Applied Physiology* 16:713-16.

24. Shephard, R. J., and Bar-Or, O. 1970. Alveolar ventilation in near-maximum exercise. *Medicine and Science in Sports* 2:83-92.

25. Storey, W. F., and Staub, N. C. 1962. Ventilation of terminal air units. *Journal of Applied Physiology* 17:391-97.

26. Tuttle, W. W. 1943. The physiological effects of heat and cold on muscle. *Athletic Journal* 24:45.

27. Wang, C. S., and Josenhans, W. J. 1971. Contribution of diaphragmatic/ abdominal displacement to ventilation in supine man. *Journal of Applied Physiology* 31:576-80.

28. Yamashiro, S. M., and Grodins, F. S. 1971. Optimal regulation of respiratory airflow. *Journal of Applied Physiology* 30:597-602.

8 Gas Transport and Internal Respiration

Thus far we have discussed the mechanical factors involved in breathing and their physiological controls; we will now consider the processes that are necessary for bringing about the ultimate goal of tissue respiration. Three processes intervene between lung ventilation and actual tissue respiration: (1) diffusion of O_2 across two very thin membranes—the wall of the alveolus and the wall of the capillary, (2) transport of O_2 via the blood to the capillary bed of the active tissues, (3) diffusion of O_2 across the capillary wall to the tissue fluids that bathe the actual consumers, the metabolizing cells. As O_2 is unloaded from the blood, CO_2 is of course being taken on for the return trip to the right heart and back to the lungs.

At this point we must consider the nature of the diffusion process and some of the laws that govern it. Let us begin by recalling from the discussion of circulatory hemodynamics, that fluids flow from point to point only because of differences in pressure, called *pressure gradients*. This is equally true for gasses. It is for this reason that physiologists usually refer to respiratory gasses in terms of pressure rather than in terms of concentration (percentage, etc.).

To illustrate this, table 8.1 gives percentages and approximate pressures of O_2 exerted in a standard atmosphere. It should be noted that the percentage concentration of O_2 is the same at 40,000 feet as at sea level; however, since one becomes unconscious in a matter of seconds at 40,000 feet altitude due to O_2 lack, it is obvious that percentage has little meaning in this situation. The atmospheric pressure of O_2, on the other hand, tells the story rather well.

PROPERTIES OF GASSES AND LIQUIDS

Basic to all gas laws is the molecular theory which states that all gasses are composed of molecules that are constantly in motion at very high velocities. A gas has no definite shape or volume, and conforms to the shape and volume of its container. Its pressure is the result of the constant impacts of its many molecules upon the walls of the container. Obviously, the pressure of a gas is increased by confining it in a smaller volume, or by increasing the activity of each molecule. Because a rise in temperature increases the velocity of molecular movement, heat also results in producing increased pressure.

Liquids, on the other hand, are composed of molecules that are much closer together, and this closeness results in their having a definite, independent volume, which varies very little with temperature or with the size and shape of the container.

TABLE 8.1

Percentage and Partial Pressures of O_2 by Altitude

Altitude	Atmospheric Pressure (mm Hg)	Percent O_2	Approximate Pressure Exerted by O_2 in the Atmosphere (mm Hg)
Sea level	760	20.93	159
10,000	523	20.93	109
20,000	349	20.93	73
30,000	226	20.93	47
40,000	141	20.93	29

For the student to understand respiratory physiology (a very important part of exercise physiology), knowledge of the laws that govern behavior of gasses is essential.

Boyle's Law. This law states that if temperature remains constant, the pressure of a gas varies inversely with its volume. If, for example, we decrease the volume by one-half, the pressure will be doubled.

Gay-Lussac's Law. If its volume remains constant, the pressure of a gas increases directly in proportion to its (absolute) temperature.

Law of Partial Pressures. In a mixture of gasses, each gas exerts a *partial pressure,* proportional to its concentration. Thus in atmospheric air with a total pressure of 760 mm Hg, O_2—which makes up 20.93 percent—has a partial pressure of 159 mm Hg: 20.93 / 100 $\times$ 760 mm = 159 mm.

Henry's Law. The quantity of a gas that will dissolve in a liquid is directly proportional to its partial pressure, if temperature remains constant.

Composition of Respiratory Gasses. The atmospheric air is composed mainly of nitrogen (N_2), oxygen (O_2), and carbon dioxide (CO_2); there are also rare gasses (argon, krypton, etc.), but these are ordinarily lumped together and included with the nitrogen fraction.

Table 8.2 illustrates the salient features of the respiratory gas exchange. It will be noted that the partial pressures of dry atmospheric air are proportional to the percentages as per the law of partial pressures; however, the alveolar air is saturated with water vapor, which contributes a partial pressure of 47 mm Hg at body temperature. The partial pres-

Table 8.2

Composition of Atmospheric Air and the Consequent Partial
Pressures of Respiratory Gasses

Gas	Percent in Dry Atmosphere	Partial Pressure in Dry Atmosphere	Partial Pressure in Alveolar Air	Partial Pressure in Mixed Venous Blood	Diffusion Gradient
Total	100	760	760	705	
H_2O	0	0	47	47	
O_2	20.93	159	100	40	60
CO_2	0.03	0.2	40	45	5
N_2	79.04	600.8	573	573	

sure of O_2 in the lungs, then, would be 20.93 percent of 760 minus 47 mm, or approximately 149 mm Hg—if we could completely exchange the air in the lungs. This, of course, is impossible because alveolar air in the lungs is a mixture of atmospheric air with air that has already participated in the respiratory exchange. For this reason, it will be noted in Table 8.2 that the actual partial pressure of O_2 in the alveolar air is 100 mm instead of the 149 mm that would be present if there were no dead space and if the lung collapsed to empty itself completely at each breath.

The importance of all this lies in the *diffusion gradients* for O_2 and CO_2 that, after all, ultimately determine the amount of gaseous exchange taking place. The diffusion gradient for O_2 is some 60 mm Hg, for CO_2 only 5 to 6 mm Hg. Since these figures obtain for normal, healthy individuals, the diffusion gradient for CO_2 is obviously sufficient to maintain the necessary homeostatic relations for CO_2 levels. This can be explained by the fact that diffusion of gasses across a membrane depends not only upon the gradient but also upon the ease with which a particular gas can penetrate the membrane. This, in turn, depends upon the solubility of the gas in the membrane (largely water). Because the solubility of CO_2 in water is some twenty or more times that of O_2, this explains the need for a greater diffusion gradient for O_2.

Acids, Bases, and pH.   Acids may be defined as compounds that yield positively charged hydrogen ions (H^+) in solution—and, conversely, bases as compounds that yield negatively charged hydroxyl ions (OH^-) in solution. A very convenient yardstick for measuring and describing degrees of acidity or alkalinity has been set up: pH, which is defined as the negative logarithm of the hydrogen ion concentration in gram molecular weight. This may be visualized as follows:

Strongest Acid										Strongest Base			
← Increasing Acidity					Neutrality					Increasing Alkalinity →			
pH = 1	2	3	4	5	6	7	8	9	10	11	12	13	14

Since this is a logarithmic scale, a very small change of pH makes a considerable change in acidity or alkalinity, and therefore pH is usually given to at least one, and usually two, decimal places. For example, the extreme fluctuations of the pH of normal blood lie within pH values of 7.30 to 7.50. The extreme values in illness have been known to go as low as 6.95 and and as high as 7.80. However, in healthy subjects, recent work has shown (8) that surprisingly low values, down to 6.80 can result from heavy anaerobic exercise. Such *short term* pH changes appeared to be well tolerated in *healthy subjects*. For a more complete treatment of pH and acid-base balance, the student is referred to a text in physiological chemistry (4).

GAS TRANSPORT BY THE BLOOD

Oxygen. Although chemical analyses have demonstrated that blood is capable of carrying only about 0.2 volume percent of O_2 (0.2 ml of O_2 per 100 ml of blood) in solution at normal atmospheric pressures, it actually transports twenty volume percent of O_2—100 times as much as will dissolve in physical solution.

The reason for this great discrepancy is the presence of hemoglobin in the erythrocytes. Hemoglobin is an iron-bearing pigment, consisting of *heme* (which contains iron) and *globin* (which is a protein). Hemoglobin has the unique characteristic of combining with O_2 quickly and reversibly, and without the necessity for help from enzyme reactions. This is not true of typical oxidation reactions, in which the O_2, once combined, is separated only with difficulty. Therefore the term *oxygenation* is used for the process, rather than *oxidation*, and the reaction can be described thus:

$$\text{Hemoglobin} + \text{Oxygen} \rightleftharpoons \text{Oxyhemoglobin}$$
$$\text{Hb} + O_2 \rightleftharpoons \text{HbO}_2$$

As is the case with all reversible reactions, if the end product on the right, HbO_2, is constantly removed, as in the lungs where oxygenated blood moves off to the tissues, the reaction continues to proceed from left to right. On the other hand, in the tissue exchange the O_2 is carried off by tissue fluids to the cells, and the reaction proceeds to the left.

It is interesting to note that if the organism depended upon dissolved O_2, an all-out effort by the cardiovascular and respiratory systems could not meet the O_2 needs of the resting metabolism, let alone the metabolism of exercise.

Carbon Dioxide. CO_2, which is the constant end product of metabolism in the cell, diffuses across the cell membrane into the tissue fluid, thence across the capillary wall into the blood plasma, where a small portion of it is transported. The larger proportion, probably ninety to ninety-five percent, diffuses from the plasma into the erythrocytes. It is transported by the erythrocyte in three forms: (1) in combination with hemoglogin, called carbamino-hemoglobin, (2) as bicarbonate, HCO_3, and (3) as dissolved CO_2, a portion of which ionizes into carbonic acid, H_2CO_3.

The exchange of CO_2, at the lungs and at the tissues, involves the following reversible reaction.

$$\text{In the Lungs} \rightarrow$$
$$HCO_3^- + H^+ \; \rightleftharpoons \; H_2CO_3 \; \rightleftharpoons \; H_2O + CO_2$$
$$\leftarrow \text{In the Tissues}$$

This is ordinarily a slow reaction; however, an enzyme, *carbonic anhydrase,* catalyzes these reactions so that they can go to completion before the blood leaves the lung or tissue capillaries.

INTERNAL RESPIRATION

Much of the story concerning internal respiration, or gas exchange in the tissues, has already been told. Two other factors, however, are basic to an understanding of the respiratory exchange.

O_2 **Dissociation Curve.** It is an interesting biochemical fact that the loading of CO_2 into the blood at the tissues considerably aids the unloading of O_2 from blood to tissues. The reverse is also true in the lungs: the unloading of CO_2 in the lungs aids the loading of O_2 into the blood.

These facts are best illustrated by the O_2 dissociation curve (fig. 8.1). If one places a straight edge vertically along the line representing a partial pressure of O_2 of 30 mm Hg (that of the tissues), the difference in hemoglobin saturation level between the points where the 40 mm CO_2 curve (blood CO_2 level) and the 80 mm CO_2 curve (active tissue level) cross this vertical line represents the difference of O_2 that the hemoglobin can hold.

This amount of O_2—in this case from approximately fifty percent to approximately thirty percent (twenty percent)—is driven off by changing CO_2 levels in the tissues. In other words, increasing the CO_2 level

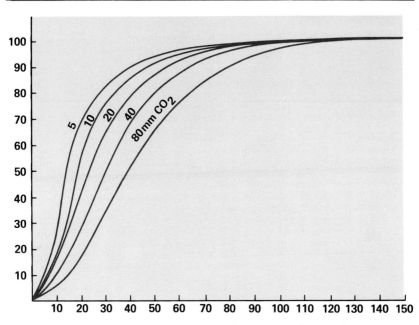

Figure 8-1. O_2 dissociation curve of blood of dogs (similar to man). The ordinate represents percentage saturation of the blood with O_2; the abscissa represents partial pressure of O_2. (From the data of Bohr, Hasselbalch, and Krogh. *Scand. Arch. Physiol.* 16:402, 1904.)

of the blood from its arterialized level of 40 mm Hg to 80 mm Hg, which probably represents the temporary local changes in blood level at the tissues, results in driving off twenty percent of the total O_2 load.

Another point regarding the O_2 dissociation curve is of very practical interest on the effect of altitude upon human respiration. It should be noted that the curve for 40 mm of CO_2, which represents the mixed venous blood (typical of the body as a whole but not of any localized tissue site), is not very steep from 100 to approximately 60 mm of O_2 partial pressure. The upper figure is typical of alveolar O_2 tension at sea level, and the lower figure represents alveolar O_2 tension at about fifteen to sixteen thousand feet above sea level, the level at which resting humans (pilots, etc.) begin having serious symptoms due to the lack of O_2. (Military regulations require the use of oxygen above 10,000 feet to provide a safety margin that allows for individual variance.) If this O_2 dissociation curve were a straight diagonal line, physical impairment would probably commence at about 90 mm of O_2 tension instead of at 60 mm or at an altitude, roughly, of 6,000 feet.

Another salient feature of the O_2 dissociation curve is that it is steep (close to vertical) when the partial pressures of O_2 are low. This fact means, of course, that small changes in partial pressure of O_2 on this part of the curve make large changes in the amount of O_2 the hemoglobin can hold, thus making large exchanges of respiratory gas efficient when the need is greatest.

Coefficient of O_2 Utilization. This term can be defined as the proportion of O_2, transported by the blood, that is given off to the tissues. Since ninety-nine percent of the transported O_2 is bound to hemoglobin, this story also can be related in terms of the O_2 dissociation curve. During resting conditions at sea level, the hemoglobin leaving the lungs is at least ninety-five percent saturated with O_2. After leaving the capillary bed of resting tissue, it is still at least seventy percent saturated. (In fig. 8.1, use the 40 mm CO_2 curve and note its intersections at the 100 mm and at the 40 mm O_2 tension lines.) Thus the hemoglobin has given off 25/95 of its O_2, or 26.3 percent, in resting conditions.

In exercise, this situation becomes much more favorable. The hemoglobin leaving the lungs is still approximately ninety-five percent saturated, but after leaving active muscle tissue, it may approach zero saturation. Thus the coefficient of oxygen utilization may increase from three to four times in exercise. It should be reiterated that this increase is facilitated by the steepness of the O_2 dissociation curve at the lower O_2 tensions (as was mentioned above).

At this point it may be well to note the combination of factors that contribute to supplying the increased oxygen demands of exercising muscle tissue. First, it will be recalled that cardiac output can increase about six times its resting value. Secondly, in combination with an increased utilization coefficient of three to four times, this means a possible increase of at least eighteen times the resting value. Third, in respect to the local situation at any given active muscle, this may be multiplied by another factor of two, due to the approximate doubling of the number of open capillaries (discussed earlier). Thus a total increase of at least thirty-six times the resting oxygen supply is possible at any active muscle group.

REGULATION OF ACID-BASE BALANCE

Even under resting conditions, the acid-base equilibrium of the body fluids is constantly challenged by the formation of CO_2 as the end product of cellular metabolism. Furthermore, when exercise work loads become severe, lactic acid is also formed, constituting an additional influence that tends to drive pH downward. Illness brings about other acidifying or alkalinizing influences. Because long-term pH changes beyond the range of 7.30 to 7.50 are inconsistent with good health, it is obvious that the human organism must be able to control acid-base balance.

Two processes are involved in this. The first line of defense against pH changes is the combination of three *buffer systems* that serve to absorb the shock, as it were, of sudden changes. Ultimately, however, *physiological changes* have to be brought about to maintain the organism in homeostasis over the longer period of time, and these physiological changes mainly involve the lungs and the kidneys.

Buffer Systems. A buffer system consists of a weak acid and a salt of that acid. The system functions as follows.

HL	NaHCO$_3$	NaL	H$_2$CO$_3$
Lactic +	Sodium $\rightarrow$	Sodium +	Carbonic
acid	bicarbonate	Lactate	acid

In this schema, lactic acid (a relatively strong acid) combines with sodium bicarbonate (salt of a weak acid) to form sodium lactate (which no longer has acid tendencies) and carbonic acid (which is a very weak acid). Thus a strong acid has been exchanged for a weak acid, and the tendency for the lactic acid to lower the pH of the blood has been greatly lessened by the buffering action of the carbonic acid, bicarbonate system.

Table 8.3 illustrates what happens when a strong acid, HCl, is added to a water solution that contains the bicarbonate buffer system. It should be noted that when the ratio of H$_2$CO$_3$ and NaHCO$_3$ is favorable (about 1:5), the addition of the first ten grams of acid brings about almost no change in relative acidity or pH. When the buffer ratio becomes less favorable, however, the addition of the same quantity of acid (300 to 310 grams) more than doubles the relative acidity, and the pH changes from 6.00 downward to 5.66. When the bicarbonate is used up, there is no longer any buffering, and the addition of ten grams of HCl (from 320 to 330) brings about a *sixfold* increase in relative acidity and, of course, a much larger drop in pH. It will be noted that the effectiveness of the buffer system depends upon the ratio of the acid to the salt.

Blood must now be considered as two fluids that need buffering: the plasma and the fluid within the erythrocytes. In the plasma, the acids to be buffered are largely *fixed acids,* so called because they are not subject to rapid excretion. They are, in general, stronger acids, such as hydrochloric, phosphoric, sulfuric, and lactic acids (the stronger acids are in very small quantities). The most important buffers in the plasma are

$$\frac{H_2CO_3}{NaHCO_3} \qquad \text{and} \qquad \frac{H\ protein}{Na\ proteinate}$$

TABLE 8.3

Effect of Buffering in Combating Acidifying Effect of
Adding Hydrochloric Acid to a Solution

HCl (gm.) Added	Buffer Ratio $H_2CO_3/NaHCO_3$	H^+ Concentration	pH	Relative Acidity
0	2.27: 11.9	0.000000057N	7.24	.57
10	2.27: 11.5	0.000000059	7.23	.59
50	2.27: 10.0	0.000000068	7.13	.68
100	2.27: 8.2	0.000000083	7.08	.83
150	2.27: 6.3	0.000000108	6.97	1.08
200	2.27: 4.4	0.000000154	6.81	1.54
250	2.27: 2.6	0.000000260	6.59	2.60
300	2.27: 0.68	0.000001000	6.00	10.
310	2.27: 0.31	0.000002200	5.66	22.
318		0.000260000	3.59	260.
320		0.000450000	3.35	450.
330		0.002700000	2.57	2,700.

Based on data from L. J. Henderson, in Best and Taylor, *Physiological Basis of Medical Practice*. Baltimore: The Williams & Wilkins Co., 1943, p. 170.

The blood proteins can act as buffer systems because, at the pH of blood, they behave as weak acids and react with the base to form a salt. In the intracellular fluids of the erythrocytes, on the other hand, the major acid to be buffered is the carbonic acid that results from the respiratory exchange. The buffer systems mainly responsible for this are hemoglobin and oxyhemoglobin, each of which can act as a weak acid or as a potassium salt, as follows.

$$\frac{H\ Hb\ O_2}{K\ Hb\ O_2} \qquad and \qquad \frac{H\ Hb}{K\ Hb}$$

Oxyhemoglobin   Hemoglobin

system   system

There are also other, less important buffer systems in both plasma and cells, such as the acid and basic sodium and potassium phosphates.

Physiological Regulation of Acid-base Balance. Although the buffering systems can resist fast changes in pH, a change does occur with the addition of an acid (or base) to the body fluids (table 8.3). These changes are corrected by two physiological mechanisms for excretion of the acid (or base): changes in respiratory function and changes in kidney function.

The function of the lungs in regulating acid-base balance is another example of the body's servomechanisms. For example, if the breath is held, the CO_2 resulting from metabolism accumulates. This has the effect of pouring acid into the tissue fluids and blood: $CO_2 + H_2O \rightarrow H_2CO_3$. This decrease in pH is interpreted as the *error signal* by the respiratory center in the medulla, which corrects the situation by increasing the rate and depth of ventilation (if possible). When the breath is held, the error signal simply grows larger and larger, until the urge to breathe overcomes the willpower to hold the breath. The rate and depth will then be greater than normal, until equilibrium has been reestablished by *blowing off* more CO_2 than is being formed: $H_2CO_3 \rightarrow CO_2 + H_2O$.

Thus the importance of the respiratory function in acid-base regulation lies in the fact that the decomposition products of carbonic acid are volatile and can be readily blown off by the lungs.

In hyperventilation, on the other hand, more CO_2 is blown off than is formed and consequently a change in the ratio of $H_2CO_3/NaHCO_3$ is brought about. The normal ratio is 1:20. If H_2CO_3 and $NaHCO_3$ are increased or decreased proportionately, no change in ratio occurs, and consequently there is no change in pH. In the case of hyperventilation, however, the H_2CO_3 decreases disproportionately because the $NaHCO_3$ remains the same, and thus a relative increase in the base occurs with a rise in pH.

If the hyperventilation is of short duration—as in preparing for an athletic event—the increased production of CO_2 during the event corrects the situation; but if hyperventilation is long-term (one hour or more), as in fever, a secondary adjustment must be made to excrete some of the bicarbonate to keep the ratio close to 1:20. This excretion of bicarbonate is done through the kidney.

The last line of defense and the one concerned with long-term changes in acid-base equilibrium is the excretion of abnormal amounts of acid or base by the kidney to maintain all the buffer systems at the proper acid-salt ratio for maintaining normal pH. When it is no longer possible to maintain these ratios, acidosis or alkalosis ensues. In severe acidosis, death ensues as a result of coma; in severe alkalosis, death may be brought about by tetany and the resulting muscle spasm of respiratory muscles.

ACID-BASE BALANCE AS A FACTOR LIMITING PERFORMANCE

The preceding discussion makes it obvious that metabolism in general provides a constant acidifying influence. When the metabolic rate is raised to seven or eight times that of the resting level, the increase in CO_2 is proportional, but ventilation can usually keep pace to maintain acid-base equilibrium. However, when the work load goes beyond aerobic capacity, lactic acid becomes the end product of metabolism, instead of CO_2. This is a much stronger acid, and it cannot be excreted quickly by respiration as could the CO_2. It has already been pointed out that under conditions of heavy anaerobic exercise the pH can drop as low as 6.80 (8).

This line of reasoning would seem to indicate that the body's ability to buffer fixed acids (such as lactic acid) should play a large part in determining the end point of anaerobic activity. Because these fixed acids are largely buffered by the bicarbonate system, the combining power of the plasma bicarbonate has been referred to as the *alkaline reserve*. Although this concept rests on a reasonably sound rationale, it is an oversimplification of the complex biochemical interactions involved in acid-base regulation, and human performance research has so far failed to show a clear-cut improvement in performance as a result of an increased alkaline reserve.

CHANGES IN LUNG DIFFUSION IN EXERCISE

The diffusion of oxygen from the alveoli to the pulmonary capillaries increases in virtually direct proportion to the effect involved in the exercise, as measured by O_2 consumption. This relationship has been demonstrated to a level at least seven or eight times that of the resting metabolism (14). In the absence of disease processes, it is very unlikely that pulmonary diffusing capacity for O_2 is a limiting factor in exercise.

The reasons for increased pulmonary diffusion are as yet not completely understood, but the increased ventilation of exercise does not seem to be a necessary factor. It has been shown that similar increases in pulmonary diffusion can occur during exercise when the ventilation is voluntarily held to resting levels (10). It seems most likely that the increase in pulmonary diffusion is the result of increased pulmonary capillary blood volume during exercise brought about by the opening of previously unopened capillaries—as discussed in the chapter on circulation.

There is evidence that highly trained athletes demonstrate better pulmonary diffusion under maximal (7) and submaximal work rates (2) than do nonathletes. This effect may be an innate, inherited characteristic of champion athletes, but it can also be brought about by the effects of a rigorous training program (7).

The recent work of Mostyn and others (6) seems to indicate that championship-level swimmers are unusually high in pulmonary diffusing capacity. Their experiments would indicate this is due to a larger-than-normal pulmonary capillary blood volume; however, a change in breathing pattern can bring about significant increases in normal nonswimmers. When subjects breathed during exercise with a *held inspiration* maneuver in which they took a fast inspiration to full capacity (one second), held the breath at full inspiration for about seven seconds, then exhaled as fast as possible, they showed a significant improvement in pulmonary diffusion. Obviously, this type of breathing is very similar to that imposed upon competitive swimmers by their environment.

Thus it would seem that in activities in which the respiratory exchange is made under unfavorable conditions such as swimming, or mountain climbing, and other activities in which the ambient atmospheric pressure of O_2 is low, the held inspiration type of breathing might provide an advantage in increasing pulmonary diffusing capacity. It is conceivable that this procedure can be of practical use to athletes who must compete at higher-than-normal elevations.

USE OF OXYGEN TO IMPROVE PERFORMANCE

It is not uncommon to see a coach administer O_2 to his athletes. This has been done by track and swimming coaches immediately before the event, and by many other coaches to hasten the recovery process—for example, between halves of a football or basketball game. Let us consider first the theoretical aspects of this procedure to determine its likely validity, and then take note of the applied research.

We must remember that the arterial blood that leaves the lungs is saturated to the extent of ninety-five to ninety-eight percent, and this degree of saturation does not seem to be changed in vigorous exercise in a normal subject at sea level. (All of this discussion will apply only to sea-level atmosphere.) If alveolar air increases its partial pressure of O_2 by a factor of three (not unreasonable in seventy to 100 percent mixtures), O_2 transport would conceivably be enhanced by two factors. (A) Hemoglobin saturation would increase by a maximum of from ninety-five to 100 percent. Because blood normally carries twenty volume percent O_2 or 20 ml of O_2 in 100 ml of blood, (in round figures) it would increase by five percent (0.05×20), for an increase of 1 ml per 100 ml of blood. (B) The O_2 in solution would increase in proportion to the increased partial pressure of O_2 (Henry's law). The amount in solution is ordinarily about 0.2 ml per 100 ml of blood. This, then, would become about 0.6 ml per 100 ml of blood, or an increase of 0.4 ml. The total potential advantage accruing in O_2 transport would therefore be something like 1.4 ml, or 1.4/20, or about seven percent.

It must be realized, however, that this discussion is predicated upon the breathing of O_2 *during* the athletic performance. If it is breathed before the performance, storage would have to occur to benefit the performance unless the subject were able to use O_2 right up to the start of the performance and then hold his breath during the performance. In this unlikely event, storage of O_2 might be thought to occur in the sense of a higher partial pressure of O_2 in the lungs at the start of the event.

Now let us review the recent research in this area under three categories: (1) O_2 before exercise, (2) O_2 during exercise, and (3) O_2 during recovery.

O_2 before Exercise.   In a well-controlled study by Miller (5), in which he administered O_2 before, during, and after a treadmill exercise, no changes in heart rate, blood pressure, blood lactate, or endurance were found when the O_2 was administered before or during recovery from the exercise. He was able to show a psychological effect from breathing air that had been marked *oxygen;* and this very likely is also the explanation for earlier studies that had shown improved performance after O_2 breathing.

O_2 during Exercise.   Available research seems to agree upon the value of O_2 administration during exercise. Miller found a significant decrease in blood lactate, and an increase in running time to exhaustion, when O_2 was administered during the treadmill run. Elbel and others (3) found significantly slower heart rates when O_2 was administered during exercise. Bannister and Cunningham (1) set exercise loads on a treadmill so that their four subjects would run to exhaustion in seven to ten minutes while breathing air. While breathing sixty-six percent O_2, all subjects were able to maintain these workloads for longer periods and three of the four subjects went beyond twenty-three minutes. They also compared the effects of twenty-one, thirty-three, sixty-six, and 100 percent O_2, and it is of interest that best results were obtained with sixty-six percent. Subjective reports of euphoria were gotten only from the sixty-six-percent mixture.

O_2 during Recovery.   Miller found no improvement in recovery for any of the measurements made as the result of breathing O_2 during recovery. Elbel et al. (3) found no significant changes in O_2 debt repayment as the result of breathing O_2 during recovery, but they found significantly slower heart rates. Their heart rate findings could be construed as hastening the recovery process, but the differences were very small, one to five beats per minute.

To summarize the case for breathing O_2 to improve performance, it seems unlikely that any *physiological* changes are brought about by breathing it before the event and (at best) only very small improvements in the recovery rate. Improved performance undoubtedly can result if O_2 is breathed *during* the event, but this can have no practical importance in athletics.

On the other hand, *psychological improvement* in performance can be brought about through suggestion (in the use of oxygen). Also, if an athlete is conditioned to the use of O_2, accidental deprivation at an important meet or game could result in a calamitous decrement in performance.

WHAT SETS THE LIMITS OF AEROBIC CAPACITY?

Aerobic capacity—the maximum O_2 consumption depends upon the transport of O_2 from the atmosphere to the mitochondria of the muscle cells. This transit involves basically four processes: (A) lung ventilation, or more precisely alveolar ventilation, (B) the interaction between pulmonary diffusion and blood transport, (C) blood transport, and (D) the interaction between tissue diffusion and blood transport.

R. J. Shephard (11, 13) has suggested the use of the O_2 *Conductance Equation* to estimate where the bottleneck to O_2 transport may lie on theoretical bases. In this approach each of the four links in the O_2 transport chain is treated as a conductance. Conductances can be added as reciprocals to give the sum of series conductances so that the total conductance which is equivalent to aerobic capacity or *maximal O_2 consumption* can be predicted in simplified form as follows:

$$\frac{1}{U_{O2}} = \frac{1}{A} + \frac{1}{B} + \frac{1}{C} + \frac{1}{D}$$

Where U_{O2} is the total conductance and A, B, C, D represent the four phases in gas transport as listed above.

When realistic estimates for maximal conductance are substituted for each of the four links in the chain then the equation looks like this (Shephard 1967a):

$$\frac{1}{U_{O2}} = \frac{1}{90} + \frac{1}{176} + \frac{1}{30} + \frac{1}{681}$$

It can readily be seen that the term C which represents blood transport has the greatest effect in setting the limit for maximal aerobic capacity. All of these data apply only to normal young subjects at sea level. Thus the theoretical application of the O_2 conductance equation suggests that the most important determinants of aerobic capacity are the interaction of cardiac output and hemoglobin level which together determine the level of blood transport. As Shephard (1967a) points out however this still leaves us with the question of the relative contributions of the cardiac musculature and of the venous return to this ceiling of performance. Experimental data tend to support the conclusions derived from the O_2 conductance equation (9).

SUMMARY

1. The important factor governing the diffusion of respiratory gasses is the difference in pressure between two points, called a *diffusion gradient.*
2. If atmospheric pressure is much below sea-level pressure, the percentage concentration of a gas (such as O_2) is meaningless because its partial pressure may be insufficient to bring about sufficient diffusion.
3. At sea level, the partial pressures of O_2 are approximately 100 mm and 40 mm Hg in the alveoli and venous blood, respectively, yielding a diffusion gradient of 60 mm Hg. For CO_2, the corresponding figures are 45 mm and 40 mm in venous blood and alveoli, respectively, with a diffusion gradient of 5 mm Hg.
4. CO_2 requires a lesser diffusion gradient than O_2 because of its greater solubility in water, and hence in the alveolar and endothelial tissues.
5. Acidity and alkalinity are expressed in pH units: 7.00 represents neutrality, higher values represent alkalinity, and lower values represent acidity.
6. Ninety-nine percent of the oxygen transport of the blood is accomplished by combination with hemoglobin; about one percent is carried in physical solution.
7. Carbon dioxide transport is accomplished largely within the erythrocytes, and in three forms: (1) carbamino-hemoglobin, (2) bicarbonate, and (3) dissolved CO_2.
8. The shape of the O_2 dissociation curve is such that gaseous exchange is greatly expedited at the lungs and at the tissues.
9. At rest, hemoglobin enters the tissues about ninety-five percent saturated and leaves about seventy percent saturated. This difference is called the *coefficient of O_2 utilization.* In exercise, comparable percentages may be 95 percent and close to 0 percent, thus effecting a great increase in O_2 utilization.
10. Acid-base balance is maintained throughout the body by buffer systems. Each is comprised of a weak acid and a salt of the acid, and functions by converting strong acids to weak acids and neutral salts.

11. When the capacity for buffering is stressed, acids and bases are excreted by the lungs and kidneys as a secondary line of defense against pH changes that may be inconsistent with the welfare of the organism.

12. As the rate of metabolism increases in exercise, the rate of diffusion for O_2 increases proportionately. This is probably brought about by the better perfusion of the lung capillaries with blood.

13. Use of O_2 to improve performance rests on sound scientific evidence only when it is used during the exercise period. A small improvement in rate of recovery seems to be possible, but this awaits corroborative evidence.

14. Both theoretical and experimental data suggest that the limits for maximal O_2 transport (*aerobic capacity*) for healthy young subjects exercising at sea level are set by the interaction of cardiac output and hemoglobin level.

REFERENCES

1. Bannister, R. G., and Cunningham, D. J. C. 1954. The effects on the respiration and performance during exercise of adding oxygen to the inspired air. *Journal of Physiology* 125:118.

2. Bannister, R. G.; Cotes, J. E.; Jones, R. S.; and Meade, F. 1960. Pulmonary diffusing capacity on exercise in athletes and nonathletic subjects. *Journal of Physiology* 152:66-67.

3. Elbel, E. R.; Ormond, D.; and Close, D. 1961. Some effects of breathing O_2 before and after exercise. *Journal of Applied Physiology* 16:48-52.

4. Hawk, P. B.; Oser, B. L.; and Summerson, W. H. 1954. *Practical physiological chemistry*. New York: McGraw-Hill Book Co.

5. Miller, A. T., Jr. 1952. Influence of oxygen administration on cardiovascular function during exercise and recovery. *Journal of Applied Physiology* 5:165-68.

6. Mostyn, E. M.; Helle, S.; Gee. J. B. L.; Bentivoglio, L. G.; and Bates, D. V. 1963. Pulmonary diffusing capacity of athletes. *Journal of Applied Physiology* 18:687-95.

7. Newman, F.; Smalley, B. F.; and Thomson, M. L. 1962. Effect of exercise, body and lung size on CO diffusion in athletes and nonathletes. *Journal of Applied Physiology* 17:649-55.

8. Osnes, J. B., and Hermansen, L. 1971. Acid base balance after maximal exercise of short duration. *Journal of Applied Physiology* 32:59-63.

9. Ouellet, Y.; Poh, S. C.; and Becklake, M. R. 1969. Circulatory factors limiting maximal aerobic exercise capacity. *Journal of Applied Physiology* 27:874-80.

10. Ross, J. C.; Reinhart, R. W.; Boxell, J. F.; and King, L. H., Jr. 1963. Relationship of increased breath-holding diffusing capacity to ventilation in exercise. *Journal of Applied Physiology* 18:794-97.

11. Shephard, R. J. 1967. Commentary on paper by A. Holmgren. *Canadian Medical Association Journal* 96:702-3.
12. ———. 1967. Physiological determinants of cardiorespiratory fitness. *Journal of Sports Medicine and Physical Fitness* 7:111-34.
13. ———. 1969. The validity of the oxygen conductance equation. *Int. Z. Angew Physiology* 28:61-75.
14. Turino, G. M.; Bergofsky, E. H.; Goldring, R. M.; and Fishman, A. P. 1963. Effect of exercise on pulmonary diffusing capacity. *Journal of Applied Physiology* 18:447-56.

9 Exercise Metabolism

The essence and the uniqueness of the study of physiology of exercise lie in its concern with physiological mechanisms not during rest but while the organism is stressed by physical activity. This physical activity may be work, physical education activity, athletics, or informal play. By observing the stress of vigorous physical activity, the exercise physiologist gains insight into physiology that is withheld when the organism is at rest. Questions pertaining to how well various organic systems can function under stress can be answered only in terms of the functional capacity an individual has in respect to his cardiovascular system, his respiratory system, his heat dissipation system, etc. An individual may show no cardiac abnormality in a physician's diagnostic examination, but this obviously does not tell us anything about his cardiac capacity for running a good time in the 440 or the mile. Functional tests are needed here, and these are in the domain of the exercise physiologist. To make these functional tests meaningful to other professions the exercise physiologist uses a vocabulary of terms that is taken from physics as well as physiology.

DEFINITION OF TERMS

Work.   Work is defined by the physicist as the product of force times the distance through which that force acts: $W = F \times D$. For example, if a man lifts a weight of 100 pounds a height of three feet, he has done work of 100 pounds times three feet, or 300 foot-pounds of work. In the metric system (which is commonly used internationally in exercise physiology, as in other sciences), the same individual, if he weighed 100 kilograms and climbed up to stand on the three-meter diving board, would have performed 100 kilograms times three meters, or 300 kilogram-meters of work. It will be noted that no mention has been made of the time it took to do the work, in either case, and this is not a relevant factor in the concept of work. The same amount of work is performed regardless of how long it takes.

Unfortunately, the physicist's definition leaves something to be desired when the muscular activity is isometric, as in the case where one "merely holds 100 pounds motionless;" here, since the distance is zero, the work must also be zero. However, other methods are available by which the effort involved can be evaluated.

Power.   If two individuals can each lift 100 pounds a distance of three feet, but one does it twice as fast as the other, we have introduced the concept of power. The man who does it twice as fast is twice as powerful. Power is usually defined in terms of horsepower, just as in rating an automobile engine.

$$1 \text{ hp} = 33,000 \text{ ft-lbs per min} = 550 \text{ ft-lbs per sec}$$

It should be noted that *power* is distinct from *strength;* power is composed of strength and speed. An athlete's power in an event (such as the shot put) can thus be increased either by improving the strength of the muscles involved—as by heavy resistance training—or by improving the speed with which the movement is made.

As an illustrative example of the calculation of horsepower, let us consider an individual performing the Harvard Step Test. In this test of physical fitness the subject lifts his body weight (150 pounds, let us say) onto a twenty-inch-high bench thirty times per minute. Thus the work done per minute would be as follows.

(handwritten margin note: convert in. to feet..)

$$W = 150 \text{ lb} \times 1\text{-}2/3 \text{ ft } (20 \text{ in}) \times 30 = 7,500 \text{ ft-lbs}$$

In terms of power, he has worked at the level of:

$$\frac{7,500 \text{ ft-lb per min}}{33,000 \text{ ft-lb per min}} = 0.227 \text{ hp}$$

A very powerful man can produce as much as three or four horsepower, but only for very short periods of time (five to ten seconds).

Energy. Energy is defined as the capacity for doing work, and can be expressed in the same units. Energy can be stored, in which case it is *potential energy;* and the energy involved in the production of work is *kinetic energy.* Because man is ultimately dependent upon food for his energy, it is obvious that energy can be transformed from one form to another. This is done in accord with the *law of conservation of energy,* which states that in the conversion of energy from one form to another energy is neither created nor destroyed. The energy in food is chemical energy, and it is converted into mechanical and heat energy by the muscles in bringing about movement and doing work.

The energy of food, which produces work, and the work itself can also be described in terms of calories (or kilocalories). One kilocalorie represents the heat required to raise the temperature of one kilogram of water one degree centigrade. To convert heat units to mechanical units:

$$1 \text{ kcal} = 3,087 \text{ ft-lb} = 427 \text{ kg M}$$

Thus a one-ounce chocolate bar that contains 150 kilocalories can theoretically produce energy for some 463,000 foot-pounds of work or enough to keep a 150-pound man doing the Harvard Step Test for more than one hour at 100 percent efficiency. (However, the actual efficiency of such an exercise is not over twenty-five percent.)

Efficiency. Efficiency is usually defined as the percentage of energy input that appears as useful work. Thus if a man requires 4,000 kilocalories input of energy to perform a muscular activity that represents 1,000 kilocalories, his efficiency would be twenty-five percent.

Most of the experimentation in this area indicates that muscular performance under favorable circumstances achieves a mechanical efficiency of twenty to twenty-five percent. It must be realized that the other energy, which does not appear as work, is not lost; it appears as heat, is dissipated, and tends to raise the body temperature during exercise.

METHODS FOR STANDARDIZING AND MEASURING WORK LOADS

In order to make meaningful measurement of the physiological processes during exercise, the exercise work load must be set up in such fashion as to be measureable and repeatable, and it should require little skill. Much of our athletic activity does not lend itself well to these requirements. Measuring the energy or work output of a football player, for instance, would be most difficult because his bursts of activity are interspersed with variable periods of relative inactivity (huddles, etc.). Furthermore, the work he does varies from moment to moment.

Three methods for establishing a standard measureable work load are in common use. Each has its advantages and disadvantages.

Bench-stepping.   The subject lifts his weight a known height (the height of the bench) and his rate can be easily set with a metronome. This activity requires minimum skill, and lends itself well to large groups, but it is subject to several sources of inaccuracy. First, the subject, particularly when he is tired, tends not to straighten his body at the hip and knee joints, and consequently he has not lifted his center of gravity the full height of the bench. Second, he is doing positive work (stepping up) and negative work (stepping down). Negative work, a relatively recent concept, requires considerably less energy expenditure than positive work, but it is difficult to assess.

Treadmill.   This instrument consists of a motor-driven conveyor belt that is large and strong enough for the subject to walk and run upon. These devices are usually constructed so that the speed of the belt and the incline are adjustable. Use of the treadmill is advantageous in using a skill with which everyone is familiar (walking or running). Furthermore, it seems to bring about a slightly better involvement of large muscle masses than any other device since the arms and shoulders can and do enter into the activity.

It has two major disadvantages. First, the subject's movements make instrumentation somewhat difficult; second, and more important, the units of work must be stated in arbitrary fashion—as running at seven mph on a ten percent incline—because much of the work is done in a horizontal direction, and this does not allow evaluation in the standard units of foot-pounds or kilogram-meters.

Bicycle Ergometer. This instrument is a stationary bicycle whose front or back wheel is driven by the subject's pedaling (fig. 9.1). The resistance against which the subject pedals is provided by a frictional band

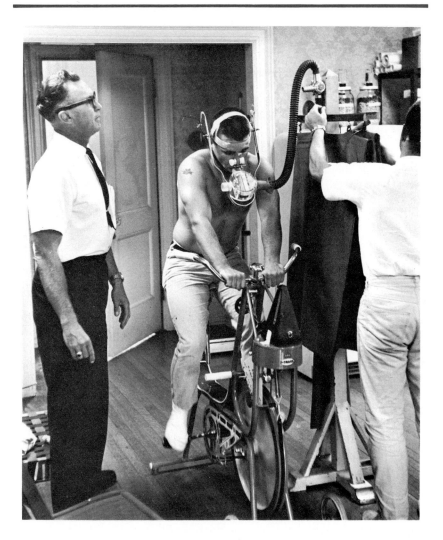

Figure 9-1. Gas collection by Douglas bag using a bicycle ergometer to establish a standard work load.

or by electromagnetic braking. The work load can be quickly and easily adjusted by changing the tension (and hence the frictional load) of the brake band or the electromagnetic load across the generator. Work is calculated easily from a scale reading, which provides the frictional resistance (force), and from a counter that records the number of times the wheel has turned and thus allows calculation of distance: $D = 2\pi rn$.

The wheel's circumference, $2\pi r$, is the distance traveled by any point on the wheel in one revolution; n is the number of revolutions during the work period. Then, since $W = FD$, the total work done may be expressed as: $W = F (2\pi rn.)$.

This piece of equipment has several advantages. First, it is relatively inexpensive or it can be built in most school workshops from a discarded bicycle. Second, the subject's upper body is relatively motionless, and thus instrumentation for electrocardiograph leads, etc., is greatly facilitated. Third, and most important, the work load is expressed in standard units of work, foot-pounds or kilogram-meters, and thus allows work comparisons more easily than the treadmill.

An international team of work physiologists compared the maximal O_2 consumption measured by the three ergometric methods in the same twenty-four healthy young subjects. They found that the terminal pulse rates and arterial lactate levels two minutes after exercise are very similar for step, bicycle and treadmill exercise (1). However, the maximal O_2 uptake in the treadmill test was seven percent greater than that in the bicycle test while the step test values were intermediate between the treadmill and bicycle ergometer values. Many other investigators have found similar results.

The consensus of opinion of an international group of experts reported to the World Health Organization (WHO) was that the "order of preference of exercise tests is considered to be as follows: upright bicycle ergometer, step test and treadmill" (32).

It must be recognized in setting work loads on the bicycle ergometer that equal work loads can have very different physiological effect if pedal frequency is allowed to vary (7, 18). Highest values of maximum O_2 consumption are gotten using a pedal RPM between sixty and seventy (17).

It is also important to consider the effects of learning and habituation upon the performance particularly when measurements such as heart rate at submaximal work loads are of concern. There is anxiety present in most subjects when confronted with a new test situation and this of course has an effect upon the observed heart rate. There is also a learning effect which results in small increases of efficiency. These effects must be controlled or balanced out in any test-retest experiment whether the exercise is on a bicycle ergometer, treadmill or stepping bench.

METHODS FOR MEASURING ENERGY OUTPUT

Direct Calorimetry. Because the human organism is essentially a heat engine, the direct approach to measurements of energy output would be to measure the heat produced by an individual's metabolic processes. This has been done in specially constructed chambers, where all metabolic heat is accumulated by the air and walls of the chamber and changes in their temperature are used to calculate the energy output. This method is called *direct calorimetry;* however, the equipment is expensive and difficult to use, and consequently is seldom used in exercise physiology.

Indirect Calorimetry. Because all of the body's metabolic processes utilize oxygen and produce carbon dioxide (either during activity or immediately after), the energy output is directly related to the quantity of these respiratory gasses. The gasses can be collected from the expired air and measured. This is a much simpler process than direct calorimetry, and it is therefore commonly used in exercise physiology. There are two methods for accomplishing indirect calorimetry: the *closed-circuit* and the *open-circuit* methods.

In the closed-circuit method illustrated in figure 9.2, the subject inspires from a face mask that is connected to an oxygen chamber (which is charged from an O_2 cylinder). His expired air is conducted back to the oxygen chamber by way of a soda lime cannister, where the CO_2 he produced is absorbed. Thus only the O_2 that remains after the respiratory exchange is returned to the oxygen chamber, and the changes in the volume of the O_2 that remains in the chamber, are recorded from breath to breath. Each peak in the kymogram in figure 9.2 represents one respiration and, by measuring the downward slope of the bottom points of the record per unit time, the value of O_2 consumed can be calculated.

This method has the advantage of simplicity, but its accuracy is not much better than plus or minus ten percent of the true value. Furthermore, no value for the CO_2 produced is obtained, and consequently the respiratory quotient (to be discussed below) must be estimated.

In the classic open-circuit method, the subject inspires directly from the atmospheric air and expires into a rubberized canvas bag, called a *Douglas bag* (fig. 9.3). After an exercise period, during which gas collection is accurately timed, samples of the expired gas are taken from the bag for analysis and the volume of expired gasses is measured by a gas

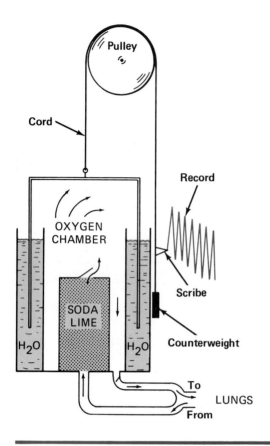

Figure 9-2. Apparatus for indirect determination of heat production by measuring oxygen consumption. The subject breathes into and from the oxygen chamber through the tubes at the bottom. The slope of the curve recorded by the movements of the upper cylinder is a measure of the rate at which oxygen is used by the subject. Arrows indicate direction of oxygen movement as the subject breathes. (From Carlson and Johnson. *The Machinery of the Body,* 1953, The University of Chicago Press, Chicago.)

meter similar to that used for metering the gas used in a home (fig. 9.3). The concentrations of O_2 and CO_2 in the atmosphere are very constant— 20.93 and 0.03 percent, respectively—and on the assumption that the remaining gasses (79.04 percent), lumped together as N_2 do not enter into physiological reactions, the volume of inspired air can be calculated from the volume of expired air as follows:

$$\frac{\text{Volume inspired}}{\text{Volume expired}} = \frac{\text{Percent of } N_2 \text{ in expired air}}{79.04}$$

or

$$\text{Volume inspired} = \frac{\text{Percent of } N_2 \text{ in expired air} \times \text{Volume expired}}{79.04}$$

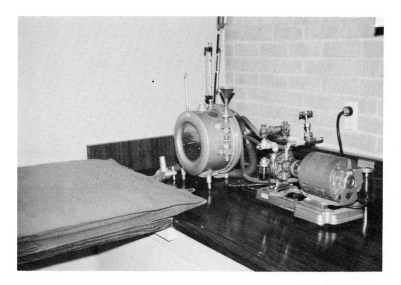

Figure 9-3. Measuring the volume of expired respiratory gases from the Douglas bag by wet-test gas meter. Gases are drawn through the meter at a constant rate by use of an electrical vacuum pump.

This calculation is necessary because the volume of CO_2 produced is not usually equal to the volume of O_2 consumed, and consequently the total volume of expired air also differs from the total inspired.

The above calculation of inspired volume from the *apparent change* in N_2 concentration is still widely used, but the assumption upon which it rests; namely that N_2 is inert physiologically, has recently been challenged. Since animal experiments had shown N_2 *retention* to occur without equivalent protein weight gain (11) Cissik, Johnson, and Rokosch (9) conducted exercise experiments which suggest that N_2 is indeed not inert and that the assumption that it is can lead to serious errors of up to thirteen percent in calculation of O_2 consumption when the inspired volume is calculated by the classic method described above. However, since the publication of this work, Luft and coworkers at the Lovelace Foundation conducted an investigation in which extreme care was observed in the measurements of temperature and the handling of gas volume correction from ATPS to STPD. Under these conditions the differences between measured inspiratory volume and that calculated by the above procedure (Haldane equation) were minute and well within the errors of measurement of the procedures employed (23). Two other studies (14, 31) have since corroborated the work of Luft et al. and on the basis of all this evidence, it appears that the Haldane equation, the calculations shown above for inspired volume, is still a valid procedure. This is indeed fortunate because the findings of Cissik et al. threw into question much of the work done over the past sixty years which had to do with open circuit measurement of O_2 consumption.

To calculate the O_2 consumed, one need only subtract the volume of O_2 remaining in the expired air (percent of O_2 expired times volume expired) from the volume of O_2 in the inspired air (20.93 times volume inspired). The same sort of calculation will also provide the volume of CO_2 produced during the exercise. This method is obviously somewhat more involved than the closed-circuit method, but the gain in precision is commensurate. In the open-circuit method, the error may be less than plus or minus 1.0 percent, compared with plus or minus ten percent for the closed-circuit. Furthermore, data are obtained for the percent of CO_2, which enables computation of R.Q.

Gas Analysis. The percentage of O_2 remaining and CO_2 produced in the expired air are analyzed either by biochemical or electronic methods. The classic biochemical method—the *Haldane apparatus* and *procedure*— uses the absorption of CO_2 by potassium hydroxide from a sample of known size. The change in volume of the sample by absorption of CO_2 is observed, and the proportion this change represents in the total volume of the sample represents the proportion or percent of CO_2 in the sample. The O_2 is then absorbed out by a strong reducing solution, and the same reasoning is applied. All of the gasses left in the sample at this point are considered N_2.

A more recent development of the biochemical (absorptiometric) method is the *Scholander apparatus* (fig. 9.4); it utilizes the same principle described above, but is a considerably faster procedure. (Both methods are capable of a precision of better than plus or minus 0.02 percent in the range of respiratory gasses.)

Still more recently, electronic methods have been developed for measuring respiratory gasses, and they have advantages in both speed and simplicity of operation. The electronic methods compare favorably with the precision of the Haldane and Scholander apparatus.

OXYGEN DEBT AND OXYGEN DEFICIT

In the normal, resting individual, the supply of O_2 to the tissues is sufficient so that a complete breakdown of glycogen occurs which results in the formation only of CO_2 and H_2O with no accumulation of lactic

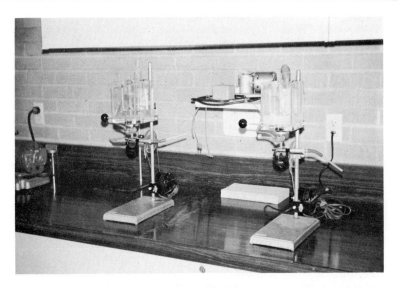

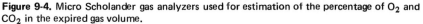

Figure 9-4. Micro Scholander gas analyzers used for estimation of the percentage of O_2 and CO_2 in the expired gas volume.

acid. This situation also applies when the rate of work is such that the metabolic demands can be met aerobically.

When exercise creates a metabolic need for greater O_2 than can be supplied by the cardiorespiratory processes, part of the energy of muscular activity is supplied by the anaerobic mechanism described in chapter two, and lactic acid accumulates as the end product of metabolism. Whenever the supply of O_2 is insufficient to meet demands, an individual is said to contract an *oxygen debt* (a term coined by A. V. Hill, a pioneer in exercise physiology).

In any exercise bout there is a transition period between rest and exercise, involving a short period during which the circulatory and respiratory adjustments lag behind.

The amount by which the O_2 supply lacks being adequate by virtue of this lag in the organisms adjustment to the rise in metabolic rate is called the *O_2 deficit*. Function of the organism under O_2 deficit conditions is made possible by several energy sources not dependent upon O_2 transport. Most important are (1) the splitting of ATP and CP, (2) anaerobic breakdown of glycogen (glycolysis) to lactic acid, and (3) use of O_2 stores such as that bound to muscle myoglobin, and blood O_2 stores as shown in figure 9.6.

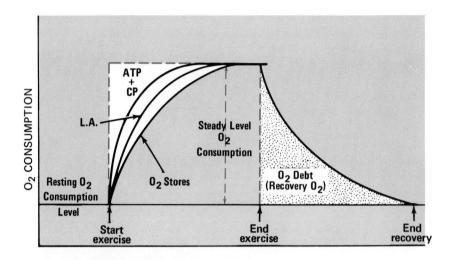

Figure 9-5. Diagram of the relationship of O_2 consumption and time before, during, and after submaximal exercise. The hatched area represents O_2 *deficit* which depends upon at least three factors: (1) breakdown of high energy phosphates ATP + CP, (2) glycolysis to form lactic acid (LA) and (3) use of O_2 stores such as oxymyohemogloben and O_2 of the venous blood. The stippled area represents the O_2 debt (the O_2 used during recovery). All values of O_2 consumption are measured above the resting value as a base line.

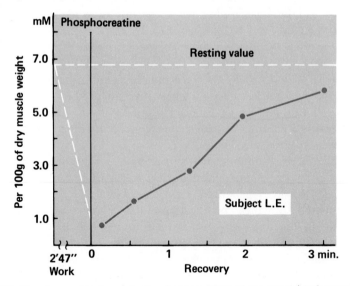

Figure 9-6. Phosphocreatine concentration (mM per 100 g of dry muscle) before and after a maximal work load. (From Hermansen, L. *Med. and Sci. Spt.* 1:32, 1969.)

O_2 *debt* is defined as the amount of O_2 taken up in excess of the resting value during the recovery period. This is ordinarily larger than the O_2 deficit since the repayment for any anaerobic metabolism beyond the initial lag must be repaid here as well as the O_2 deficit.

In light exercise where a steady level of O_2 consumption is attained as in figure 9.6, the O_2 debt may be due entirely to the O_2 deficit at the beginning of exercise. At the end of exercise then, there must be a recovery period during which the O_2 debt is repaid. This is the reason why the heart and the ventilation rates remain elevated after exercise ceases.

When an exercise represents a true overload in which a steady state cannot be achieved, the duration of the effort (or the level of performance) is limited by the athletes ability to sustain an O_2 debt. In maximum work load situations where energy supply is predominately from anaerobic sources, duration is limited to one to two minutes and recovery may take forty-five minutes or even longer.

To illustrate the O_2 debt concept, let us consider a typical experiment on the bicycle ergometer.

Time	Activity	Total Liters of O_2 Consumed	Liters of O_2 Consumed per Minute
8:00-8:05	Resting (seated on bicycle)	1.50	.30
8:05-8-10	Riding (@ 10,000 ft.-lb./min.)	16.50	3.30
8:10-8:40	Recovery (seated on bicycle)	14.00	.47

Calculations (in liters)

1. Total gross O_2 cost = O_2 during + O_2 recovery
= 16.50 1. + 14.00 1. = 30.50 1.

2. Total net O_2 cost = O_2 during + O_2 recovery − O_2 for equivalent period of rest (35 min)
= 16.50 1. + 14.00 1. − (35 × 0.30) = 20.1

3. Net O_2 cost per min of ride = $\dfrac{20.00 \text{ l.}}{5 \text{ min}}$ = 4 1./min

4. Net O_2 intake during ride = O_2 during − O_2 for equivalent rest period
= 16.50 − (5 × 0.30) = 15.1

5. Net O_2 intake during per min = $\dfrac{15.00 \text{ l.}}{5 \text{ min}}$ 3 1./min

6. O_2 debt incurred per min = net O_2 cost per min of ride − net O_2 intake during per min
= 4.00 1. − 3.00 1. = 1 1./min

7. Total O_2 debt incurred = 5 × 1.00 1. = 5 1.

It is clear that such an individual had a metabolic demand for four liters of O_2 per minute, three liters of which he was able to provide by aerobic mechanisms and one liter of which was provided by anaerobic mechanisms. This constituted an O_2 debt that was repaid during the recovery period by consumption of more O_2 per minute than his resting state would have demanded, until the O_2 debt was paid. The length of time for monitoring recovery O_2 consumption is determined by observations of heart rate and minute-by-minute O_2 consumption. When these values have returned to their pre-exercise values, recovery is complete.

LACTACID AND ALACTACID O_2 DEBT AND NEW CONCEPTS

Under overload conditions (work loads greater than aerobic capacity) it had been established in the older literature that for every liter of O_2 debt, the lactic acid level increased by seven grams. However, the classic work of Margaria, Edwards, and Dill (24) had shown that for the first 2.5 liters of O_2 debt no increase in lactate could be demonstrated. On this basis, O_2 debt was thought to have two components: *lactacid* which was represented by proportional increases in blood lactate and *alactacid* for which no lactate increase was found. Furthermore, Margaria et al., also demonstrated a great difference in the repayment of these two components of the O_2 debt. The alactacid debt was repaid at a rate approximately thirty times faster than the lactacid debt. Thus the fast component (alactacid) was ascribed to replacement of O_2 and energy stores and the slow or lactacid component was thought to be used to remove lactate from the blood.

While the two components of O_2 debt with respect to rate of repayment are well verified, unfortunately the *lactacid-alactacid* explanation of the physiology involved has proved to be an oversimplification. It is now clear that many processes besides the elimination of lactate may be involved in the delayed return of O_2 uptake to the resting value after cessation of exercise (which we call O_2 debt):

1. During exercise, O_2 stores of the body are greatly reduced and part of the recovery O_2 is used to:
   a. restore muscle myoglobin to resting values
   b. restore venous oxyhemoglobin levels
   c. replenish O_2 dissolved in tissue fluids
2. The rise in body temperature resulting from vigorous exercise creates a demand for more O_2.
3. Neither heart rate nor cardiac output return immediately to resting values and thus excess O_2 is required for cardiac metabolism.

4. The same is true for pulmonary function.
5. The output of catecholamines is probably still above resting values and this augments O_2 consumption.
6. The high energy phosphate breakdown (see fig. 9.6) must be reversed at a considerable cost of O_2 consumption (22).

To further complicate the relationship of lactate level to O_2 debt as measured by excess recovery O_2, Rowell and co-workers have shown that even during moderate exercise as much as fifty percent of the lactate production may be removed by hepatic splanchnic tissues (27). Obviously, this precludes any neat seven gram lactate per liter O_2 debt relationship as had been suggested by earlier workers. Thus a lactate build up in the blood would be unlikely at any but the heaviest work loads as shown in figure 9.7.

TRAINING EFFECT ON ANAEROBIC METABOLISM AND O_2 DEBT

In football, baseball, basketball and probably in most of the athletic activities which find favor in our country, one of the important determinants of success is *anaerobic capacity,* the ability to get moving quickly

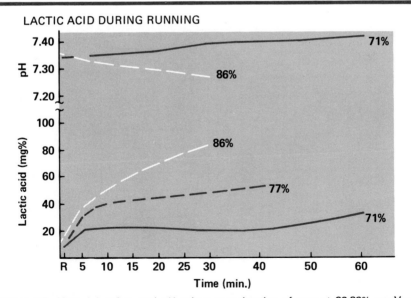

Figure 9-7. Mean LA values and pH values over duration of runs at 82-89% max$\dot{V}_{O_2}$, 74-79% max$\dot{V}_{O_2}$ and 67-74% max$\dot{V}_{O_2}$. (From Nagle, F. *Med. and Sci. Spt.* 2:185, 1970.)

for short distances. Relatively few sports events in the USA require a sustained effort longer than thirty to sixty seconds and consequently the vast majority of events depend upon anaerobic capacity which has been given very little attention by researchers in physiology of exercise.

Until recently, we did not even have a simple means for measurement of this important parameter. Fortunately, a simple and practical method has been developed by Margaria, Aghemo and Rovelli (25). The test consists of measuring the vertical component of the maximal speed with which an individual can run up an ordinary staircase. The test is fully described in the laboratory manual designed to accompany this text (13).

Figure 9.8 shows the very sizable improvements which occur in the ability to contract an O_2 debt as the result of training swimmers for 100 and 200 meter swimming events (16). Figure 9.9 shows the effects of swim training on the lactate concentration after maximum exercise. These results which show the trainability for anaerobic events have been supported by Cunningham and Faulkner (12) who also found an improvement in O_2 debt of nine percent and post exercise blood lactate of seventeen percent after training with interval sprints.

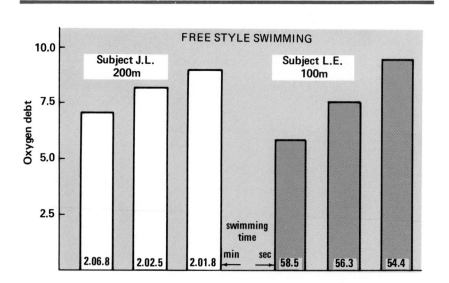

Figure 9-8. O_2 debt in relation to the actual time of performance. Note the increasing O_2 debts with improvement in performance (lower times). (From Hermansen, L. *Med. and Sci. Spt.* 1:37, 1969.)

INTERMITTENT WORK

At this point it is of interest to examine some recent work by Astrand and Christensen and their coworkers (5, 6, 8); it may bear on our discussion of O_2 debt, and it seems to have large implications for the planning of training regimens. In one experiment, for example, a well-trained subject was able to work for thirty minutes at a very high work load (4.4 liters of O_2 per minute) by alternating five seconds of work with five seconds of rest. This appeared to be something like a steady state in that very little lactic acid accumulated. Even for a highly trained athlete, a work load of that size done continuously would result in a large O_2 debt.

In another experiment a subject alternately ran ten seconds and rested five seconds, for a total of thirty minutes and 6.67 kilometers. His O_2 intake for the thirty-minute period averaged 5.0 liters per minute (his maximum capacity was 5.6 liters per minute). His actual O_2 uptake for the twenty minutes of running was 101 liters, and his uptake during the accumulated rest periods was 49 liters. Subtracting a resting O_2 con-

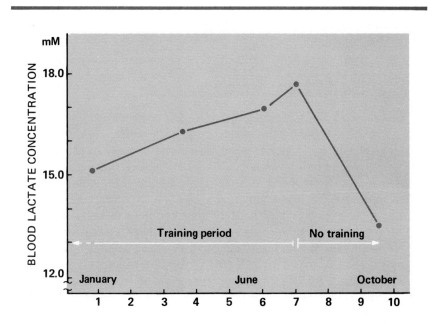

Figure 9-9. Blood lactate concentration (peak value) after maximal exercise (100 m swimming) during the training period and after two and a half months with no training. (From Hermansen, L. *Med. and Sci. Spt.* 1:37, 1969.)

sumption of 4.0 liters for the ten minutes of rest from the total forty-nine liters leaves a tremendous O_2 debt of forty-five liters, which had been eliminated in some fashion during the five-second rest periods. The largest O_2 debts ordinarily reported after continuous work run from fifteen to twenty liters of O_2. These experimenters suggest that O_2 is stored as oxymyohemoglobin in the muscles during the rest periods to support metabolism during the work periods without resort to the anaerobic mechanisms. This is an interesting possibility and provides a scientific basis for interval training of athletes.

MAXIMAL O₂ CONSUMPTION AS A MEASURE OF PHYSICAL FITNESS

The maximal O_2 consumption for any individual is a good criterion of how well various physiological functions can adapt to the increased metabolic needs of work or exercise. At least the following functions are involved and contribute to the magnitude of an athlete's ability to maintain a steady state:

1. Lung ventilation
2. Pulmonary diffusion
3. O_2 and CO_2 transport by the blood
4. Cardiac function
5. Vascular adaptation (vasodilatation of active and vasoconstriction of inactive tissues)
6. Physical condition of the involved muscles

The method for measuring maximal O_2 consumption (aerobic capacity) involves working the subject at ever-increasing work loads during each of which his steady level O_2 consumption is measured (usually by open circuit spirometry). When an increase in work load fails to elicit a significant increase in O_2 consumption the highest value attained represents the maximum O_2 consumption as shown in figure 9.10.

Any of the ergometric methods discussed earlier can be used. The test can be administered either on a continuous or discontinuous protocol. In the discontinuous method the subject is worked at each load until a steady O_2 level is attained (at least five minutes) with rest periods between work loads sufficient to allow recovery. Unfortunately, this method usually involves at least two or three visits to the laboratory and requires a great deal of technician and lab time in addition. Fortunately, the results obtained by the continuous method where the load is increased every minute or every two minutes are closely comparable to those obtained in the discontinuous method (2). This procedure can be consummated in one half hour visit to the laboratory. The error of the measure-

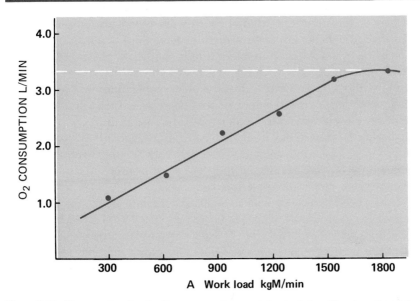

Figure 9-10. Diagram showing the O_2 consumption work load relationship when the subject was tested at repeated five-minute workbouts with rest intervals. The maximum O_2 consumption is indicated by the dash line at 3.30 L/min.

ment of aerobic capacity has been reported to be of the order of 2.5 percent (29).

Saltin and Astrand (28) tested ninety-five male and thirty-eight female members of the Swedish national teams and found the mean maximal O_2 uptake for the best fifteen males to be 5.75 L/min and the best ten females 3.6 L/min. The highest values found were 6.17 L/min and 4.07 L/min for the male and female, respectively. It is of interest that the highest values were achieved by the cross country ski team.

A clever experiment was designed by Klissouras (20) to determine to what extent aerobic capacity is determined genetically. He tested fifteen monozygous and ten dizygous twins and found that in these young boys aged seven through thirteen the variability in aerobic capacity was determined ninety-three percent by genetic factors. In a subsequent experiment (21) in which comparisons were made of a trained versus untrained monozygous twin, the trained twin was found to be superior in aerobic capacity by thirty-seven percent; but the absolute value after training was still only in the average category leading to the conclusion that while training can bring about substantial improvement, the ceiling is set by genetic factors.

O_2 Pulse.   The measurement of maximal O_2 consumption requires on the part of the subject, a willingness to work to exhaustion plus a sufficiently conditioned musculature to fully load the O_2 transport systems. In sedentary middle aged or older adults neither of these conditions is apt to be satisfied. Furthermore, exhaustive physical tests are not completely without hazard for sedentary older populations where unrecognized heart disease may complicate matters. Under such conditions, considerable information can be derived from measuring O_2 pulse at a standardized submaximal level that can be attained by all members of the group to be tested. O_2 pulse is derived by simply dividing O_2 consumption by the heart rate at the time of measurement and thus has the dimension of O_2 transport per heart beat.

It has been shown that at any given work rate the subject with the greatest maximum work capacity (aerobic capacity) has the highest O_2 pulse and conversely the lowest work capacity is associated with the lowest O_2 pulse, etc. (30). O_2 pulse under exercise conditions is, of course, largely determined by stroke volume and A-V O_2 difference (26).

RESPIRATORY QUOTIENT

The relationship of CO_2 produced to the O_2 consumed—RQ, the *respiratory quotient*—is an important physiological concept because it provides information that tells which foodstuff is being used for energy supply, if the subject is resting or in a steady state of moderate exercise.

$$RQ = \frac{\text{Vol } CO_2 \text{ produced}}{\text{Vol } O_2 \text{ consumed}}$$

Thus, if carbohydrate is completely oxidized to CO_2 and H_2O, the relationship can be described as:

$$C_6H_{12}O_6 + 6O_2 \rightarrow 6CO_2 + 6H_2O$$

And it follows that $RQ = \dfrac{6 \ CO_2}{6 \ O_2} = 1.00$ if one volume of CO_2 is pro-

duced for each volume of O_2 consumed. If fat is used as a source of energy, however, the ratio is somewhat different. The fats and oils of our foods are largely mixtures of palmitin, stearin, and olein. These substances are of similar chemical compositions, and their oxidation can be simplified as follows.

$$2C_{51}H_{98}O_6 + 145O_2 \rightarrow 102CO_2 + 98H_2O$$

$$RQ = \frac{102}{145} = 0.70$$

Since the exact structure of the extremely large protein molecules has not yet been completely elucidated, the RQ for protein metabolism is estimated from known amino acid structures as approximately 0.80. However, protein plays a very small part in energy metabolism and, because its participation can be closely estimated from urine analysis, it is not important for the present discussion.

Consequently, if a subject is in a steady state, a reasonably valid deduction of the foodstuff being oxidized can be made on the basis of the observed value of the RQ. For example, if analysis of the respired gasses yielded an RQ of 1.00, the subject could be considered to be utilizing only carbohydrate for energy, and a value between 0.70 and 1.00 would indicate a mixture of fat and carbohydrate being burned. The exact amounts of each of the latter can be determined mathematically or from a suitable table (15, p. 659).

However, during exercise in which a steady state is not attained, RQ does not truly reflect the percentage of fat and carbohydrate utilized. If the work load is partially anaerobic, lactic acid accumulates, and this causes a temporary metabolic acidosis which is compensated by a respiratory alkalosis brought about by *blowing off* more CO_2 than is forming metabolically. This compensatory hyperventilation has been found to be closely related to excess lactate formed during anaerobic exercise (19). In heavy exercise, it is common to find RQs above 1.00 and as high as 1.30. On the other hand, during recovery the RQ is usually below .70, showing that lactate is being removed from the circulation, and is bringing about a temporary alkalosis that is compensated by hypoventilation in recovery.

Issekutz and Rodahl (19) have developed an interesting concept of *excess CO_2*, which is calculated: Excess CO_2 equals total CO_2 minus 0.75 times O_2. This calculation has the effect of telling us how much CO_2 was produced above that predicted from O_2 consumption for an average metabolic RQ of 0.75. In one male and one female subject they found a linear relationship between excess CO_2 and minute ventilation. The author has confirmed this with 29 subjects, and the correlation between these two measures was found to be high, $r = 0.836$ (see fig. 9.11)

It is the author's belief, in agreement with Issekutz and Rodahl that excess CO_2 (or excess RQ) is a very good measure of the percentile participation of the anaerobic processes in the total energy expenditure. Furthermore, because RQ is available in every open-circuit metabolic experiment, the tedious process of doing blood lactate analyses may be obviated, especially if the high correlation ($r = 0.92$) between lactate and excess CO_2 found by Issekutz and Rodahl is corroborated by other workers.

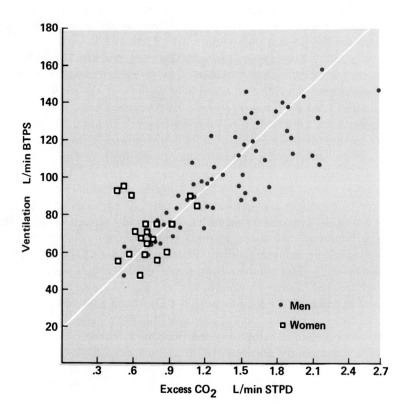

Figure 9-11. Relationship between ventilation (minute volume) and excess CO_2 production.

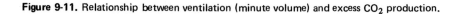

NEGATIVE WORK

So far, the main concern has been with work loads involving predominantly concentric contraction in which the muscle shortens to do work; this can be called *positive work.*

But effort is also involved in the muscular activity of resisting lengthening, as in eccentric contraction, and the physicist's definition of work can no longer be applied. It has become common usage to refer to the work done by eccentric contraction as *negative work*, and to compute it as if it were positive: $W = F \times D$. However, the work calculated in this fashion cannot be used interchangeably with the work of positive work; the energy involved per unit work is quite different.

This was ingeniously demonstrated by Abbott, Bigland, and Ritchie (1) who coupled two bicycle riders in opposition, one of whom pedaled concentrically while the other pedaled eccentrically. Although the forces developed exactly balanced each other, the O_2 consumption of the subject doing positive work was 3.7 times higher. Asmussen (3) confirmed this, and plotted negative and positive work loads versus O_2 consumption (fig. 9.12). Although negative work was linearly related to O_2

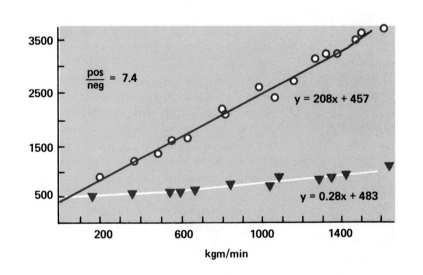

Figure 9-12. The oxygen consumption in ml./min. of a man bicycling "uphill" and "downhill" on a motor-driven treadmill plotted against the rate of work in kgm./min. (From Asmussen. "Experiments on Positive and Negative Work," in *Ergonomics Society Symposium on Fatigue,* 1953. Courtesy of H.K. Lewis, London.)

consumption, the ratio of the slope lines was 7.4 for their rate of pedaling. For varying rates of pedaling, the ratio of O_2 consumption for positive/negative work varied from three to nine, the ratio increasing with the speed of pedaling. Thus it would seem that positive work is from three to nine times more costly in terms of energy expenditure than negative work.

SUMMARY

1. Some of the terms needed for discussing work metabolism intelligently are as follows. (A) *work:* $W = F \times D$; (B) *power* (in hp): 1 hp = 33,000 ft-lbs/min; (C) *energy* (in kcal): 1 kcal = 3,087 ft-lbs; (D) *efficiency* (in ratio or percentage):

$$E = \frac{\text{Work output}}{\text{Energy input}}$$

2. Three methods are commonly used for setting up standard work loads: *bench-stepping, treadmill,* and *bicycle ergometer.*

3. The two methods for measuring energy expenditures are *direct* and *indirect calorimetry;* the latter uses either the *closed-circuit* or the *open-circuit* method.

4. Muscular work can be performed *aerobically,* if the energy source (glycogen) is completely oxidized to CO_2 and H_2O, or *anaerobically,* if the biochemical breakdown of glycogen ends at the lactic acid stage.

5. When exercise begins, there is a lag in the response of the O_2 transport systems. The amount by which the O_2 supply lacks being adequate until the O_2 transport catches up with the demand is called O_2 *deficit.*

6. O_2 *debt* is defined as the amount of O_2 taken up in excess of the resting value during the recovery period. This constitutes the repayment of the O_2 deficit plus any anaerobic metabolism which may have occurred.

7. Anaerobic capacity is a very important determinant of success in many American athletics. Improvement in this parameter can be brought about by appropriate training directed to short, sprint-type activity.

8. When equal loads of continuous and intermittent work are compared, much lower O_2 debts seem to result from intermittent work. Storage of O_2 as oxymyohemoglobin has been postulated to explain this phenomenon.

9. If physical fitness is defined as physical working capacity, the best single measure of this factor is maximal O_2 consumption.

10. Under resting and steady-state exercise conditions, the *respiratory quotient* (RQ) accurately reflects the foodstuff being utilized.

11. During exercise that cannot be performed aerobically, RQ seems to reflect the percentual participation of aerobic processes.

12. Work in which muscular contraction is eccentric is called *negative work.* Depending upon the rate, negative work can be performed from three to nine times more economically than *positive work.*

REFERENCES

1. Abbott, B. C.; Bigland, B.; and Ritchie, J. M. 1952. Physiological cost of negative work. *Journal of Physiology* 117:380-90.
2. Andersen, K. L.; Shephard, R. J.; Denolin, H.; Varnauskas, E.; and Masironi, R. 1971. *Fundamentals of exercise testing*. Geneva: World Health Organization.
3. Asmussen, E. 1953. Experiments on positive and negative work. In *Ergonomics society symposium on fatigue, eds*. W. F. Floyd and A. T. Welford. London: Lewis & Co.
4. Astrand, I. 1960. Aerobic work capacity in men and women with special reference to age. *Acta Physiologica Scandinavica* 49 (suppl. 169).
5. Astrand, I., Astrand, P. O.; Christensen, E. H.; and Hedman, R. 1960a. Intermittent muscular work. *Acta Physiological Scandinavica* 48:448-53.
6. Astrand, I.; Astrand, P. O.; Christensen, E. H.; and Hedman, R. 1960b. Myohemoglobin as an oxygen-store in man. *Acta Physiologica Scandinavica* 48:454-60.
7. Bannister, E. W., and Jackson, R. C. 1968. The effect of speed and load changes on oxygen intake for equivalent power outputs during bicycle ergometry. *Int. Z. Angew. Physiologie* 24:284-90.
8. Christensen, E. H.; Hedman, R.; and Saltin, B. 1960. Intermittent and continuous running. *Acta Physiologica Scandinavica* 50:269-86.
9. Cissik, J. H.; Johnson, R. E.; and Rokosch, D. K. 1972. Production of gaseous nitrogen in human steady-state conditions. *Journal of Applied Physiology* 32:155-59.
10. Consolazio, C. F.; Johnson, R. E.; and Pecora, L. J. 1963. *Physiological measurements of metabolic functions in man*. New York: McGraw-Hill Book Co.
11. Costa, G. 1960. Hypothetical pathways of nitrogen metabolism. *Nature* 188:549-52.
12. Cunningham, D. A., and Faulkner, J. A. 1969. The effect of training on aerobic and anaerobic metabolism during a short exhaustive run. *Medicine and Science in Sports* 1:65-69.
13. deVries, H. A. 1971. Laboratory experiments in physiology of exercise. Dubuque, Ia. Wm. C. Brown Company Publishers.
14. Fox, E. L., and Bowers, R. W. 1973. Steady state equality of respiratory gaseous N_2 in resting man. *Journal of Applied Physiology* 35:143-44.
15. Hawk, P. B.; Oser, B. L.; and Summerson, W. H. 1947. *Practical-physiological chemistry*. Philadelphia: The Blakiston Company.
16. Hermansen, L. 1969. Anaerobic energy release. *Medicine and Science in Sports* 1:32-38.
17. Hermansen, L., and Saltin, B. 1969. Oxygen uptake during maximal treadmill and bicycle exercise. *Journal of Applied Physiology* 26:31-37.
18. Hess, P., and Seusing, J. 1963. Der Einfluss der Tretfrequenz und des Pedaldruckes auf die Sauerstoff aufnahme die Untersuchungen am Ergometer. *Int. Z. Angew Physiol.* 19:468-75.

19. Issekutz, B. Jr., and Rodahl, K. 1961. Respiratory quotient during exercise. *Journal of Applied Physiology* 16:606-10.
20. Klissouras, V. 1971. Heritability of adaptive variation. *Journal of Applied Physiology* 31:338-44.
21. ———. 1972. Genetic limit of functional adaptability. *Int. Z. Angew Physiol.* 30:85-94.
22. Knuttgen, H. G., and Saltin, B. 1972. Muscle metabolites and oxygen uptake in short term submaximal exercise in man. *Journal of Applied Physiology* 32:690-94.
23. Luft, U. C.; Myhre, L. G.; Coester, W. K.; and Loeppky, J. A. 1973. Reevaluation of the open circuit method for measuring metabolic rate with regard to the alleged metabolic production of gaseous nitrogen. *Specialized Physiological Studies in Support of Manned Space Flight.* Report to NASA Manned Spacecraft Center, Houston, Texas.
24. Margaria, R.; Edwards, H. T.; and Dill, D. B. 1933. The possible mechanisms of contracting and paying the O_2 debt and the role of lactic acid in muscular contraction. *American Journal of Physiology* 106:689-715.
25. Margaria, R.; Aghemo, P.; and Rovelli, E. 1966. Measurement of muscular power (anaerobic) in man. *Journal of Applied Physiology* 21:1662-64.
26. Musshoff, K.; Reindell, H.; Stein, H.; and Konig, K. 1959. Die Sauerstoff aufnahme pro Herzschlag (O_2 puls) als Funktion des Schlagvolumens, der Arterio-venosen Differenz Des Minuten volumens und Herzvolumens. *Zeitschrift fur Kreislaufforschung* 48:255-77.
27. Rowell, L. B.; Kraning, K. K.; Evans, T. O.; Kennedy, J. W.; Blackmon, J. R.; and Kusumi, F. 1966. Splanchnic removal of lactate and pyruvate during prolonged exercise in man. *Journal of Applied Physiology* 21:1773-83.
28. Saltin, B., and Astrand, P. O. 1967. Maximal oxygen uptake in athletes. *Journal of Applied Physiology* 23:353-58.
29. Taylor, H. L.; Buskirk, E.; and Henschel, A. 1955. Maximal oxygen intake as an objective measure of cardiorespiratory performance. *Journal of Applied Physiology* 8:73-80.
30. Wasserman, K.; Van Kessel, A. L.; and Burton, G. G. 1967. Interaction of Physiological mechanisms during exercise. *Journal of Applied Physiology* 22:71-85.
31. Wilmore, J. H., and Costill, D. L. 1973. Adequacy of the Haldane transformation in the computation of exercise VO_2 in man. *Journal of Applied Physiology* 35:85-89.
32. World Health Organization. 1968. Exercise tests in relation to cardiovascular function. WHO Tech. Report Series no. 388. Geneva, Switzerland.

10 The Endocrine System and Exercise

There are essentially two systems for coordinating the physiological functions of the human organism: the *nervous system* provides the mechanism for bringing about quick homeostatic responses, and the *endocrine system* may be thought of as functioning in the long-term picture of metabolic control. There is also a high degree of interrelationship between the functions of the two systems for each affects the function of the other. It is obvious that the endocrine secretion affects the nervous system through vascular channels that bathe nerve tissue. The effects of the nervous system upon the endocrines seem to be brought about by hypothalamic effects upon the master gland, the *pituitary*, but the exact method of control is not yet completely understood.

The endocrine system of ductless glands includes the pituitary, adrenals, thyroid, parathyroid, sex glands, and the pancreas. All of these glands have very important physiological functions, but only the first three apply directly enough to the physiology of exercise to be considered in this text.

THE SELYE THEORY OF STRESS

It has long been known that stressful situations call forth various physiological responses; however, Hans Selye, a Canadian endocrinologist, was the first to observe and report the fact that regardless of the form the stressor might take the response was always the same: a *stress syndrome* (concurrent symptoms that characterize a disease) consisting of: (1) adrenal enlargement, (2) thymus and lymphatic involution (shrinkage), and (3) bleeding ulcers of the digestive tract. This same stress syndrome was found to result from such diverse stressors as illness, traumatic injury, heavy exercise, or emotional upset.

Furthermore, this triad of symptoms, which Selye (18) called the *general adaptation syndrome*, seems to go through three stages in time: (1) the alarm reaction, (2) the stage of resistance, and (3) the stage of exhaustion. Thus the alarm reaction (AR) elicits the typical triad of symptoms, but if the stressor is of long duration, the organism enters the stage of resistance (SR), during which the stress syndrome or GAS seems to disappear, but the resistance of the organism to stress is greater. Finally, after the acquired adaptation is lost, the stage of exhaustion (SE) is entered, the original stress syndrome reappears, and death eventually ensues from the exhaustion of *adaptational energy*.

Selye defined stress as the "state manifested by a specific syndrome which consists of all the nonspecifically induced changes within a biologic system," or, more simply, as the "rate of wear and tear in the body." The reaction of the organism to stressors, regardless of type, therefore involves the same stress syndrome in which the pituitary gland is alerted by the hypothalamus. The pituitary secretes the adrenocorticotrophic hormone (ACTH), which stimulates the adrenal cortex to secrete its glucocorticoids (mainly cortisone and cortisol), which produce the syndrome described above in which the lymphatic tissues shrink (glucocorticoids are anti-inflammatory) and ulceration occurs in the digestive tract.

Concomitantly, the alarm reaction can be brought about by the coordinating efforts of the nervous system. This system also seems to act by secreting hormones, but it acts more directly on the tissues, e.g., at the nerve endings. The nerve endings of the sympathetic nervous system are of two types: *adrenergic,* so called because their stimulation is thought to release the catecholamines, adrenalin and noradrenalin, and *cholinergic,* whose stimulation seems to bring about release of acetylcholine.

IMPLICATIONS OF THE SELYE THEORY FOR HEALTH AND PHYSICAL EDUCATION

The cortex (outer rind) of the adrenal glands secretes many hormones, and each of the hormones may have several effects; however, our discussion will be confined to two classes of corticoids (hormones from the adrenal cortex): *pro-inflammatory corticoids* (PC) and *anti-inflammatory corticoids* (AC). In general, the PC corticoids of Selye belong to the group of hormones referred to by physiologists as *mineralocorticoids* because they affect mineral metabolism-causing sodium retention and potassium excretion. The most important of this group are aldosterone and desoxycorticosterone. The anti-inflammatory corticoids belong to the group physiologists call *glucocorticoids* because they can increase blood sugar levels. The most important of these are cortisone and cortisol.

In many diseases the processes of inflammation may be essential to wall off infectious agents that are invading the tissues, preventing their spread throughout the entire organism. On the other hand, it is Selye's contention that some diseases are simply an overreaction of the organism to a stressor that is not serious enough to merit a strong reaction of PC corticoids. In these cases, the disease is merely a manifestation of overactivity of the PC corticoids, and it can be relieved or ameliorated by AC corticoids, such as cortisone. Some of the diseases in which maladaptation of the adrenal cortex is thought to play a part are high blood pressure, various heart diseases, rheumatoid arthritis, and allergic reactions.

One of the most important implications of Selye's work lies in his hypothesis that every individual inherits a certain amount of *adaptation energy* that cannot be appreciably changed. If we accept this hypothesis, and Selye's hypothesis that heavy muscular work constitutes a strong stressor, we should be forced to the conclusion that heavy exercise (athletics) might well shorten life, for when adaptation energy runs out the organism enters the stage of exhaustion, and death ensues.

Fortunately, however, the story is not that simple. As pointed out by Michael (11), the available evidence indicates that exercise produces a degree of protection against stress (the resistance stage of Selye?). The author has provided evidence for a tranquilizer effect of exercise which acts both acutely and chronically (4). Electromyographic experiments in the laboratory have shown that as little as 15 minutes of moderate exercise will reduce nervous tension for at least an hour afterward and physical conditioning over a period of time results in a chronically reduced tension level. Thus it might be postulated that although adaptation energy is used up faster during the workout, the rest of the day is under less stress and therefore we might expect a significant net gain in the "stress of life."

Indeed, Selye's concept of deviation appears entirely compatible with the author's viewpoint. Selye points out that humans seldom if ever die of old age; they die because of the weakness or uneven wear of one organ or system. For this reason, he emphasizes the importance of the stress quotient:

$$\frac{\text{Local stress in any one part}}{\text{Total stress in the body}}$$

He suggests that when stress is disproportionately great on one organ or system, deviation—changing the type of activity to better distribute the stress—may be beneficial.

Selye's GAS theory seems to provide a rational basis for answering many of the perplexing questions that have plagued medical science. It also poses many questions for investigation by exercise physiologists.

MEASUREMENT OF STRESS

An important outcome of Selye's work is the new insight into changes resulting from stress that can be measured objectively, indirectly allowing quantitative measurement of stress itself. Ideally, we would like to measure stress directly, by observing the changes in adrenal size and activity—the method used with animals, where the subjects of experimentation can be sacrificed. In human experiments this is not possible; so indirect measures have been devised.

The end product of metabolism of the adrenal corticoids is the kidneys' excretion into the urine of 17-ketosteroids. Thus the measurement of urinary 17-ketosteroids affords one method for evaluating stress. This method suffers from the fact that voiding of urine cannot be related in time to the actual formation of the corticoids with any precision. Also the 17-ketosteroids may reflect testicular function.

A simpler method that has achieved some popularity is based on the often observed fact that increased adrenal cortical function results in a decreased number of circulating eosinophils (eosinopenia). Eosinophils are leucocytes (white blood cells) that stain deeply with eosin dye, and they can therefore be easily identified under the microscope. Stressors of emotional and traumatic nature have been shown to reduce significantly the level of circulating eosinphils if repeated measurements are made and if the normal diurnal variation is taken into account (7, 13, 16, 17). On this basis a clinical test for the adequacy of adrenocortical reserve has been devised. It seems to be generally accepted that administration of 25 mg of ACTH should bring about a fall of at least fifty percent in circulating eosinophils if the adrenal cortical reserve is normal (8). Unfortunately, this test is also not specific for adrenal cortical function since the same response results from epinephrine secreted by the adrenal medulla.

EXERCISE AND STRESS

There is a growing body of evidence (3, 9, 21) which indicates that exercise alone unless carried to complete exhaustion does not produce a typical stress response. The psychological and emotional components of athletic activity appear to be much more important in producing a stress response than does the work load of exercise per se.

Hill et al. (9) showed the importance of psychological factors on adrenal cortical activation in a series of experiments with a college racing crew. Corticoid output on practice days, when physical exercise work load was comparable to race and time trial days was not increased over the control days on which there was no rowing. There was, however, evidence of significant adrenal cortical stimulation during the time trial and race days where emotional involvement occurred. Thus it is extremely important for the physical educator and coach to recognize the difference in stress level between a physical conditioning program (very little) and that of the competitive athletic situation where stress can be very high. This also points out the foolishness of evaluating health values of physical conditioning by comparing samples of competitive athletes against nonathletes.

That exercise can improve the response to stress in rats has been demonstrated by Bartlett (1). It had previously been shown that stress made laboratory animals *thermolabile* (more reactive to temperature change). The body temperature change in rats exposed to a low temperature (5° C.) was found to be significantly less if they had been conditioned by three to ten minutes of daily exercise for twelve days.

Even more important, Selye (19) has shown that animals can be made less vulnerable to experimental heart attacks brought on by sensitization (salt and hormone) and subsequent stress if they are conditioned by physical exercise. Furthermore, he feels that conditioning by the moderate stress of a reasonable program of physical exercise sets up a ". . . cross-resistance to various forms of pathogenic stress. By exercising intelligently a man can train his heart to resist attacks that might otherwise kill him. It doesn't matter if he has been training with calisthenics and is later attacked not by physical but emotional stress. . . . Cross-resistance will help his heart stand off the attack in any case."

In an experiment on college women, Ulrich (22) found that with varsity basketball players the stress level was lower after a game (eosinophil count) than it was when they had been prepared for a game that did not materialize. It would seem that the physiological effects of emotional stress can be worked off by vigorous physical activity.

FUNCTION OF THE ADRENAL CORTEX IN TRAINING AND CONDITIONING

Exercise has been shown to cause significant drops in the eosinophil count even when little emotional involvement occurs, as in an experimental gymnasium exercise program (24). It has also been shown that the emotional involvement alone can bring about this drop in eosinophil count (15). Thus the adrenal cortex increases its function in response to both the physical and the emotional components of exercise, and it seems reasonable to assume that the effects are additive. Experience would seem to bear out this conclusion in that a competitive athletic event seems to be more stressful if a large emotional component is present as in a league championship game compared with a scrimmage.

There seems to be unanimity in the literature that the *onset* of a heavy work program (or training program) elevates corticoid secretion; however, data for the effects of a *prolonged* training program have only recently been made available (2, 5, 14). In rats and hamsters there is a highly significant hypertrophy of the adrenals that seems to require three weeks to occur. The secretion of corticoids paralleled the adrenal hypertrophy for approximately three weeks, and then fell off toward pretraining levels, while the hypertrophy was maintained at the higher level. The hypertrophy of the adrenal was found to be almost entirely due to growth of the cortex; the medulla showed only a small increase in size. The return to normal level of adrenal cortical function is the result of adjustment to the exercise demands and not to exhaustion (2, 6).

It is important to recognize one very important difference between animal and human experiments with respect to adrenal cortical function. Humans can be exercised through their voluntary efforts, whereas animals such as rats and hamsters must ordinarily be coerced through tying weights to their tails in survival swimming or by administering electric shocks to motivate their treadmill running. Thus animal training and conditioning experiments are necessarily traumatic and the adrenal response may be in part due to the trauma. Steadman and Sharkey (20) have provided evidence on human subjects which corroborates the animal studies in that nonexhaustive exercise increased adrenal cortical activity only during a period of familiarization (two weeks) after which a return to normal was found.

Prokop (14) has shown (with hamsters) that a maximum training load of two-thirds maximum provides the best training stimulus for the adrenal gland. It is of interest that this is also the load that best develops muscular strength. Prokop also pointed out that this two-thirds maximum load must not be increased by *extracurricular additive stress*, or overtraining will result.

Prokop provides a very interesting analogy between the three phases of Selye's GAS and the phases involved in the athlete's training regime. Although no experimental evidence is provided for this concept, it corresponds to the facts observed by coaches and athletes during the training process.

PHASE OF G.A.S.	PHASE OF TRAINING REGIME
1. Alarm reaction	1. The phase of *adaptation* in which training is initiated and progresses toward peak performance (5-12 weeks)
2. Resistance	2. *Completed adaptation* or achievement of peak condition (3-6 weeks)
3. Exhaustion	3. *Readaptation* or the loss of peak condition (starts 8-16 weeks after beginning of training)

It would seem there are two types of athletes if we classify athletes by their endocrine function in the training regime: the *sympathicotonic*, who achieves his peak rapidly but can hold it for only relatively short periods, and the *vagotonic*, who achieves his peak more slowly but can hold it longer.

Overtraining and the resulting "staleness" can also be best explained in terms of adrenal function and the GAS of Selye. If when an athlete enters the readaptation phase of Prokop (SE of Selye), he is encouraged to work harder to maintain his peak—fighting the natural endocrine cycle, as it were—he will show signs of adrenal exhaustion, such as hypertension, increased nervous tension, and a less effective metabolism that results in impaired performance. The fact that Prokop has been able to treat staleness by administering corticoids lends further support to his analogy between the GAS and the training regime.

THE ADRENAL MEDULLA AND EXERCISE

The adrenal medulla may be thought of as a part of the sympathetic nervous system, functionally and anatomically, because its secretory cells embryologically arise from the same source as do the postganglionic neurons of the sympathetic system. The function invoked by secretion of the hormones of the adrenal medulla, the *catecholamines* (*adrenalin* and *noradrenalin*), is entirely similar to the function brought about by activity of the sympathetic nervous system. Both lead to the reactions characterized by Cannon as *fight or flight,* in which the organism is prepared for action by release of energy (calorigenic activity), rise in blood pressure, rise in blood sugar and heart rate, etc.

The work of Vendsalu (23) indicates that the plasma level of noradrenalin is greatly increased during exercise while that of adrenalin is only slightly augmented. He also furnished data showing that this increase is not due to increased secretion by the adrenal medulla, and must consequently be attributed to increased output by the nerve endings of adrenergic fibers of the sympathetic nervous system during the exercise workouts. His work also indicates that the vasoconstriction required to maintain blood pressure in postural changes is largely due to the activity of noradrenalin.

Recent evidence shows that urinary catecholamine excretion (12) and plasma catecholamine levels (10) are increased approximately in proportion to the percentage of maximal work capacity which is being utilized in human subjects.

A summary of the available evidence indicates that, of the two medullary hormones, noradrenalin is the more important for vasoconstrictor activity and adrenalin seems to have greater activity in raising blood sugar and metabolic rates.

THE THYROID GLAND

The main function of the thyroid gland is the manufacture of its hormone, *thyroxine,* from iodine and an amino acid, *tyrosine.* This formation of thyroxine is stimulated by the thyrotrophic hormone from the anterior pituitary gland. Control of its formation is by a typical physiological servomechanism. Decreased levels of thyroxine in the blood circulating through the anterior pituitary gland increase the output of thyrotrophic hormone, which in turn increases the output of thyroxine by the thyroid gland. This servomechanism also works in reverse.

Thyroxine is carried in the blood in loose combination with the plasma protein. For this reason the function of the thyroid gland is usually measured by making the protein-bound iodine (PBI) radioactive and measuring the degree of radioactivity.

The most important effect of thyroxine is to increase cellular metabolism. Because this increase in cellular metabolism is general, and not restricted to any one type of tissue, it results in increases in the body's basal metabolic rate (BMR). In fact, BMR was used to evaluate thyroid function before the more accurate PBI test was introduced. Thyroxine also increases the work of the heart and brings about increased blood pressure. The nervous system becomes hyperreactive with increased thyroxine and hyporeactive if its secretion rate is low.

Probably the most important facet of thyroid function for the physical educator is its effect upon weight gain or loss. A relative lack of thyroxine (hypothyroidism) can result in a forty percent decrease in BMR, and hyperthyroidism can raise the BMR to about double its normal value. Consequently, hypothyroidism usually leads to obesity, and hyperthyroidism to weight loss. It must be noted, however, that glandular malfunction is only rarely the cause of weight problems, and is, of course, diagnosed only by the physician.

SUMMARY

1. Two interrelated systems coordinate physiological functions: the *nervous system*, for quick coordinations, and the *endocrine system*, for slower, longer-lasting effects.
2. Selye's *theory of stress* postulates a specific syndrome of physiological effects of stress that are nonspecifically induced.
3. The *general adaptation syndrome* (GAS) of Selye proceeds through three stages: (1) the alarm reaction, (2) the stage of resistance, and (3) the stage of exhaustion.
4. Physical education and athletics can play an important part in lowering the stress quotient, defined as:

$$\frac{\text{Local stress in any one part}}{\text{Total stress in the body}}$$

5. Stress can be measured by evaluation of urinary 17-ketosteroids or by the decrease in circulating eosinophils.
6. There is evidence that physical exercise may reduce stress under certain conditions. Selye's work also seems to indicate that exercise may condition the individual better to withstand stress of all kinds.
7. Many of the phenomena observed in training and conditioning athletes can be explained in terms of Selye's GAS.
8. The hormones produced by the adrenal medulla—the *catecholamines, adrenalin* and *noradrenalin*—bring about physiological changes entirely similar to those brought about by activity of the sympathetic nervous system: (1) increased heart rate and stroke volume, (2) increased blood pressure, (3) increased blood sugar, and (4) increased release of energy.
9. Changes in thyroid activity can reduce BMR by as much as forty percent in hypothyroidism, and may increase it twofold in hyperthyroidism.

REFERENCES

1. Bartlett, R. G., Jr. 1956. Stress adaptation and inhibition of restraint-induced (emotional) hypothermia. *Journal of Applied Physiology* 8:661-63.
2. Buuck, R. J., and Tharp, G. D. 1971. Effect of chronic exercise on adrenocortical function and structure in the rat. *Journal of Applied Physiology* 31:880-83.
3. Connell, A. M.; Cooper, J.; and Redfearn, J. W. 1958. The contrasting effects of emotional tension and physical exercise on the excretion of 17-Ketogenic steroids and 17-Ketosteroids. *Acta Endocrinologica* 27:179-94.
4. deVries, H. A., and Adams, G. M. 1972. Electromyographic comparisons of single doses of exercise and meprobamate as to effects on muscular relaxation. *American Journal of Physical Medicine* 51:130-41.
5. Frenkl, R., and Csalay, L. 1962. Effect of regular muscular activity on adrenocortical function in rats. *Journal of Sports Medicine and Physical Fitness* 2:207-11.
6. ———. 1970. On the endocrine adaptation to regular muscular activity. *Journal of Sports Medicine and Physical Fitness* 10:151-56.
7. Gabrilove, J. L. 1950. The level of circulating eosinophils following trauma. *Journal of Clinical Endocrinology and Metabolism* 10:637-40.
8. Gofton, J. P.; Graham, B. F.; McGrath, S. D.; and Cleghorn, R. A. 1953. Evaluation of changes in eosinophil levels in studies of adrenocortical function and stress. *Journal of Aviation Medicine* 24:123-26.
9. Hill, S.; Goetz, F. C.; Fox, H. M.; Murawski, B. J.; Krakauer, L. J.; Reifenstein, R. W.; Gray, S. J.; Reddy, W. J.; Hedberg, S. E.; St. Marc, J. R.; and Thorn, G. W. 1956. Studies on adrenocortical and psychological response to stress in man. *AMA Archives of Internal Medicine* 97:269-98.

10. Kotchen, T. A.; Hartley, L. H.; Rice, T. W.; Mougey, E. H.; Jones, L. G.; and Mason, J. W. 1971. Renin, norepinephrine and epinephrine responses to graded exercise. *Journal of Applied Physiology* 31:178-84.

11. Michael, E. D., Jr. 1957. Stress adaptation through exercise. *Research Quarterly* 28:50-54.

12. Neal, C.; Smith, C.; Dubowski, K.; and Naughton, J. 1968. 3-Methoxy-4-Hydroxymandelic acid excretion during physical exercise. *Journal of Applied Physiology* 24:619-21.

13. Persky, H. 1953. Response to stress: evaluation of some biochemical indices. *Journal of Applied Physiology* 6:369-74.

14. Prokop, L. 1963. Adrenals and sport. *Journal of Sports Medicine and Physical Fitness* 3:115-21.

15. Renold, A. E.; Quigley, T. B.; Kenard, H. E.; and Thorn, G. W. 1951. Reaction of the adrenal cortex to physical and emotional stress in college oarsmen. *New England Journal of Medicine* 244:754-57.

16. Roche, M.; Thorn, G. W.; and Hills, A. G. 1950. The level of circulating eosinophils and their response to ACTH in surgery. *New England Journal of Medicine* 242:307-14.

17. Schoen, I.; Strauss, L.; and Bay, M. W. 1953. Evaluation of the eosinophil count in patients undergoing major surgery. *Surgery, Gynecology and Obstetrics* 96:403-8.

18. Selye, Hans. 1956. *The stress of life.* New York: McGraw-Hill Book Co.

19. ———. 16 October 1961. Unmasking of faces of stress. *Medical Tribune.*

20. Steadman, R. T., and Sharkey, B. J. 1969. Exercise as a stressor. *Journal of Sports Medicine and Physical Fitness* 9:230-35.

21. Suzuki, T.; Otsuka, K.; Matsui, H.; Ohukuzi, S.; Sakai, K.; and Harada, Y. 1967. Effects of muscular exercise on adrenal 17-Hydroxycorticosteroid secretion in the dog. *Endocrinology* 80:1148-51.

22. Ulrich, A. C. 1956. Measurement of stress evidenced by college women in situations involving competition. Doctoral dissertation, University of Southern California [Physical Education], 1956.

23. Vendsalu, A. 1960. Studies on adrenalin and noradrenalin in human plasma. *Acta Physiologica Scandinavica* 49, suppl. 173.

24. Wake, R. F.; Graham, B. F.; and McGrath, S. D. 1953. A study of the eosinophil response to exercise in man. *Journal of Aviation Medicine* 24:127-30.

Part Two

PHYSIOLOGY APPLIED
TO PHYSICAL EDUCATION

11 Physical Fitness

Hardly a day goes by without a newspaper reference to physical fitness or the lack of it. We hear frequently from the medical profession that obesity is our most common disease, that we suffer from a softness brought about by our highly mechanized lives, and that our complex civilization is producing ever-increasing levels of nervous and mental disease. On the other hand, sports writers have a field day after our Olympic successes enthusiastically rebutting allegations of *our* lack of physical fitness because our *athletes* demonstrated superb fitness.

Herein lies one of the greatest fallacies of American physical education. We do indeed develop outstanding athletes to represent us in international competition, but they are in no way typical of the population. It is unfortunate that the spectator sports—football, basketball and baseball—occupy such a prominent place in physical education, for there is little opportunity to pursue them in adult life. In fact, this emphasis is probably also responsible for the neglect of our less physically talented children; our culture encourages them to be spectators rather than participants.

Despite all the interest shown in physical fitness, by laymen and professionals alike, we are not yet prepared to offer a universally acceptable definition of the term, much less an operational definition. It must be realized that not all definitions can be couched in terms of absolutes; sometimes a definition must be arbitrary, and arrived at by consensus. Thus a nautical mile is based on an absolute measure, one minute of latitude; but the statute mile, which we use much more frequently, is an arbitrary 5,280 feet. It is necessary that we define physical fitness arbitrarily so that we may proceed with an operational definition, and with the most important work of all: improving physical fitness at all levels of our population.

The best possible definition of physical fitness encompasses the work that has been performed and accepted by the two professions most interested in this area: physical education and medicine. Thus physical educators have developed many fine test batteries, which include such test items as running, jumping, throwing, pull ups, push ups. These test batteries, which are categorized as tests of *motor fitness*, attempt to measure the following *elements* of physical fitness: (1) strength, (2) speed, (3) agility, (4) endurance, (5) power, (6) coordination, (7) balance, (8) flexibility, and (9) body control.

On the other hand, the concept of *physical working capacity* (PWC) has gained wide acceptance among physiologists, pediatricians, cardiologists, and other members of the medical profession. Physical working capacity may be defined as the maximum level of metabolism (work) of which an individual is capable. PWC is measured by objective and accurate means (maximal O_2 consumption), and simpler but valid methods are available for predicting PWC from the submaximal heart rate tests described below.

Much could be gained by wider usage of the PWC concept in the physical education profession. First, a unification of thought between physical education and medical professions would be most beneficial to both professions. Second, PWC testing would provide a motivating factor for students in physical activity classes who are not well enough endowed in the skill aspects to compete successfully in athletics with their peer groups.

That the PWC concept is not widely used in physical education is probably due to three factors:

1. Physical educators' inability to perform these analyses
2. Lack of facilities
3. Classes that are too large to permit sufficient attention to individual testing

We suggest that some of the tests described in this chapter (*e.g.*, the Astrand-Ryhming Nomogram) require only one inexpensive piece of equipment, the bicycle ergometer, and ought to be at least a part of every corrective physical education program. It is also to be hoped that eventually an enlightened public will demand a smaller size for physical education classes, at which time PWC testing should become an integral part of the general program.

An individual's PWC is ultimately dependent upon his capacity to supply oxygen to the working muscles. This in turn means that PWC probably evaluates, directly or indirectly, at least the following elements of physical fitness: (1) cardiovascular function, (2) respiratory function, (3) muscular efficiency, (4) strength, (5) muscular endurance, and (6) obesity. The last item, obesity, becomes a factor because the final score in maximal O_2 consumption is usually expressed in milliliters of O_2 per kilogram of body weight.

It is readily seen that PWC and motor fitness testing are needed in a well-rounded physical education curriculum. The relative importance of the elements tested by the two major components varies with the age group under consideration, and this factor will be considered in a later portion of this chapter.

MEASUREMENT OF PWC BY MAXIMUM O_2 CONSUMPTION

Work by human muscular effort can be produced by aerobic and anaerobic metabolic processes as discussed earlier. However, anaerobic processes, when fully loaded, can function only for approximately forty seconds. For this reason it is really *aerobic capacity* that we measure when we measure PWC, and it is sometimes referred to in these terms.

The best approach to the measurement of PWC is to have a subject perform successive work bouts of from three to six minute duration and of increasing intensity with adequate rest periods between successive bouts. During each work bout the O_2 consumption is measured and, when the O_2 consumption fails to rise with increased load, this *maximum O_2 consumption* value is a measure of the subject's aerobic capacity or PWC.

The work load can be provided by treadmill, bicycle ergometer, or even by bench-stepping. The O_2 consumption must be measured by the open-circuit system because most closed-circuit systems cannot handle maximum lung ventilations without seriously restricting the air flow to the subject; the open-circuit system is also considerably more accurate. For details on this testing, the reader is referred to other sources (5, 10).
in which the work loads are selected to produce heart rates of approxi-

It is obvious that this technique requires laboratory facilities, and, even more seriously, it is not usable for large groups or classes. For these reasons the author has validated simpler techniques that are applicable to physical education class work. These methods are discussed in the following section.

ESTIMATION OF PWC FROM HEART RATE AT SUBMAXIMAL LOADS

It has long been known that heart rate rises linearly with increasing work loads (within limits). Furthermore, the rate of rise in heart rate for the same increments of work has been used in several different methods for evaluating PWC. Figure 11.1 illustrates this principle for two middle-age men, one in good athletic condition, the other in the untrained condition.

PWC-170 Test. Sjostrand (26) and Wahlund (28) used this principle to evaluate physical working capacity. It was modifed by Adams (1) for use on elementary and junior high school boys and girls in order to compare the physical fitness of California and Swedish children. This test consists of two consecutive six-minute bicycle ergometer rides in which the work loads are selected to produce heart rates of approximately 140 and 170 per minute. The working capacity is calculated by plotting (on graph paper) the heart rate against the work load at the end of each trial. A straight line is drawn through the two points to intersect the line of 170 beats per minute. The estimated amount of work that corresponds to a heart rate of 170 is then recorded as the individual's PWC-170. The heart rate of 170 is used because this is generally accepted

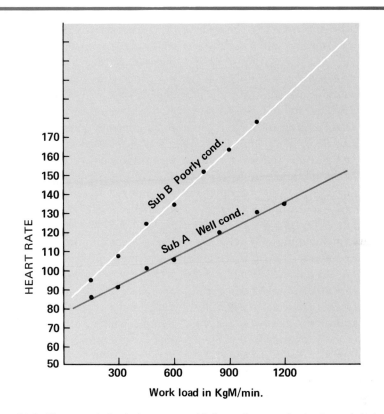

Figure 11-1. The rate of rise in heart rate with increasing exercise load as a function of physical condition.

as the level above which no significant increase in work load occurs. Use of this principle for the unconditioned subject in figure 11.1 would thus give an estimated PWC-170 of 975 kilogram-meters per minute.

This PWC-170 test has been found to correlate rather well with the measured maximal O_2 consumption of college men in the author's laboratory: $r = 0.88$. The standard error of prediction of maximal O_2 consumption from the PWC-170 test was found to be plus or minus 9.4 percent, which seems to be an entirely acceptable value for this type of test (10). The test eliminates all of the laboratory technique of maximal O_2 consumption tests, but is still unsuitable for use with large groups.

Astrand-Ryhming Nomogram. This test utilizes the same basic principle as the PWC-170. Astrand and Ryhming (4) found, when working at a load that required fifty percent of maximal O_2 consumption, that the heart rate for a group of healthy male subjects averaged 128 after six minutes of work. The corresponding heart rate for female subjects was 138. When their subjects worked with a heavier load, thus demanding an oxygen consumption of seventy percent of their aerobic capacity, the average heart rate was 154 for males and 164 for females. The standard deviation was eight or nine beats per minute.

Astrand and Ryhming used these data to develop a nomogram (fig. 11.2) for predicting maximal O_2 consumption from heart rate for one six-minute submaximal work load. They found that the accuracy of prediction varied with the level of the work load selected. On the bicycle ergometer at 900 kilogram-meters per minute, the standard error of prediction for men was plus or minus 10.4 percent, and at 1,200 kilogram-meters per minute it was plus or minus 6.7 percent. The author found a correlation of 0.74 between predicted maximal O_2 consumption by the Astrand-Ryhming method and maximal O_2 consumption as measured in his laboratory. These data yielded an error of prediction of plus or minus 9.3 percent, which agrees with their figures. Table 11.1 provides the nomogram data for young men in more easily used form.

This has proved a very usable method for small groups, and it requires about ten minutes per subject. Norms which are given in table 11.2 have been provided (3). The test can be performed with no equipment other than a stop watch (for taking heart rate) since the nomogram includes step-test data as well as data for bicycle ergometer use.

It should be pointed out that errors of prediction in this method are larger with unconditioned, sedentary groups than the reported errors, and also that ambient temperatures, which impose a heat stress upon the individual being tested, will obviously invalidate the procedure. For subjects over twenty-five years of age an age correction factor must be applied (27).

Harvard Step Test.   The two tests we have described utilize heart rate *during* exercise as a criterion of PWC. Exercise on a bicycle ergometer is best suited for this approach since the subject's upper body is relatively stationary. To eliminate the need for a bicycle ergometer tests have been devised that use bench-stepping and heart rate *after* exercise (during recovery). The principle is that the better the physical working capacity of the individual, the greater the proportion of the cardiac cost that is paid during exercise, the smaller the recovery cardiac cost (see chapter five), and the lower the rate during recovery.

The Harvard step test is probably the most widely used test, and it was devised for use with large groups. It is simple and easily administered; however, its error of prediction of maximal oxygen consumption

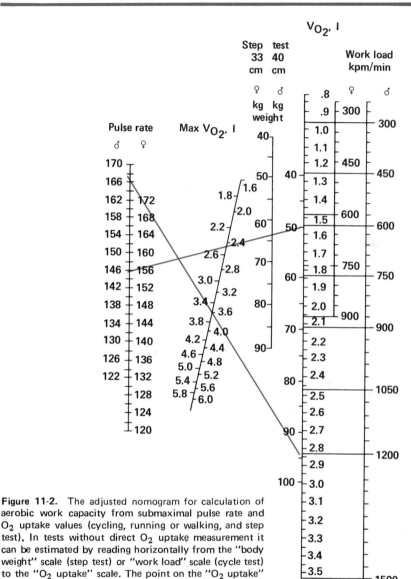

Figure 11-2. The adjusted nomogram for calculation of aerobic work capacity from submaximal pulse rate and O_2 uptake values (cycling, running or walking, and step test). In tests without direct O_2 uptake measurement it can be estimated by reading horizontally from the "body weight" scale (step test) or "work load" scale (cycle test) to the "O_2 uptake" scale. The point on the "O_2 uptake" scale (VO_2, 1) shall be connected with the corresponding point on the "pulse rate" scale and the predicted maximal O_2 uptake read on the middle scale. A female subject (61 kg) reaches a heart rate of 156 at step test; predicted maximum VO_2 = 2.41. A male subject reaches a heart rate of 166 at cycling test on a work load of 1,200 kpm./min.; predicted maximum VO_2 = 3.61 (exemplified by dotted lines). From I. Astrand. *Acta Physiologica Scandinavica,* 49 [suppl. 169] 1960.)

TABLE 11.1

Calculation of Maximum Oxygen Uptake from Pulse Rate and
Work Load on a Bicycle Ergometer

Working Pulse	Maximum Oxygen Uptake Liters/min					Working Pulse	Maximum Oxygen Uptake Liters/min				
	300 kpm/ min	600 kpm/ min	900 kpm/ min	1200 kpm/ min	1500 kpm/ min		300 kpm/ min	600 kpm/ min	900 kpm/ min	1200 kpm/ min	1500 kpm/ min
120	2.2	3.5	4.8			148		2.4	3.2	4.3	5.4
121	2.2	3.4	4.7			149		2.3	3.2	4.3	5.4
122	2.2	3.4	4.6			150		2.3	3.2	4.2	5.3
123	2.1	3.4	4.6			151		2.3	3.1	4.2	5.2
124	2.1	3.3	4.5	6.0		152		2.3	3.1	4.1	5.2
125	2.0	3.2	4.4	5.9		153		2.2	3.0	4.1	5.1
126	2.0	3.2	4.4	5.8		154		2.2	3.0	4.0	5.1
127	2.0	3.1	4.3	5.7		155		2.2	3.0	4.0	5.0
128	2.0	3.1	4.2	5.6		156		2.2	2.9	4.0	5.0
129	1.9	3.0	4.2	5.6		157		2.1	2.9	3.9	4.9
130	1.9	3.0	4.1	5.5		158		2.1	2.9	3.9	4.9
131	1.9	2.9	4.0	5.4		159		2.1	2.8	3.8	4.8
132	1.8	2.9	4.0	5.3		160		2.1	2.8	3.8	4.8
133	1.8	2.8	3.9	5.3		161		2.0	2.8	3.7	4.7
134	1.8	2.8	3.9	5.2		162		2.0	2.8	3.7	4.6
135	1.7	2.8	3.8	5.1		163		2.0	2.8	3.7	4.6
136	1.7	2.7	3.8	5.0		164		2.0	2.7	3.6	4.5
137	1.7	2.7	3.7	5.0		165		2.0	2.7	3.6	4.5
138	1.6	2.7	3.7	4.9		166		1.9	2.7	3.6	4.5
139	1.6	2.6	3.6	4.8		167		1.9	2.6	3.5	4.4
140	1.6	2.6	3.6	4.8	6.0	168		1.9	2.6	3.5	4.4
141		2.6	3.5	4.7	5.9	169		1.9	2.6	3.5	4.3
142		2.5	3.5	4.6	5.8	170		1.8	2.6	3.4	4.3
143		2.5	3.4	4.6	5.7						
144		2.5	3.4	4.5	5.7						
145		2.4	3.4	4.5	5.6						
146		2.4	3.3	4.4	5.6						
147		2.4	3.3	4.4	5.5						

Modified from I. Astrand's *Acta Physiologica Scandinavica* 49 (suppl. 169) 1960
by P.-O. Astrand in *Work Test with the Bicycle Ergometer*. Varberg, Sweden: Monark,
1965.

in the author's laboratory was plus or minus 12.5 percent. The test requires only a stepping bench or benches (twenty inches high and eighteen
inches deep) adequate for the number of subjects (who are to step
simultaneously), a stop watch for each observer, and a metronome.

TABLE 11.2

Norms for Maximum O_2 Consumption (Aerobic Working Capacity)

Women					
Age	Low	Fair	Average	Good	High
20-29	1.69	1.70-1.99	2.00-2.49	2.50-2.79	2.80+
	28	29-34	35-43	44-48	49+
30-39	1.59	1.60-1.89	1.90-2.39	2.40-2.69	2.70+
	27	28-33	34-41	42-47	48+
40-49	1.49	1.50-1.79	1.80-2.29	2.30-2.59	2.60+
	25	26-31	32-40	41-45	46+
50-65	1.29	1.30-1.59	1.60-2.09	2.10-2.39	2.40+
	21	22-28	29-36	37-41	42+
Men					
Age	Low	Fair	Average	Good	High
20-29	2.79	2.80-3.09	3.10-3.69	3.70-3.99	4.00+
	38	39-43	44-51	52-56	57+
30-39	2.49	2.50-2.79	2.80-3.39	3.40-3.69	3.70+
	34	35-39	40-47	48-51	52+
40-49	2.19	2.20-2.49	2.50-3.09	3.10-3.39	3.40+
	30	31-35	36-43	44-47	48+
50-59	1.89	1.90-2.19	2.20-2.79	2.80-3.09	3.10+
	25	26-31	32-39	40-43	44+
60-69	1.59	1.60-1.89	1.90-2.49	2.50-2.79	2.80+
	21	22-26	27-35	36-39	40+

Lower figure = ml of O_2/kg. body weight.
From I. Astrand, *Acta Physiologica Scandinavica*, 49 (suppl. 169), 1960.

Subjects are lined up in front of the stepping bench (thirty inches of width are allowed for each), and there is one observer for each subject. The person in charge counts cadence to a metronome set at 120 counts per minute: up—two—three—four, etc. On *up*, the subject places one foot on the bench; on *two*, he brings the other foot up and *straightens his back and legs;* on *three*, he steps down with the foot that was placed on the bench first; and on *four*, he returns to the starting position. Thus he completes one step every two seconds, or thirty steps per minute. The subject leads off with the same foot each time, although one or two changes may be made in the course of the five-minute stepping period.

If the subject falls behind the cadence because of exhaustion, he is stopped twenty seconds after falling behind the pace. When the subject stops (either at completion at five minutes or due to exhaustion) he sits down quietly, and the observer restarts the stopwatch, having recorded the duration of the stepping. The observer then takes the pulse rate at the carotid artery in the neck from sixty to ninety seconds after exercise. On the basis of the duration and the recovery pulse rate, the score (in arbitrary units) is taken from table 11.3. Interpretation of the score is as follows: below 50, poor; 50 to 80, average; above 80, good.

Progressive Pulse Rate Test.   A test devised by Cureton (7) has been used in the author's laboratory for several years. In this test the stepping bench is seventeen inches high and the stepping is done as in the Harvard step test except that there are five one-minute bouts with increasing rates: 12, 18, 24, 30, and 36 steps per minute. After each one-minute stepping bout (and within ten seconds), the recovery heart rate is taken for two minutes. The subject then rests, until his pulse stabilizes within eight to twelve beats of his standing, normal rate, before he starts the next-higher load. The pulse rates are plotted on a chart as in table 11.4.

This test was found to correlate with measured maximal O_2 consumption, $r = 0.71$, and the standard error of prediction was plus or minus 13.7 percent (10). It has several advantages over the Harvard Step Test:

1. It does not stress the subject as severely, and consequently it results in less muscular soreness.
2. It is more easily motivated because of its method of scoring.
3. Most important, it starts with low work loads, and the test can be terminated at any work load under which performance drops sharply.

Cureton (7) has furnished the norms for men aged twenty-six to sixty which are provided in table 11-4. The author has developed norms for college age men which are provided in the lab manual designed to accompany this and other textbooks in exercise physiology (12). The author has also developed norms for the older men and women (over sixty) in the course of his work in gerontology (13). Norms for boys and girls of elementary and secondary school age would be highly desirable since the test offers significant advantages.

Cooper 12-minute Run-Walk Test.   Cooper (6) developed a twelve-minute modification of the original Balke fifteen-minute run-walk field test which he validated on 115 young air force men (mean age equaled twenty-two). He found that his test results on the distance covered in twelve minutes correlated .897 with measured maximal O_2 consumption. To achieve good results with this test, motivation must be high; as Cooper

TABLE 11.3

Scoring for the Harvard Step Test

Duration of Effort (Minutes)	Total Heart Beats 1 to 1½ Minutes in Recovery											
	40-44	45-49	50-54	55-59	60-64	65-69	70-74	75-79	80-84	85-89	90-94	95-99
	Score (Arbitrary Units)											
0 - ½	6	6	5	5	4	4	4	4	3	3	3	3
½-1	19	17	16	14	13	12	11	11	10	9	9	8
1 -1½	32	29	26	24	22	20	19	18	17	16	15	14
1½-2	45	41	38	34	31	29	27	25	23	22	21	20
2 -2½	58	52	47	43	40	36	34	32	30	28	27	25
2½-3	71	64	58	53	48	45	42	39	37	34	33	31
3 -3½	84	75	68	62	57	53	49	46	43	41	39	37
3½-4	97	87	79	72	66	61	57	53	50	47	45	42
4 -4½	110	98	89	82	75	70	65	61	57	54	51	48
4½-5	123	110	100	91	84	77	72	68	63	60	57	54
5	129	116	105	96	88	82	76	71	67	63	60	56

From *Physiological Measurements of Metabolic Function in Man* by Conzolazio et al. Copyright © 1963. McGraw-Hill Book Company. Used by permission.

TABLE 11.4

Scoring the Progressive Pulse Rate Test · Adult Men (26-60 Years) · Rating Scale for Progressive Pulse Rates

Classification	Total 2 Min Pulse Count after 12 Steps/Min	Total 2 Min Pulse Count after 18 Steps/Min	Total 2 Min Pulse Count after 24 Steps/Min	Total 2 Min Pulse Count after 30 Steps/Min	Total 2 Min Pulse Count after 36 Steps/Min	Standard Score	Percentile
Excellent	71	77	84	98	105	100	99.9
	80	86	94	109	118	95	99.7
	89	95	104	119	130	90	99.2
	97	105	114	130	143	85	98.2
Very good	106	114	124	141	156	80	96.7
	115	123	134	152	168	75	93.3
	123	132	144	162	181	70	88.4
Above average	132	142	154	173	193	65	81.6
	141	151	164	184	209	60	72.6
	149	160	175	195	218	55	61.8
Average	158	169	185	206	231	50	50.0
	167	178	195	217	244	45	38.2
	175	188	205	227	256	40	27.4
Below average	184	197	215	238	269	35	18.4
	193	206	225	249	281	30	11.5
	201	216	235	260	294	25	6.7
Poor	210	225	245	271	306	20	3.6
	219	234	255	281	319	15	1.8
	227	243	265	292	332	10	.82
Very poor	236	252	276	303	344	5	.35
	245	262	286	314	357	0	.14
Mean	157.9	169.3	184.6	205.8	231.0		
Sigma	28.9	30.8	33.6	36.03	41.9		
Number	115	114	113	112	96		
Range	100-226	100-238	120-306	120-309	120-370		

From Cureton, T. K. "The Nature of Cardiovascular Condition in Normal Humans." Journal of Association of Physical and Mental Rehabilitation 12:41-49, 1958.

pointed out "this study indicates that in young, well motivated subjects, field testing can provide a good assessment of maximum O_2 consumption; but the accuracy of the estimate is related directly to the motivation of the subjects."

Doolittle and Bigbee (14) used the test on 153 ninth grade boys and found the validity to be equally good for them ($r = 0.90$) and the test-retest data correlated $r = 0.94$. They also found the twelve-minute run-walk to be a more valid test for this age group than a 600-yard run-walk test ($r = 0.62$).

Maksud and Coutts (19) found the test equally reproducible with boys aged eleven to fourteen but the validity correlation with maximum O_2 consumption was lower ($r = 0.65$).

MOTOR FITNESS TESTS

Many excellent tests of motor fitness have been devised. The elements of motor fitness are so many, however, and some are so difficult to define, that each motor performance test battery must be considered a compromise between the ideal of measuring all identifiable elements and the practical need to choose a number of representative elements, which allows measurement in reasonable amounts of time. Obviously, testing programs that intrude unnecessarily on instructional time cannot be tolerated.

For this reason, only examples of some of the best compromises will be offered here. For illustrative purposes, an example of the approach used by the armed forces during World War II, and one example of test batteries for school-age children, will be offered.

Army Air Force Physical Fitness Test. The items for this test were selected to evaluate the motor fitness elements of muscular strength and endurance, cardiorespiratory endurance, speed, coordination, and power. The test items selected were sit-ups, pull-ups, and a 300-yard shuttle run (five lengths of sixty yards each). It was the author's experience during World War II that several hundred men could be tested per hour by four experienced physical training instructors. This test is one of the best for handling very large groups of adult men.

AAHPER Youth Fitness Test Battery. After the much publicized results of the Kraus-Weber test (18) and other research findings pointed out the need for a national concern about fitness, a committee of members of the national research council of the AAHPER was set up, under the direction of Paul A. Hunsicker. As a result of this group's work on the Youth Fitness Project, the Youth Fitness test was developed, designed for boys and girls from the fifth through the twelfth grade. National norms are available for these age groups (and also for college men and women and young adults from eighteen to thirty (2). This test battery consists of the following items (all for grades five through twelve).

1. Pull-up, for boys; modified pull-up for girls
2. Sit-up for boys and girls
3. Shuttle run for boys and girls
4. Standing broad jump for boys and girls
5. Fifty-yard dash for boys and girls
6. Softball throw for distance for boys and girls
7. 600-yard run and walk for boys and girls
   Additional tests in aquatics are recommended where facilities permit.

Interestingly, Olree et al. (21) showed that three of the items correlated 0.925 with the results of the entire test. Thus a great saving in time can be effected by using only those three items: (1) pull-ups, (2) sit-ups, and (3) fifty-yard run, with only a small loss in intelligence of less than fifteen percent.

PHYSICAL FITNESS EVALUATION AS A FUNCTION OF AGE GROUPS

It is obvious that the various criteria of physical fitness do not have equal importance for all age groups, and several criteria that seem likely to be very important for middle-age and elderly age groups have not yet been mentioned. Because very little experimental work has been done to identify the most important elements of physical fitness for the older age groups, much of what follows is based upon the author's survey of medical and physical education opinion.

There seems little doubt that the motor fitness elements discussed above are important in elementary and secondary school age children. Physical working capacity is at least of equal importance for secondary school age groups, and possibly of somewhat lesser importance for those on the elementary level since the latter are active in vigorous physical activity by nature. It would, however, be difficult to justify many of the elements of motor fitness as necessary or essential for middle-age and elderly populations. For example, it is unlikely that a matron or a businessman needs high levels of speed, strength, or agility.

For the older age brackets a much better case can be made for the importance of (1) normality of body weight, (2) cardiovascular fitness, (3) respiratory fitness, (4) ability to achieve neuromuscular relaxation, and (5) flexibility. The value of the first four elements is probably self-evident; the last, flexibility, becomes more important as the aging process proceeds because connective tissues tend to lose their elasticity with age, and this in turn seems to be related to many of the aches and pains of old age. Considerable evidence exists that maintenance of range of motion exerts a beneficial effect in this regard. Table 11.5 lists the factors of greatest importance in physical fitness by age groups.

TABLE 11.5

Suggested Values of the Components of Physical Fitness
By Age Groups (In Order of Importance)

Prepuberty	Adolescence	Young Adult	Older Adult
Motor fitness	Motor fitness	PWC	PWC
PWC	PWC	Body weight	Body weight
	Body weight	Relaxation	Flexibility
		Flexibility	Relaxation

BASIC PRINCIPLES FOR IMPROVEMENT OF PHYSICAL FITNESS

Of the five major components of physical fitness (table 11.5), only motor fitness and physical working capacity will be discussed at this point (the other factors are considered in detail in later chapters). The details for improvement of the various elements involved may differ, but, in general, basic principles emerge that govern the overall process.

Overload Principle. Whether we are concerned with strength, muscular endurance, or circulorespiratory factors, improvement in function occurs only when the system involved is challenged. Improvement occurs when, and only when, the work load is greater than that to which an individual is accustomed.

Progression. A systematic approach, in which the work loads are increased gradually and according to plan, must be integrated with the application of the overload principle. If the starting work loads are not suitable to the status of the individual or the mean level of the group, undue fatigue or exhaustion results that may interfere with progress. The increments in work load should be planned so that even the top level of a group is challenged and so that the lowest levels are not discouraged. If the range of the group is too large to permit this, it should be broken down into two or more groups.

Sweat Is Not a Dirty Word in Physical Fitness. As with all human endeavor, we seldom get anything worthwhile for nothing; there is no physical-conditioning Santa Claus. Achievement of high levels of physical working capacity is accomplished only by endurance work sufficient in intensity and duration to challenge the circulorespiratory system. With normal ambient temperatures, these levels of intensity and duration are usually not achieved until sufficient heat from within the body is developed to bring about sweating.

The Fun Approach. Physical educators must be realists. Although physical conditioning may require work and sweat, there is no reason why the process should be unpleasant. It is the author's contention that the conditioning process is best brought about by *fun* methods, that very high levels of intensity and duration can be brought about through *play* activities. Physical fitness is more easily motivated in this fashion and more likely to continue as a lifelong habit.

Many recreational activities can bring about rapid improvement in PWC. In general, the best activities are those that include (1) vigorous running, (2) lifting of body weight, and (3) quick changes in direction. Some of the better activities, from the standpoint of circulorespiratory fitness, are tennis, badminton, handball, volleyball (if properly played), soccer, and rugby.

It should be pointed out that even the best activities may not produce much benefit unless they are *vigorously pursued.* For example, such excellent activities as tennis or badminton may be unproductive unless worthy opponents are selected. Furthermore, some activities which are not ordinarily vigorous enough to merit mention (such as swimming) can be excellent conditioners if the intensity and duration bring about the necessary rise in the metabolic rate.

Interval Training Approach. When the situation is such that the fun approach is difficult or impossible, or if an individual's tastes run to a more formalized or structured approach, a vigorous calisthenics or jogging program is the answer. In any kind of structured approach the interval training concept can be used to good advantage. It has been shown that great total work loads can be tolerated if they are broken up into bouts of short duration (chapter 9). Improvement in endurance factors is brought about not so much by increasing the total work as by decreasing the rest intervals.

For example, if no other form of activity were available, even stair climbing could be effectively utilized by applying the interval training approach. We might set ten trips as the beginning total work load, with twenty-second rest periods between trips. As improvement occurs, the rest period could be reduced to fifteen seconds, and so on. When the entire ten-trip work load can be accomplished without rest, the total can be increased to fifteen trips, with twenty-second rest interval reintroduced.

Time Required for Improvement in Physical Fitness. A frequent question in the current revival of interest in physical fitness is "How much can we really accomplish in two thirty-minute periods per week (or five fifteen-minute periods)? As an answer to this question, three classes in weight training and conditioning consisting of 67 male college students were tested at the beginning and end of a semester on three motor fitness test items: the standing broad jump, push-ups, and the 300-yard shuttle run. A subgroup of twenty-three was also tested on the Indiana Motor Fitness Index IV. The training procedure consisted of one thirty-minute period per week of weight training and one thirty-minute period per week of interval running. Highly significant improvements were found in all test items, and ninety-five percent of those tested on Index IV improved their fitness ratings with a mean gain of 23.4 standard score units (9). (This is not to say that two thirty-minute workouts per week provide optimum results; three to five workouts a week usually provide the best rate of improvement.)

SPECIFICS FOR CONDITIONING THE CARDIOVASCULAR AND RESPIRATORY SYSTEMS

Intensity. Frequent references are made to the work of Karvonen and coworkers (17) in which they showed that a subject must work to at least sixty percent of his heart rate range to get a training effect if the effort lasts thirty minutes a day for four to five days per week. This means that a man with a resting heart rate of seventy and a maximum of 190 (for a young man) who thus has a heart rate range of 120 beats must work at a minimum of

$$70 + (.60 \times 120) = 142 \text{ beats/min}$$

Although this work was done on only six subjects their conclusions have in general been supported by others (16, 24).

For older men (mean age, seventy), the author has found the intensity threshold for a training effect to be only forty percent of heart rate range. It is of interest that even vigorous walking of sufficient duration (forty minutes) can achieve threshold value and bring about significant training effects in middle aged (23) and old men (11).

Shephard (25) compared the importance of intensity, duration, and frequency and found that intensity was the main factor, but that training was also influenced by the frequency of exercise and marginally by its duration.

Duration of Workout. Optimal training effects probably require a training duration of at least twenty to thirty minutes. At the present time this estimate can be supported only on somewhat equivocal data (25, 29) and much expert opinion. Further research in this area is needed.

Frequency of Workouts. There is also little definitive evidence here. One well controlled study by Pollock, Cureton and Greninger (22) showed that training four times per week is superior to two times per week in improving working capacity, cardiovascular fitness and body composition. These findings are in general agreement with those of Shephard (25) who found five times per week superior to either three or one per week.

THE AEROBICS SYSTEM OF COOPER

Dr. K. H. Cooper developed a physical fitness program for U.S. Air Force personnel (8) which was subsequently offered to the public as a paperback book titled *Aerobics*. The need for such information is well defined by the sales—over two million— of the book. The popularity of Cooper's aerobics system is probably due to his recognition of the need for a *systematic* approach to personal physical fitness which the average sedentary middle-aged American would find feasible. The point system he developed is based on the rate of O_2 consumption demanded by various activities at various intensities thus the name *aerobics*. For example, running the mile under 6:30 requires about six times the O_2 consumption that walking a mile in twenty minutes does. Thus one point for the twenty-minute mile and six points for the six-minute mile, with proportional values assigned in between the two extremes. His work led him to believe that a minimum of thirty points per week were required to achieve and maintain desirable levels of fitness. One of the significant advantages in his system lies in the use of O_2 consumption as the common denominator because this allowed extrapolation of his data to many other types of physical activity such as cycling, swimming, handball, etc., so that an individual could earn his thirty points in any one of these activities or even by mixing them up (after the basic conditioning process).

There have been many criticisms of his system, some valid, most unjustified. The most valid criticism (20) is that the point system as established by Cooper does not in fact award equal points for equal energy expended, being somewhat low for some athletic activities such as soccer. Also it must be recognized that twenty minutes of effort is not four times as effective as five minutes nor are four sessions per week twice as effective as two as has been shown by Shephard (25).

In summary, however, we must recognize the very large contribution that Cooper's work has made to the acceptance of physical fitness concepts by the lay public.

POTENTIAL PHYSIOLOGICAL CHANGES RESULTING FROM TRAINING

It has been found in many well-controlled experiments that very significant physiological changes are brought about by conditioning previously sedentary subjects. One of the better experiments (15) showed for example that sixteen weeks of training (cross country running and interval training) three times a week produced the following benefits:

1. Fifty-two percent increase of total work output at exhaustion
2. Decrease in heart rate at a submaximal task from 170 to 144 beats per minute
3. Maximal O_2 uptake improved by 16.2 percent
4. Maximal cardiac output improved by almost two liters/min
5. Stroke volume increased by 13.4 percent
6. The A-V oxygen difference increased significantly
7. Lower blood lactate levels at a given submaximal load
8. Significant improvements in mechanical efficiency at the higher submaximal work loads.

Pursuit of Excellence. We do not begin life with an equal innate capacity for mental or physical achievement. Consequently, we cannot pursue excellence in physical fitness on an absolute scale; everyone should, however, strive for the highest level of physical fitness within the limitations of his physical potential. Then, and only then, can he begin to live a full life.

SUMMARY

1. Physical fitness can be conceptualized in two ways: (1) the *motor fitness* concept in which the elements of performance are measured and (2) the *physical working capacity* concept in which the capacity for O_2 transport is evaluated.
2. The following elements constitute motor fitness: (1) strength, (2) speed, (3) agility, (4) endurance, (5) power, (6) coordination, (7) balance, (8) flexibiilty, and (9) body control.
3. *Physical working capacity* (PWC) is determined by the following physiological components: (1) cardiovascular function, (2) respiratory function, (3) muscular efficiency, (4) strength, (5) muscular endurance, and (6) maintenance of proper body weight.
4. Evaluation of PWC is best accomplished by *measuring* maximum O_2 consumption. PWC can also be *estimated* from submaximal tests if errors of measurement ranging from ten to fifteen percent are acceptable as a trade off for the savings of time and effort by both subject and investigator.

5. The relative importance of the elements of physical fitness changes with increasing age. Motor fitness which is important to children is no longer of great importance to adults. For middle-aged and older adults the maintenance of (1) high levels of PWC, (2) appropriate body weight, (3) good flexibility, and (4) a relaxed musculature are much more important since these factors contribute to good health.

6. Improvement of physical fitness rests upon at least the following general principles: (1) the system to be conditioned must be overloaded, (2) systematic progression must be applied, (3) circulorespiratory fitness is only achieved by workouts where intensity and duration are sufficient to bring about a sweating response in normal climates, and (4) motivation can be significantly improved if *fun* type activities can be injected into the routines.

7. The best information at the present time suggests that successful conditioning depends upon: (1) achieving an *intensity* which requires at least sixty percent of the potential heart rate response, (2) a duration of at least twenty to thirty minutes workout, and (3) a minimum of three workouts per week.

8. The Cooper *Aerobics approach* is based on sound principles and offers the significant advantage of being based on the common denominator of oxygen consumption which allows formulation of the point system so that many different activities can be used in the conditioning process.

9. Physiological benefits derived from a conditioning program which improves physical fitness include at least the following: (1) large increases in physical working capacity, (2) significant gains in aerobic capacity (*maximum O_2 consumption*), (3) increased capacity for cardiac output brought about by increases in both strike volume and O_2 extraction, (4) submaximal work loads can be accomplished at lower heart rates and more efficiently (lower O_2 consumption).

REFERENCES

1. Adams, F. H.; Bengtsson, E.; Berven, H.; and Wegelius, C. 1961. The physical working capacity of normal school children. *Pediatrics* 28:243-57.
2. American Association for Health, Physical Educaton and Recreation. 1958. *Youth fitness test manual*. Washington, D. C.
3. Astrand, I. 1960. Aerobic work capacity in men and women with special reference to age. *Acta Physiologica Scandinavia* 49, suppl. 169.
4. Astrand, P. O., and Ryhming, I. 1954. A nomogram for calculation of aerobic capacity (physical fitness) from pulse rate during submaximal work. *Journal of Applied Physiology* 7:218-21.

5. Consolazio, C. F.; Johnson, R. E.; and Pecora, L. J. 1963. *Physiological measurements of metabolic functions in man.* New York: McGraw-Hill Book Co.

6. Cooper, K. H. 1968. A means of assessing maximal O₂ intake. *Journal of the American Medical Association* 203:201-04.

7. Cureton, T. K. 1958. The nature of cardiovascular condition in normal humans (part 3). *Journal of the Association for Physical and Mental Rehabilitation* 12:41-49.

8. Department of the Air Force. 15 March 1968. USAF physical fitness program. Air Force Pamphlet AFP 50-40 (Test).

9. de Vries, H. A., and Bartlett, K. T. 1962. Effects of a minimal time conditioning program upon selected motor fitness measures of college men. *Journal of the Association for Physical and Mental Rehabilitation* 16:99-102.

10. de Vries, H. A., and Klafs, C. E. 1965. Prediction of maximal O₂ intake from submaximal tests. *Journal of Sports Medicine and Physical Fitness* 5:207-14.

11. deVries, H. A. 1970. Physiological effects of an exercise training regimen upon men aged 52-88. *Journal of Gerontology* 25:325-36.

12. ———. 1971. Laboratory experiments in physiology of exercise. Dubuque, Ia.: Wm. C. Brown Co. Publishers.

13. ———. 1974. *Fitness after fifty.* Englewood Cliffs: Prentice-Hall.

14. Doolittle, T. L., and Bigbee, R. 1968. The twelve-minute run-walk: a test of cardiorespiratory fitness of adolescent boys. *Research Quarterly* 39:491-95.

15. Ekblom, B.; Astrand, P-O.; Saltin, B.; Stenberg, J.; and Wallstrom, B. 1968. Effect of training on circulatory response to exercise. *Journal of Applied Physiology* 24:518-28.

16. Faria, I. E. 1970. Cardiovascular response to exercise as influenced by training of various intensities. *Research Quarterly* 41:44-50.

17. Karvonen, M. J.; Kentala, E.; and Mustala, O. 1957. The effects of training on heart rate. *Annales Medicinae Experimentalis et Biologiae Fenniae* 35:307-15.

18. Kraus, H., and Hirschland, R. P. 1954. Minimum muscular fitnes in school children. *Research Quarterly* 25:178-88.

19. Maksud, M. G., and Coutts, K. D. 1971. Application of the Cooper twelve-minute run-walk test to young males. *Research Quarterly* 42:54-59.

20. Massie, J.; Rode, A.; Skrien, T.; and Shephard, R. J. 1970. A critical review of the aerobics points system. *Medicine and Science in Sports* 2:1-6.

21. Olree, H.; Stevens, C.; Nelson, T.; Agnerik, G.; and Clark, R. T. 1965. Evaluation of the AAHPER youth fitness test. *Journal of Sports Medicine* 5:67-71.

22. Pollock, M. L.; Cureton, T. K.; and Greninger, L. 1969. Effects of frequency of training on working capacity, cardiovascular function, and body composition of adult men. *Medicine and Science in Sports* 1:70-74.

23. Pollock, M. L.; Miller, H. S.; Janeway, R.; Linnerud, A. C.; Robertson, B.; and Valentino, R. 1971. Effects of walking on body composition and cardiovascular function of middle aged men. *Journal of Applied Physiology* 30: 126-30.

24. Sharkey, B. J., and Holleman, J. P. 1967. Cardiorespiratory adaptations to training at specified intensities. *Research Quarterly* 38:698-704.

25. Shephard, R. J. 1968. Intensity, duration and frequency of exercise as determinants of the response to a training regime. *Internationale Zeitschrift für Angewandte Physiologie Einschliesslich Arbeitphysiologie* 26:272-78.

26. Sjostrand, T. 1947. Changes in the respiratory organs of workmen at an ore smelting works. *Acta Medica Scandinavica* suppl. 196-687-99.

27. Von Dobeln, W.; Astrand, I.; and Bergstrom, A. 1967. An analysis of age and other factors related to maximal oxygen uptake. *Journal of Applied Physiology* 22:934-38.

28. Wahlund, H. 1948. Determination of the physical working capacity. *Acta Medica Scandinavica* suppl. 215.

29. Yeager, S. A., and Brynteson, P. 1970. Effects of varying training periods on the development of cardiovascular efficiency of college women. *Research Quarterly* 41:589-92.

12 Metabolism and Weight Control

It was pointed out in chapter eleven that weight control is a major component of physical fitness for adults; it is a less important factor in the physical fitness of children, but only because children are usually more active. We immediately recognize the desirability of normal weight in respect to appearance, and in physical performance obesity is a distinct disadvantage because a large proportion of the body weight, which does not contribute to performance, must nevertheless be moved at a definite cost in terms of energy. Thus an athlete who carries an excess twenty pounds of fat would compete on equal terms with athletes of normal weight only if they were forced to carry twenty-pound weights about their middle, and the rules of athletic participation have not yet provided such an equalizer for the fat man.

Most important of all, obesity has been shown to be associated with increased incidence of diabetes, gallstones, high blood pressure, and heart disease. Man has learned only very recently to produce food in super abundance, and only in the industrially advanced cultures; consequently, obesity as an endemic problem is also relatively new. As with most emerging health problems, passage of time is required before the facts can be sifted from the misinformation and the "old wives' tales." It is the purpose of this chapter to synthesize the experimentally established facts into a practical approach to the problem of weight control.

PHYSIOLOGY OF WEIGHT GAIN AND WEIGHT LOSS

First, we must recognize the fact that the human organism is a heat exchange engine, and, although "wondrously and fearfully" constructed, must obey all the physical laws that govern energy exchange. The net energy exchange that expresses the process of metabolism most simply can be written:

Caloric balance = Kilocalories from food − (Kilocalories of basal
metabolism + Kilocalories of work metabolism + Kilocalories
lost in excreta)

It can be seen that if the energy intake exceeds the energy outgo, an individual is in positive energy balance. Since the law of the conservation of energy tells us that energy can neither be gained nor lost but only changed in form, we must look for this energy to be deposited in the form of body fat, which is indeed what happens. One gram of fat produces (or can be considered equal to) approximately 9.3 kilocalories. Allowing for the water content and connective tissue in fat tissue, then one pound of fat will be deposited in the body when an excess of approximately 3,500 kilocalories has been consumed.

Conversely, if the energy spent is greater than the energy consumed, there is a negative caloric balance. For a negative balance of 3,500 kilocalories, a pound of fatty tissue would have been lost.

A most important point here is that the metabolism equation does not dictate the *rate* at which weight can be gained or lost. Obviously a pound of weight is lost if we go into a negative caloric balance of 3,500 kilocalories at a rate of 100 kilocalories per day for thirty-five days or 350 kilocalories for ten days. In the first case we lose one pound in thirty-five days, and in the second case one pound in ten days. Many people have been discouraged from using exercise to reduce weight because of misleading salesmanship which stated the need for thirty-six hours of walking or other ridiculously heavy work loads to lose one pound of weight. It is indeed undesirable, as well as impossible, to lose one pound per day in this fashion. However, by applying only a very low level of salesmanship and *sound physiology*, we might say that walking an extra half hour per day would result in a weight loss of five pounds per year; and it is the *long haul* that counts.

Metabolism of Carbohydrate, Fat, and Protein. It may be asked how it comes about that fatty tissue is deposited—in keeping with the energy balance equation—if a person eats a balanced diet that consists of all three basic foodstuffs, or even a pure carbohydrate or protein diet. The discussion in chapter two and figure 2.2 illustrate the fact that the three different foodstuffs have a common path in the final stages of their metabolic breakdown.

In the case of a negative caloric balance, as exists during dieting, it is easy to understand how stored fat may be utilized as a source of energy. In fact, the fatty tissues that are found beneath the skin between the muscles and padding the viscera are in a constant state of flux. Neutral fat from the blood constantly replenishes the fat stores of the various fat cells, which release them when they are needed for energy purposes.

When a positive energy balance exists, synthesis of fat tissue from the excess carbohydrate or protein occurs in the liver, from whence it is transported to the fat cells. Some synthesis of fat from glycerol and fatty acids also occurs in the fat tissue cells themselves. In this fashion, weight gain (of fatty tissues) occurs when the food intake (energy) is greater than the energy output.

Although the basic laws of energy balance are always applicable, evidence is accumulating that people vary in the methods by which they metabolize food (9), and because of this there are differences in the efficiency with which food is converted into energy. Differences in the efficiency of food utilization probably account for the fact that some people can "eat like a horse" and remain thin, while others "eat like a bird," but become obese.

WHAT IS NORMAL WEIGHT?

Overweight and *underweight* are widely used terms, and this use implies that we know what constitutes normal weight for a given individual. Ordinarily, normal weight is predicted from tables that have been developed by insurance actuaries and that provide minimum, average, and maximum weights for any given age, height, and sex. But does such a table really tell us what one's proper weight may be? We could answer this question in the affirmative only if the data from which the tables were calculated were taken from a population of people whose weights were normal, and obviously this situation does not exist.

By the use of such age-height-weight tables, gross errors are not uncommon in assessing normal weight. For example, a man six-foot tall, with a very light skeletal framework, might be thirty to forty pounds overweight at 200 pounds, whereas an extreme mesomorph (heavy skeleton and musculature) might be at his best weight for athletic competition at 200 pounds.

Furthermore, age-height-weight tables commonly allow small increments in body weight with increasing age, and this concept also has been challenged (4). Air force standards have been recommended that do not allow weight increases with age; these tables essentially retain the current recommended weight for ages twenty-six through thirty as applicable to all ages. This is a more logical approach to the prediction of normal weight because of evidence that during each decade after age twenty-five the body loses about three percent of its metabolically active cells. If this loss of tissue is replaced, it is probably replaced by fat tissue, so that even if an individual maintains constant weight as he grows older he probably carries an increasing proportion of fat tissue. Obviously, it is the proportion of fat tissue in the body's composition rather than the reading on a scale that is of paramount importance.

According to US Air Force standards, 115 percent of the standard weight is defined as overweight. For young males, *obesity* is frequently defined as the condition in which more than twenty percent of the body weight is composed of fat tissue.

When fifty-one male USAF personnel were compared by these two standards (24), it was found that fifteen who were not fifteen percent over the standard weight were nevertheless obese (more than twenty percent body fat). Furthermore, six cases who would have been considered overweight by the tables were found to have less than twenty percent body fat, and consequently were not really obese. Thus twenty-one of the fifty-one cases would have been incorrectly classified by use of the age-height-weight tables alone. This clearly illustrates the need for estimation of body composition, rather than a complete reliance upon tables of averages. It should be obvious that overweight due to a preponderance of bone and muscle does not have the same significance as overweight due to fatty tissue. Fortunately, methods have been devised for this discrimination.

METHODS FOR ESTIMATION OF BODY COMPOSITION

Underwater Weighing. It is common knowledge that fat people float better than thin people, and this is because fat tissue is less dense than other tissue (except lung tissue). Consequently, underwater weighing, which provides measures of body density and specific gravity, can also provide reasonably accurate estimates of the proportions of *lean body weight* and *body fat tissue* (12).

In this procedure the subject is completely submerged. Then, by Archimedes' principle, an individual's specific gravity is calculated:

$$\text{Specific gravity} = \frac{\text{Dry weight}}{\text{Loss of weight in water}}$$

This value must be corrected for residual lung volume, which is determined by a nitrogen wash-out of the lungs. With the corrected specific gravity, one may enter tables to arrive at the percent of body fat (5). The normal body fat percentage for young men has been estimated at from ten to fourteen percent by various investigators; the normal value for young women is slightly higher.

Measurement of Body Volume. Specific gravity of the human body can also be calculated if its volume is known.

$$\text{Specific gravity} = \frac{\text{Weight of body (dry)}}{\text{Weight of equivalent volume of water}}$$

This technique also involves complete submersion of the subject, with measurement of the water displacement by introduction of the subject's body into a small tank whose shape is such that small volume changes make large changes in water level. The tank is called a *volumeter*, and the measurement must be corrected for volume of residual air (1).

Hydrometric Method. This method depends upon the principle that the proportion of fat-free body weight that is water can be assumed to be constant, at approximately seventy-two percent; therefore, any of the chemical methods by which the dilution of a solute by the body water can be calculated can yield data on the total body water and, indirectly, the fat-free body weight. This is usually done by having a subject drink a measured amount of *heavy water*, deuterium oxide. Since this heavy water is handled by the human body in exactly the same way as regular water, the amount of deuterium oxide excreted in the urine can be used as the basis for calculation of total body water. The calculation for fat-free body weight is simply:

$$\text{Fat-free weight} = \frac{\text{Total body water}}{0.72}$$

The methods discussed thus far require considerable time and laboratory facilities. Simpler methods have been proposed that depend upon skinfold measures to estimate subcutaneous fat tissue or upon a combination of anthropometric measures to estimate the size of the bony framework. These methods are of a lower order of accuracy, but are nevertheless far better criteria of the degree of obesity or normality of body weight than age-height-weight tables.

Estimation of Body Fat from Skinfold Measures. Much of the early work in this area was done by Cureton (7). More recent work by Sloan, Burt, and Blythe (22) provides a very simple method for predicting body density from two skinfold measurements: over the iliac crest and on the back of the arm. They found that the error in body density measurements that was introduced into the determination of body fat by estimating body density from these two skinfold measurements is plus or minus three percent of body weight. The use of additional skinfold measurements did not increase the accuracy. They reported that percentages of body fat in three groups of college-age women ranged from twenty to twenty-five percent.

Estimation of Body Fat from Anthropometric Measures. Although Behnke and his collaborators have provided much of the basic conceptualization that underlies the relationship between anthropometric measures and body composition (2), the simplest method for estimation of fat-free body weight has been provided by Von Dobeln (23) for use on flying personnel, Swedish and American. He found relationships between height, bi-styloid radio-ulnar breadth (width of wrist), and femoral condylar breadth (width of knee), with measured density represented by:

$$FFW = 15.1 \ (L^2 \times R \times F \times 100)^{0.712}$$

(L = height in meters; R = sum of the right and left bi-styloid radio-ulnar breadths in meters; F = sum of right and left femoral condylar breadth in meters; and FFW = fat-free body weight in kilograms.)

Since these data are applicable to college-age men, table 12.1 is provided to simplify the estimation of FFW. The reported standard error of this method for young, healthy subjects is about plus or minus four percent, compared with less than two percent for direct measurements of density and nine percent when FFW is estimated from height alone.

GAINING WEIGHT

The purposeful gaining of weight is a problem for a relatively small segment of our population; however, some persons desire to pad a slender or frail frame for purposes of appearance, and sometimes to provide a greater mass for body-contact sports, such as football. It is obvious from the foregoing that this can be accomplished simply by ingesting more calories (in the form of food) than are spent in energy every day. For some individuals this constitutes a problem because their energy output may be prodigious due to a restless (nervous) temperament. Furthermore, this approach to the problem results in deposition of fat tissue that —beyond the normal values mentioned earlier—is not desirable.

The best method for gaining weight for any normal, healthy young individual consists of an exercise program designed to provide muscular hypertrophy with a minimum of energy expenditure. This type of exercise is best provided by professionally directed weight training, and almost invariably results in weight gains—of muscle tissue, not fat. This approach, if undertaken in moderation, is suitable for girls as well as boys.

Girls frequently express concern over the possibility of becoming muscular, but sex differences prevent this from happening in all but the most extreme exercise programs. Even in extremely heavy resistance exercise programs, there is little evidence to support the belief that girls may develop large muscles. It is more likely that excessively muscular girls are seen in association with heavy resistance sports because of a selective process: they choose to participate in sports in which they will excel.

REDUCING WEIGHT

Although the theory underlying weight reduction is beautifully simple, the practice for many millions of Americans is definitely not a simple process after obesity has set in. This is probably due to the interaction of psychological (emotional) and social problems with the basic physiology underlying the obesity.

From the standpoint of energy metabolism, obesity is necessarily the end result of a *positive energy balance*. Although this is a great over-

TABLE 12.1

Fat-free Body Weight (Kg) Determined from Anthropometric Measurements (Cm.)

Height	(Right + Left Femoral Condylar Breadth)					×	(Right + Left Bi-styloid Radio-ulnar Breadth)				
	170	180	190	200	210	220	230	240	250	260	270
160	43.0	44.8	46.6	48.3	50.0	51.7	53.4	55.0	56.6	58.2	59.8
1	43.4	45.2	47.0	48.7	50.5	52.2	53.8	55.5	57.1	58.7	60.3
2	43.8	45.6	47.4	49.2	50.9	52.6	54.3	56.0	57.6	59.3	60.9
3	44.2	46.0	47.8	49.6	51.4	53.1	54.8	56.5	58.1	59.8	61.4
4	44.6	46.4	48.2	50.0	51.8	53.5	55.3	57.0	58.7	60.3	62.0
5	45.0	46.8	48.7	50.5	52.2	54.0	55.8	57.5	59.2	60.8	62.5
6	45.3	47.2	49.1	50.9	52.7	54.5	56.2	58.0	59.7	61.4	63.0
7	45.7	47.6	49.5	51.3	53.2	54.9	56.7	58.5	60.2	61.9	63.6
8	46.1	48.0	49.9	51.8	53.6	55.4	57.2	59.0	60.7	62.4	64.1
9	46.5	48.4	50.3	52.2	54.1	55.9	57.7	59.5	61.2	62.9	64.7
170	46.9	48.9	50.8	52.7	54.5	56.4	58.2	60.0	61.7	63.5	65.2
1	47.3	49.3	51.2	53.1	55.0	56.8	58.7	60.5	62.2	64.0	65.8
2	47.7	49.7	51.6	53.5	55.4	57.3	59.1	61.0	62.8	64.5	66.3
3	48.1	50.1	52.1	54.0	55.9	57.8	59.6	61.5	63.3	65.1	66.9
4	48.5	50.5	52.5	54.4	56.4	58.3	60.1	62.0	63.8	65.6	67.4
5	48.9	50.9	52.9	54.9	56.8	58.7	60.6	62.5	64.3	66.2	68.0
6	49.3	51.3	53.3	55.3	57.3	59.2	61.1	63.0	64.9	66.7	68.5
7	49.7	51.7	53.8	55.8	57.7	59.7	61.6	63.5	65.4	67.2	69.1
8	50.1	52.2	54.2	56.2	58.2	60.2	62.1	64.0	65.9	67.8	69.6
9	50.5	52.6	54.6	56.7	58.7	60.7	62.6	64.5	66.4	68.3	70.2
180	50.9	53.0	55.1	57.1	59.1	61.1	63.1	65.0	67.0	68.9	70.7
1	51.3	53.4	55.5	57.6	59.6	61.6	63.6	65.6	67.5	69.4	71.3
2	51.7	53.8	56.0	58.0	60.1	62.1	64.1	66.1	68.0	70.0	71.9
3	52.1	54.3	56.4	58.5	60.6	62.6	64.6	66.6	68.6	70.5	72.4
4	52.5	54.7	56.8	58.9	61.0	63.1	65.1	67.1	69.1	71.1	73.0
5	52.9	55.1	57.2	59.3	61.5	63.6	65.6	67.6	69.6	71.6	73.5
6	53.3	55.5	57.7	59.9	62.0	64.1	66.1	68.2	70.2	72.2	74.1
7	53.7	56.0	58.1	60.3	62.4	64.5	66.6	68.7	70.7	72.7	74.7
8	54.1	56.4	58.6	60.8	62.9	65.0	67.1	69.2	71.2	73.3	75.3
9	54.5	56.8	59.0	61.2	63.4	65.5	67.6	69.7	71.8	73.8	75.8
190	55.0	57.2	59.5	61.7	63.9	66.0	68.2	70.3	72.3	74.4	76.4
1	55.4	57.7	59.9	62.2	64.4	66.5	68.7	70.8	72.9	74.9	77.0
2	55.8	58.1	60.3	62.6	64.8	67.0	69.2	71.3	73.4	75.5	77.5
3	56.2	58.5	60.8	63.1	65.3	67.5	69.7	71.8	74.0	76.0	78.1
4	56.6	59.0	61.2	63.6	65.8	68.0	70.2	72.4	74.5	76.6	78.7
5	57.0	59.4	61.7	64.0	66.3	68.5	70.7	72.9	75.0	77.2	79.3

From W. Von Dobeln, "Fat-free Body Weight of Swedish Air Force Pilots," *Aerospace Medicine* 32:67-69, 1961.

simplication, it will aid temporarily in understanding the problem. From this point of view, only three alternative methods are available for the reduction of weight:

1. Increased energy expenditure and constant food intake
2. Decreased food intake and constant energy expenditure
3. A combination of methods 1 and 2

The first method can be accomplished by exercise programs, the second by diet.

Since the easiest *cure* for obesity is prevention, let us consider the etiology of this health problem. A few years back it was fashionable to place the blame for obesity upon endocrine malfunction; this was a popular theory in that an obese person could absolve himself of blame. Medical research, however, has not substantiated this theory; on the contrary, evidence is accumulating that indicts our sedentary way of life as the real cuprit.

Greene (10), who studied 350 cases of obesity, found inactivity was associated with the onset of obesity in 67.5 percent of the cases, and that a history of increased food intake was found in only 3.2 percent. Pariskova (18), who analyzed the body composition of 1,460 individuals of all ages, concluded: "One of the most important factors influencing body composition is the intensity of physical activity, and this is true in youth, adulthood, and old age." In a study by Corbin and Pletcher, using 16 mm movie films to evaluate the activity level of elementary school children, it was shown that body fatness was significantly correlated ($r = -.520$) with lack of physical activity but not with caloric intake ($r = .155$) (6). Many other investigations, too numerous to cite, provide indirect support for the belief that lack of physical activity is the most common cause of obesity. Thus a clear-cut case can be made for the importance of habitual, lifelong, vigorous physical activity as a preventive measure against obesity.

That planned exercise such as jog-walk combinations is a feasible method for weight reduction in the obese even in the absence of any dietary restriction has been well demonstrated by Moody, Kollias, and Buskirk (16). Obese college age women lost on the average 5.3 pounds over an eight-week period in which they participated in about an hour of jogging-walking on the average of four times per week. Skinfold measurements suggested that the weight loss was the result of a much larger loss of fatty tissue with a concommitant gain of solid tissue (fat free weight). This latter observation is very important to note because the converse is true when weight is lost by fasting (3). Fasting has been shown to result in weight losses which are sixty-five percent due to losses of lean body tissue and only thirty-five percent due to loss of fat. This observation may explain the wrinkling and sagging tissues so often seen to accompany large weight losses by fasting or severe dietary restrictions.

Can we infer from the above that exercise is also the best means for treating the severely obese? Not necessarily. Although exercise can certainly make a contribution, medical supervision is necessary to protect the severely obese person from overstrain of the cardiovascular system, connective tissues, etc. For the moderately obese (ten to thirty percent above predicted normal weight), a combination of diet and exercise is probably the optimal procedure.

Misconceptions in Exercise and Weight Control. Despite the evidence that has been cited in favor of exercise as a means of weight control, it has in recent years been popular to ridicule this practice. Data are presented that illustrate the need for thirty-five miles of running, or thirty-six hours of walking—or some other ridiculous amount of physical activity—to lose one pound of weight. Two outstanding authorities in the area of nutrition, Mayer and Stare (14), have given the lie to such statements; and they have also provided experimental evidence to rectify other misconceptions. They have pointed out that it is neither necessary nor desirable to expend the energy required to lose one pound in one exercise bout; further, that "a half hour of handball or squash a day would be equivalent to 19 pounds per year."

Another general misconception is that exercise is not effective in weight reduction because appetite is automatically increased in direct proportion to the increased activity. Mayer et al. (15) have shown that while appetite follows activity in the range of normal activity in animals, this is not so in the low levels of activity. Figure 12.1 illustrates their work, and shows that sedentary animals (those most apt to be obese) actually display a decrease in appetite with an increase of up to one hour of daily exercise. Mayer and his collaborators have also shown that this principle applies to humans.

Metabolic After-effects of Exercise. The increase in metabolic rate incurred during physical activity is the main cause of energy loss. As long ago as 1933, the work of Margaria, Edwards, and Dill (13) mentioned an increased *resting* metabolic rate that lasted for several hours after completion of exercise, and that could not be attributed to repayment of oxygen debt.

This increased metabolic rate was further investigated in the author's laboratory (8). In a controlled experiment it was found that the resting metabolic rate was from 7.5 to twenty-eight percent higher four hours

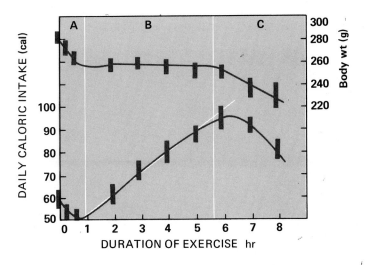

Figure 12-1. The relationship between activity and appetite and the effects upon body weight in animals. (From Mayer, et al. *American Journal of Physiology* 177:544, 1954.)

after a vigorous workout than at the same time of day on *nonexercise* control days. This higher metabolic rate was shown to persist for at least six hours after exercise, and this effect of exercise—over and above the energy cost of the exercise itself—would have resulted in a weight loss of four or five pounds per year if the individuals tested had exercised daily. Figure 12.2 illustrates the results of the experiment.

What Kind of Exercise Is Best? To be effective in reducing weight, exercise must be of the vigorous, endurance type in order that energy expenditure may be maximized. In designing such an exercise program, the following six factors must be considered.

1. The exercise must allow *gradual progression* from low levels to higher levels of energy expenditure.
2. Participants must be protected from injury to bony and connective tissues in the early stages.
3. The exercise must be vigorous enough to result in increased body heat, as evidenced by sweating.
4. Intensity of the exercise should be as high as possible, and should last for at least thirty minutes. Maximal energy output cannot be obtained if the musculature is quickly exhausted by a few quick maximal repetitions, as in weight lifting.

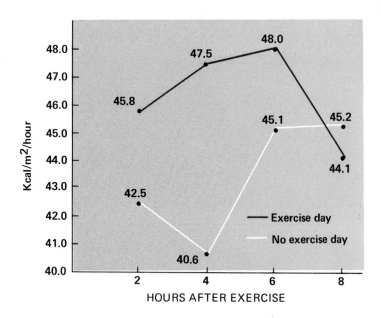

Figure 12-2. Metabolic after effects of a vigorous workout compared with a similar day in which no workout was taken. Each experimental point represents the mean of at least six observations for each of two middle-age male subjects.

5. Soreness should be prevented, or relieved, by the procedures described in chapter fifteen.
6. After a minimum level of fitness is achieved, the program should be built around activities that are enjoyable, and thus self-motivating.

Passmore and Durnin (19) have provided a rather complete survey of the energy requirements of various activities. Some of their data are provided in table 12.2.

Dieting to Lose Weight. Severe dietary restriction is a procedure that requires medical supervision; it cannot be properly treated in this text. Moderate dietary restriction, which results in weight losses of one or two pounds per week, can be accomplished by estimation of the daily energy expenditure and maintenance of a daily food intake of 500 to 1,000 kilocalories per day below the expenditure level. These figures are readily available in various texts on nutrition.

Some interesting new concepts about the physiology of weight reduction deserve comment here. It has been shown (11) that rats trained to eat their entire daily food ration in one to two hours gain more weight

TABLE 12.2

Energy Requirements of Various Activities

No. of Subjects	Age	Sex	(kg)	Activity	kcal/ min
12	32	M	66	Lying at ease	1.4
16	34	M	66	Sitting at ease	1.6
7	38	M	64	Standing at ease	1.9
112	young	M	..	Sitting, playing cards	2.4
3	19	M	64	Driving car	2.8
1	..		68	Volleyball	3.5
1	29	M	63	Golf	5.0
2	20	M	69	Archery	5.2
1	23	M	69	Dancing (rhumba)	7.0
4	..	M	68	Canoeing (4 mph.)	7.0
7	19	M	70	Tennis	7.1
3	..	M	73	Horseback riding (trot)	8.0
3	..	M	73	Horseback riding (gallop)	10.0
4	25	M	65	Cross-country running	10.6
1	..	M	71	Cycling (13.1 mph.)	11.1
1	21	M	68	Swimming (backcrawl)	11.5
1	21	M	90	Swimming (crawl, 45 yd./min.)	11.5
1	..	F	57	Skiing (level, hard snow; moderate speed)	15.9
1	..	F	68	Skiing (uphill, hard snow; maximum speed)	18.6

Based on data from R. Passmore and J. V. G. A. Durnin, "Human Energy Expenditure," *Physiological-Reviews* 35:801-35, 1955.

than animals eating ad libitum. It was further demonstrated that the trained rats increased the rate at which their adipose tissue incorporated food breakdown products into lipids (fats) by twenty-five times.

This work was extended and applied to the medical treatment of obesity in humans by Gordon, Goldberg, and Chosy (9). They initiated treatment in obese patients with a forty-eight-hour fast (to break the metabolic pattern of augmented lipogenesis), then instituted a 1,320-kilocalorie diet that consisted of 400 kilocalories of protein, 720 kilocalories of fat, and 200 kilocalories of carbohydrate. This diet was given in six feedings daily, corresponding to breakfast, midmorning, lunch, midafternoon, supper, and bedtime; all feedings were approximately similar in size. They report that results have been encouraging, and they have been surprised that no patient has complained of hunger at any time, although some have lost as much as 100 pounds.

If these results can be generalized, it would seem that concentrating a large part of the daily food intake into one large meal has unfavorable metabolic consequences (increased lipogenesis, or fat deposition). Furthermore, skipping breakfast seems undesirable. Indeed, if these data are substantiated by other investigators, a change in American eating patterns is indicated.

WATER RETENTION IN WEIGHT REDUCTION PROGRAMS

Obese people are very frequently discouraged by the results of their dieting; after one, two, or even three weeks of semistarvation the scale still reads the same. If they have honestly adhered to a negative caloric balance, the reason for this phenomenon is probably water retention. It has been shown that even though body tissues are being oxidized and the end products excreted, weight may not demonstrate this loss because sufficient water is retained by the tissues to offset the weight of the oxidized tissues. This water retention cannot continue indefinitely, however, so that the predicted weight change eventually occurs although it may not follow the day to day caloric deficit (17). Figure 12.3 illustrates the phenomenon.

The physiology of this water retention seems to be explained by the fact that the water formed as a by-product of the metabolism of the body's fat stores is not excreted immediately via the kidney in obese subjects because of an increased level of antidiuretic hormones.

Gordon, Goldberg and Chosy (9) have also demonstrated the *water binding effect* of consumption of an appreciable quantity of concentrated carbohydrate food. A severely obese man, who had been losing weight successfully, was given an 800-gram carbohydrate, 4,000-kilocalories per day diet for two days. He promptly gained eighteen pounds, which required three weeks to lose. The weight gained was shown to be water.

It is extremely important that anyone embarking upon a diet to lose weight be aware of these facts so as not to be discouraged when results are delayed by water retention.

SPOT REDUCING

Women are frequently encouraged to use localized exercises to reduce fatty stores in the areas of greatest fat deposition, usually buttocks, hips, and thighs. Schade et al. (20) conducted an experiment on twenty-two overweight college women in which one group used *spot reducing exercises* and the other general exercise. The researchers concluded there was

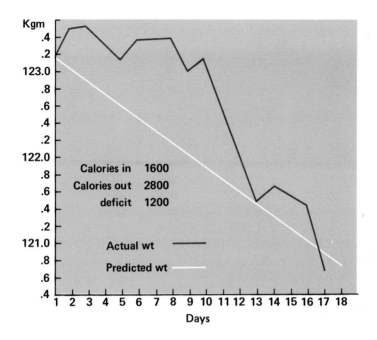

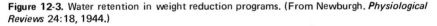

Figure 12-3. Water retention in weight reduction programs. (From Newburgh. *Physiological Reviews* 24:18, 1944.)

no significant difference in the effect of spot and generalized exercise on fat distribution in their subjects.

The best evidence available seems to indicate that in negative caloric balance situations the fat comes off the area of greatest concentration, regardless of how the exercise is performed.

THE LONG HAUL CONCEPT OF WEIGHT CONTROL

It should be emphasized that weight control is best performed as a matter of childhood habit formation, which then automatically takes care of the *long haul*. This habit formation should include the development of physical skills that will permit, indeed encourage and motivate, regular participation in a vigorous activity. Such sports as tennis, badminton, handball, skiing, and horseback riding are ideally suited to lifetime needs since they are vigorous, enjoyable, and can be performed with a minimum of cooperation by other persons. A person who develops these skills and participates in them regularly—at least twice, and preferably three or four times a week—will seldom have to be unduly concerned about his diet. With normal moderation in eating, including a gradual decrease in caloric intake with age above twenty-five years, he will in all likelihood have no problem with obesity.

When obesity gets a start due to inactivity or overeating, it is wise to get started with corrective efforts as early as possible. The corrective measures, exercise and diet, should be set up with habit formation in mind. Thus one cannot set up a habit pattern that involves any of the many popular *crash diets;* when normal weight is regained, a change is necessary, and all too often the change is a reversion to the prediet obesity-causing regimen. A series of cycles of weight gain and loss is then set up, and discouragement ensues, with complete loss of control.

On the other hand, a sensible approach would involve a dietary restriction of only 300 to 500 kilocalories per day, with a progressive buildup of exercise such as an hour of tennis or horseback riding (another loss of 400 to 600 kilocalories). In this fashion, pleasurable habits can be formed that require no changes and that do not cause the distress of semistarvation on a crash diet. The process may take a little longer, but it will be infinitely more successful.

If the effectiveness of exercise for losing weight is questioned, the layman can most readily see the answer not in research but in the empirical wisdom of the experience of mankind. Obesity is practically unknown among vigorous, healthy athletes, ditch-diggers, heavy laborers, many of whom daily consume prodigious amounts of food.

MAKING WEIGHT IN ATHLETICS

In many sports, such as wrestling and boxing, competition is organized into divisions by body weight; also, some states set up high school and junior high school athletics on the basis of a classification system that depends—at least in part—on the weight of the athletes. It does not require a great deal of sophistication, in coach or athlete, to see the advantages of competing in the lowest possible weight class.

For mature athletes, *making weight* is not a large health problem because experience has taught them what their normal weight should be; however, the author has seen many extreme cases of weight loss by high school athletes—on occasion as much as fifteen pounds in a boy whose normal weight was 150 or 160 pounds. This practice should be condemned in the strongest terms, for these short-term weight losses can be obtained only by drastic changes in water metabolism (sweating it off, plus water restriction), and there are attendant changes in kidney and cardiovascular function (whose consequences are still difficult to evaluate). In secondary school athletes, a five percent weight loss is certainly the outside limit of prudence and it is quite likely that even this amount (without medical supervision) is too great for some boys.

SUMMARY

1. Besides the aesthetic disadvantages, obesity has been shown to be associated with many degenerative diseases.
2. Weight gain and loss follow the laws of themodynamics. A positive energy balance results in a gain in weight, and a negative energy balance results in a loss.
3. Carbohydrate, fat, and protein follow the same final pathway in their metabolism, and thus fat and protein can substitute for carbohydrate in furnishing energy. All three foodstuffs, if eaten in excess, can result in deposition of fat tissue.
4. Estimation of what constitutes normal or proper body weight is subject to great inaccuracy unless measurements of body composition are made. Scale readings are relatively meaningless unless we know the proportion of the reading that is due to fatty tissues.
5. A gain in weight is best accomplished by heavy resistance, low-repetition type exercise, such as weight training, in which weight gain is brought about through muscular hypertrophy.
6. Weight loss can be accomplished by increased activity (exercise) or dietary restriction. If the weight is not grossly abnormal, a progressive exercise program, although slower, is the sounder approach.
7. Moderate increases in activity level, contrary to popular opinion, do not result in increased food intake if the individual has been sedentary previously.
8. Vigorous exercise not only creates an immediate increase in metabolism, it also brings about a longer-lasting (six- to eight-hour) rise in resting metabolism, which further contributes to weight loss.
9. Considerable evidence indicates that concentrating the daily food consumption into one or two large meals results in a greater tendency toward obesity.
10. In dieting to lose weight, a temporary water retention (up to three weeks) may obscure the true fat-tissue loss that is occurring.
11. *Spot reducing* rests on no sound physiological basis; rather, the best available evidence indicates that regardless of the part of the anatomy exercised, weight loss first occurs in the largest fat deposits.

12. Maintaining normal weight should be a long-term process that involves hygienic habit formation. *Crash diets* are usually foredoomed to failure because they do not accomplish habit formation.
13. *Making weight* in athletics must be considered potentially hazardous for adolescents. Weight losses for this purpose should never exceed five percent (short term), and even these losses should be effected under competent supervision.

REFERENCES

1. Allen, T. H. 1963. Measurement of human body fat: a quantitative method suited for use by aviation medical officers. *Aerospace Medicine* 34:907-9.
2. Behnke, A. R. 1963. Anthropometric evaluation of body composition through life. *Annals of the New York Academy of Sciences* 110:450-64.
3. Benoit, F. L.; Martin, R. L.; and Watten, R. H. 1965. Changes in body composition during weight reduction in obesity. *Annals of Internal Medicine* 63:604-12.
4. Beyer, D. H. 1961. Weight control—a new air force program. *Aerospace Medicine* 32:814-17.
5. Consolazio, C. F.; Johnson, R. E.; and Pecora, L. J. 1963. *Physiological Measurements of metabolic functions in man.* New York: McGraw-Hill Book Co.
6. Corbin, C. B., and Pletcher, P. 1968. Diet and physical activity patterns of obese and non-obese elementary school children. *Research Quarterly* 39:922-28.
7. Cureton, T. K. 1947. *Physical fitness appraisal and guidance.* St. Louis: C. V. Mosby Company.
8. deVries, H. A., and Gray, D. E. 1963. After effects of exercise upon resting metabolic rate. *Research Quarterly* 34:314-21.
9. Gordon, E. S.; Goldberg, M.; and Chosy, G. J. 1963. A new concept in the treatment of obesity. *Journal of the American Medical Association* 186: 50-60.
10. Greene, J. A. 1939. A clinical study of the etiology of obesity. *Annals of Internal Medicine* 12:1797-1803.
11. Hollifield, G., and Parson, W. 1962. Metabolic adaptations to a "stuff and starve" feeding program. *Journal of Clinical Investigation* 41:250-53.
12. Keys, A., and Brozek, J. 1953. Body fat in adult man. *Physiological Reviews* 33:245-325.
13. Margaria, R.; Edwards, H .T.; and Dill, D. B. 1933. The possible mechanisms of contracting and paying the O_2 debt and the role of lactic acid in muscular contraction. *American Journal of Physiology* 106:689-715.
14. Mayer, J., and Stare, F. J. 1953. Exercise and weight control: frequent misconceptions. *Journal of the American Dietetic Association* 29:340-43.
15. Mayer, J.; Marshall, N. B.; Vitale, J. J.; Christensen, J. H.; Mashayek, M. B.; and Stare, F. J. 1954. Exercise, food intake and body weight in

normal rats and genetically obese adult mice. *American Journal of Physiology* 177:544.

16. Moody, D. L.; Kollias, J.; and Buskirk, E. R. 1969. The effect of a moderate exercise program on body weight, and skinfold thickness in overweight college women. *Medicine and Science in Sports* 17:75-80.

17. Newburgh, L. H. 1944. Obesity and energy metabolism. *Physiological Reviews* 24:18.

18. Pariskova, J. 1964. Impact of age, diet and exercise on man's body composition. In *International Research in Sport and Physical Education*, eds. E. Jokl and E. Simon. Springfield, Ill.: Charles C. Thomas Publisher.

19. Passmore, R., and Durnin, J. V. G. A. 1955. Human energy expenditure. *Physiological Reviews* 35:801-35.

20. Schade, M.; Hellebrandt, F. A.; Waterland, J. C.; and Carns, M. L. 1962. Spot reducing in overweight college women. *Research Quarterly* 33:461-71.

21. Shock, N. W., and Yiengst, M. J. 1955. Age changes in basal respiratory measurements and metabolism in males. *Journal of Gerontology* 10:31-40.

22. Sloan, A. W.; Burt, J. J.; and Blyth, C. S. 1962. Estimation of body fat in younger women. *Journal of Applied Physiology* 17:967-70.

23. Von Dobeln, W. 1961. Fat-free body weight of Swedish air force pilots. *Aerospace Medicine* 32:67-69.

24. Wamsley, J. R., and Roberts, J. E. 1963. Body composition of USAF flying personnel. *Aerospace Medicine* 34:403-5.

13 Prophylactic and Therapeutic Effects of Exercise

The nature of the illnesses that beset our American population has in recent years undergone a transition from a predominance of infectious diseases to the present predominance of degenerative diseases. This change represents an implicit compliment to the medical profession for its contributions, both in research and clinical practice, toward the virtual control and the imminent eradication of a large portion of the formerly dreaded infectious scourges.

The increase of such degenerative diseases as cardiovascular accidents (heart attacks and strokes), hypertension, neuroses, and malignancies offers a challenge not only to medicine but to physical education as well. It seems that as improvements in medical science allow us to escape the decimation of such infectious diseases as tuberculosis, diptheria, poliomyelitis, we live longer, but we fall prey to the degenerative diseases at a slightly later date. Whether this involvement with the degenerative problems is a necessary concomitant of our living longer or the result of our simultaneous change in life style cannot yet be answered.

Along with our newly acquired control over the infectious diseases, we have made at least three other changes that seem likely to affect adversely our physical and mental well-being:

1. We have learned to produce more food than we need, and we eat commensurately.
2. We have learned to control our environment with very little expenditure of physical energy.
3. We have so constituted our society that most of us are subjected to unusual stresses, for which our biological responses are inadequate or, indeed, deleterious.

Where our grandfathers labored hard and long physically in agriculture or in industry, our present generation not only uses automobiles to go to the corner drugstore; we have power lawn mowers for the man of the house and automatic washers and dishwashers for the lady, and Junior gets a motor scooter at the earliest possible age. On weekends we stage athletic spectacles in which our population gets its exercise vicariously by watching its hired athletes get a workout. The result of this sedentary life style appears to be the growth of degenerative diseases, and an increasing involvement with neuroses and psychoses for which our grandparents just did not have time.

No one in his right mind advocates a return to the long, tedious drudgery of manual work, but we cannot deny there is a need to learn how to adjust in better fashion to our newly found leisure time. The *fun* of exercise, sport, and physically vigorous recreation must replace the *tedium* of hard work that kept our grandfathers physically fit. Herein is the challenge to concerted effort by the medical and physical education professions.

When two events are related in time we are tempted to assign a causal relationship; thus the decreased need for physical activity and the increased incidence of degenerative disease, having come about during the same period of time, are thought to be related as cause and effect. From the scientific point of view, much experimental evidence, derived under controlled conditions, is necessary to support such a contention. On the other hand, we do not need 100 percent certainty in order to start applying theories that have much empirical support and no apparent disadvantages; and this is the case for exercise as a *prophylactic* (preventive) or *therapeutic* (corrective) agent against degenerative disease. Furthermore, zeal and dedication to the vigorous life are badly needed qualities in professional physical educators. The remainder of this chapter will review the evidence for the benefits of physical exercise.

THE CARDIOVASCULAR SYSTEM AND EXERCISE

Physical Activity and Coronary Heart Disease. Since W. W. II, several large scale statistical surveys have been conducted to evaluate the relationships between activity level and coronary heart disease.

Probably the most widely known study was conducted by Morris et al. (28) on bus drivers and conductors of the London Transport Authority. They found, among 31,000 drivers and conductors, that the drivers suffered significantly more coronary heart disease than the conductors. Since the drivers might be considered sedentary, while the conductors (of double deck busses) did considerable walking and stair-climbing, it would seem that men in active jobs suffer less coronary heart disease. However, we cannot deduce from this that the exercise involved was the causative factor, because it is possible that coronary-prone people selected the driver jobs.

Taylor and his colleagues at the Laboratory of Physiological Hygiene at the University of Minnesota conducted a similar study on American railway employees (40). They found that in 191,609 man-years of risk, and 1,978 reported deaths, the age-adjusted deaths for arteriosclerotic heart disease were 5.7, 3.9, and 2.8 for clerks, switchmen, and section men, respectively. Since the clerks' jobs were sedentary, the switchmen's moderately active, and the section men's very active, these data support those of Morris et al.

In the Framingham, Massachusetts study a team of investigators from the US Public Health Service classified men as to their habitual level of physical activity (25). In the ten years following the physical activity assessments, 207 men developed some manifestation of a coronary attack and those who had been classified as most sedentary in each age group had an incidence almost twice that of the group who were at least moderately active.

Brunner (6) studied 5,279 men and 5,229 women in the Israeli Kibbutzim. The Kibbutzim are run as communes and consequently offered the advantage of allowing the comparison of physical activity effects uncontaminated by the effects of income, diet, etc., since all members regardless of the nature of their work have the same income and eat in the same communal dining room. He found the incidence of the anginal syndrome, myocardial infarction, and fatalities due to coronary heart disease was 2.5 to four times higher in sedentary than in their physically active workers.

Many more studies could be cited to support the need for physical activity as a prophylactic measure against coronary heart disease. A good review of the literature on this subject is available (15).

Exercise and Coronary Circulation.　　Eckstein (13) operated on 117 dogs to produce various degrees of narrowing of the circumflex coronary artery. This simulated the narrowing brought about in coronary disease by deposition of cholesterol in the intima of the coronary arteries. When the dogs with constricted arteries were exercised, coronary blood flow capacity increased significantly by virtue of increased collateral circulation.

Raab (31, 32) provided considerable data on the importance of the autonomic control of the heart. The rate and metabolism of the heart are established as the result of a balance between the parasympathetic system (vagus nerve) and the sympathetic system (accelerator nerve). This balance is established in the midbrain and is mediated through release of neurohormonal (chemical) transmitters. The sympathogenic effects are brought about by the catecholamines, epinephrine and norepinephrine, and the vagal effects are brought about through acetylcholine.

In general, athletic training brings about vagal preponderance, as indicated by the slower heart rate in the athlete both at rest and under any given work load. A state of nervous excitement (emotional upset) causes a sympathogenic preponderance. The sympathogenic catecholamines were shown (by Raab) to have undesirable effects on the myocardium, such as an excessive increase in O_2 consumption. Raab et al. (32) demonstrated that the combination of coronary constriction (as in atherosclerosis) and a sympathogenic supply of catecholamines brings about the typical EKG changes of coronary disease. He felt that this neurohormonal imbalance (sympathetic preponderance) is caused jointly by "(1) hypothalamic-stimulating emotional socioeconomic pressures, and (2) a deficiency of vagal and sympathoinhibitory counter regulation resulting from lack of physical exercise."

In a recent experiment by Heusner et al. (19), it was shown that similar myocardial damage can be produced by: (1) epinephrine injection, (2) anoxia, (3) severe emotional stress, (4) and *severe* exercise. Most interestingly they also showed that appropriate physical conditioning can protect against the stressor effect of extreme anxiety or emotional stress.

Results from two different laboratories agree in showing increased coronary tree size to result from physical conditioning in rats (38, 41). Stevenson et al. extended their investigation to include the question of the effect of intensity and frequency upon the increase in coronary vessel size. They found that moderate exercise (twice weekly) had a more beneficial effect than extremely severe exercise (four hours per day, four days per week) (38).

Exercise Effect on Blood Pressure. One of the better experiments in this area was performed by Boyer and Kasch (5) who found that six months of participation in their San Diego State fitness program resulted in decreases of systolic pressure of almost 12 mm Hg and 13 mm Hg in diastolic values in twenty-three hypertensive men.

Changes in the Blood Accompanying Stress and Exercise. Thus far we have discussed the effects of stress and exercise upon the blood vessels and muscle tissue of the heart; however, another factor is thought to be of considerable importance in the etiology of heart disease: the *physicochemical properties* of the blood that courses through these coronary vessels. It is obvious that changes in the blood that lead to quicker coagulation or clotting time might also be more likely to result in thrombus formation, the plugging of a coronary artery in a heart attack.

The work of Schneider and Zangari (36) demonstrated the effects of stress upon the blood. Anxiety, tension, fear, anger, and hostility were associated with shorter clotting times, increased viscosity, and blood pressure. It was suggested that this pattern was appropriate as a protective reaction when the organism was under attack because excessive blood loss would be prevented by the shortened clotting time and O_2 transport would be enhanced by the increased viscosity. If this pattern were used chronically, however—as seemed to be the case in their hypertensive subjects—it could prove detrimental by favoring intravascular thrombosis and by increasing the work of the heart (because of the increased viscosity of the blood).

Increases of *total blood volume* (TBV) which had been reported earlier were considered equivocal because of methodological questions but recent evidence has now been presented to confirm the fact that endurance training can increase the blood volume by as much as six percent (30). The increased TBV was found to be due to increased plasma volume, while red cell volume did not change significantly.

Use of Physical Conditioning in Cardiac Rehabilitation. Hellerstein studied 656 middle aged men of whom 254 had coronary heart disease (CHD); the remainder were coronary prone (18). Detailed evaluation of a subgroup of 100 men with coronary disease showed that they were able to perform muscular effort more efficiently after training, i.e., with lower heart rates, lower blood pressure and greater aerobic capacity. Ischemic electrocardiographic changes were decreased in two-thirds of the subjects after conditioning.

In Israel, Gottheimer has had many years experience in the use of physical conditioning for cardiac rehabilitation (17). In observations of 1,103 patients with ischemic heart disease over a five-year period in which they gradually trained toward high level sports performance he found evidence for (1) reduced heart rate at rest and after exercise, (2) more efficient breathing, (3) EKG abnormalities having either disappeared or diminished, and (4) normalized blood pressures. But most importantly, the mortality rate was reduced to 3.6 percent over five years compared with twelve percent in a similar population of physically inactive postinfarction patients in Israel.

Mechanisms by Which Physical Conditioning May Reduce Occurrence or Severity of CHD. Fox and Haskell (14) have suggested the following mechanisms by which physical activity may have a beneficial effect upon CHD:

1. Increased coronary vascularization.
2. Improvement of myocardial function as evidenced by (A) bradycardia, (B) increase in stroke volume, (C) increased cardiac output, (D) longer diastolic period available for coronary perfusion, (E) reduction in heart chamber size at any given work load, (F) myocardial hypertrophy, (G) decrease in systemic arterial pressure, and (H) redistribution of blood flow to more active muscles.
3. Serum lipids—lowering levels of cholesterol and serum triglycerides.
4. A favorable effect upon blood clotting and fibrinolysis.
5. Blood pressure effects.
6. Reduction of obesity.
7. Psychic benefits.

LIPID METABOLISM AND EXERCISE

The lipids include the *typical fats,* which are esters of fatty acids and glycerol (triglycerides), and *sterols* such as cholesterol (as well as other categories). Our interest in these members of the lipid family stems from the fact that both are found in the deposits that narrow the lumen of arteries in atherosclerosis. Whether there is a causal relationship is not yet known; however, the physician's concern with the blood cholesterol level as a predisposing factor to heart disease is well known, and it is based on statistical evidence that indicates a strong relationship (though possibly not causal) between cholesterol level and heart disease. For these reasons, the effect of exercise on blood triglyceride and cholesterol is of interest.

Taylor (39) reports experiments in which it was shown that substantial amounts of fat can be added to the diet without raising cholesterol levels if the level of physical activity is also increased.

Rochelle (34) has demonstrated that vigorous physical exercise (a two-mile run) five days a week for five weeks produced a significant decrease in plasma cholesterol.

It has also been shown that ingestion of a high-fat meal results in significantly higher levels of fat in the blood than does ingestion of a low-fat meal (7). Exercise performed immediately after ingestion of the high-fat meal was found to decrease this hyperlipemia significantly.

Holloszy et al. (20) have shown that six months of physical conditioning by calisthenics and distance running reduced serum triglycerides by forty percent. However this effect appeared to last only about two days. Thus it may be inferred from their work that serum triglycerides can be maintained at a significantly lower level by exercise, but the exercise must be done at least every other day.

Gollnick and Taylor have shown (16) liver cholesterol was significantly lower in exercised rats than in unexercised controls regardless of diet. On the same diet the exercised rats also had about fifty-five percent less lipid in their livers than pair-fed controls.

Malinow and Perley (26) injected radioactive isotope labelled cholesterol into human subjects and showed that the rate of cholesterol oxidation was much greater during light exercise than at rest.

Montoye has provided an excellent survey (27) of the research findings in this area. He points out: "In various populations, blood cholesterol, body fatness, percentage of calories from fat, total fat intake, all appear to vary together, and are inversely related to physical activity."

PULMONARY FUNCTION EFFECTS

Beneficial effects of conditioning include significant improvement in functional residual capacity, residual volume, vital capacity and the ratio of residual volume/total lung capacity (4). It has also been shown that lung diffusion is better in trained than in untrained young men and women (21).

OXYGEN TRANSPORT EFFECTS

The benefits to the systems which determine the capacity for oxygen transport have been supported by experiments too numerous to cite. In general, improvements in maximal O_2 consumption from appropriate physical conditioning have been shown to occur in all ages and both sexes. Improvements reported have ranged from five to thirty percent. Differences in training effect would be expected according to the fitness level at the start of an experiment and the intensity-duration-frequency characteristics of the training regimen.

EFFECTS ON BONES, JOINTS, AND CONNECTIVE TISSUE

It is well known that disuse of the skeletal system results in its atrophy with the eventual development of osteoporosis. Loading of the bones of the skeletal framework is necessary for normal bone metabolism which consists of both anabolic and catabolic processes as in other living tissues. In bone, both mineral and organic metabolic processes are involved and a recent study using swine has provided evidence that the stress of exercise exerts a conservatory influence on both the mineral and the collagenous (organic) components of bone (2).

Recent work from several independent investigations has shown the importance of physical conditioning on connective tissues such as ligaments. It was shown in rats that the strength of ligaments of the knee joint improves with physical activity (1, 45). Tipton and coworkers have performed a series of experiments in which the same ligament strength results were shown in larger animals (dogs) and in addition they demonstrated that the collagen content and fiber bundle size were significantly greater in trained dogs (42). Interestingly, they also showed the beneficial exercise effects on ligament strength after surgical repair. This, of course, has important implications for the postsurgical treatment of knee injuries in athletes. In another investigation Tipton et al. questioned whether these effects were hormonal since connective tissues are known to be responsive to hormonal effects. They found that the mechanical stresses of training can act independently of the hormonal effect which was verified.

In the author's laboratory, Chapman (8) showed that the resistance to movement in a joint can be significantly reduced both in the old as well as the young.

EFFECTS OF EXERCISE ON CANCER IN ANIMALS

Rigan (33) has provided a summary of the research reports for the years 1920 until 1963 that relate to the effects of exercise on cancer. Evidence was reported to show an inverse relationship between physical activity and the cancer death rate in men. In various animal experiments over these forty years, the following observations were reported.

1. Caloric restriction inhibited the growth rate of malignancies.
2. In mice, two hours of daily exercise reduced the incidence of mammary gland carcinoma.
3. Three studies indicated a retarded tumor growth rate in exercised mice.
4. Tumor growth rate was reported to be inhibited in rats when they were injected with saline solution that had bathed excised rat muscle fatigued by exercise.

More recent evidence has been supplied by Colacino and Balke (9) who found only half the number of tumors in exercising mice compared with controls when both groups had been subjected to carcinogenic agents. Since there were no differences in food intake or weight, their study supports the older work with respect to the effect of exercise on tumor growth.

It must be emphasized that none of these studies provides evidence of a direct cause-and-effect relationship between exercise and cancer. Exercise is *not* being advanced as a panacea for cancer prevention; however, if a life of hygienic exercise can make a contribution—no matter how small in a statistical sense—to the prevention of this dread disease, this information (even though causal relationships are not scientifically validated) may be extremely important.

EXERCISE AND RESISTANCE TO DISEASE

Advocates of the vigorous life have long felt that physical training and conditioning should provide a degree of resistance to infectious disease, but the absence of scientific evidence upon which to base such a theory has been most frustrating. There is still no definitive evidence from which valid conclusions can be drawn, but the work of Zimkin (44) and his colleagues suggests that this is a fruitful area for further research. Their work used Selye's general adaptation syndrome (see chapter ten) as a point of departure, and they hypothesized that the stage of resistance was nonspecific as to the type of stress, and would therefore have prophylactic significance.

They tested this hypothesis by developing a *stage of resistance,* using exercise as the stressor. It was found that physical exercise materially increased the body's resistance to infection. They reported experiments that showed agglutination titre and phagocytic activity (both advantageous in the prevention of illness) were increased much more in trained animals than in untrained.

Very importantly, they found that the training effects required optimum intensity and duration of work. Too much work not only failed to produce the desired resistance but might, in some cases, result in decreased resistance.

It is difficult to evaluate this work because no statistical treatments are offered, and in almost all cases the original work is in Russian. A very interesting field of research is suggested, however, and corroboration of their results could have large implications for physical education and for medicine.

EFFECTS OF EXERCISE ON NEUROMUSCULAR TENSION (RELAXATION)

The importance of the ability to achieve neuromuscular relaxation is emphasized by the many references to this topic in popular literature. More than 300 million dollars are spent yearly in the United States on tranquilizers to quiet jangled nerves. Many books and articles have been written on the subject; and physical educators often voice the opinion that a good workout can relieve nervous tension. Until very recently, however, very little scientifically acceptable evidence had been submitted that relates exercise and relief of residual neuromuscular tension.

State of Neuromuscular System Related to Anxiety and Tension. Overwhelming evidence supports the concept of a neuromuscular manifestation of various psychologically induced *anxiety* and *tension* states. The classic work, and much of the evidence, has been provided by Edmund Jacobson (22, 23, 24), who was the first to recognize this relationship and to apply it to the need for making objective measurements of previously unmeasurable symptoms. Thus by making electronic measurements of the activity of the skeletal muscles, (electromyography or EMG) it was possible to gain an objective insight into subjects' emotional states, nervousness, etc. Later investigators have supported the work of Jacobson, and, on the basis of the work of Sainsbury and Gibson (35) and Nidever (29), it would appear that sampling even one or two representative muscles in the resting state can provide good evidence on the state of the entire organism at any given moment. Significant relationships have been shown to exist between these EMG measurements on selected skeletal muscles and such clinical states as headache, backache, mental activity, emotional states, etc.

The author has shown that integrated EMG activity of the biceps brachii is more than doubled when a resting subject undergoes eyestrain by reading fine print (10). Surprisingly, intermittent, loud, irritating noise caused no significant increase in neuromuscular tension. Possibly we have become inured to noise.

Improvement of Relaxation by the Teaching of Kinesthesis. Improvement through training in ability to achieve voluntary relaxation, both at rest and in activity, has been demonstrated. Jacobson applied the principles of teaching kinesthetic perception (24) with electromyographically demonstrable success. The method depends upon teaching a subject to recognize progressively decreasing levels of voluntary muscular tension until his perceptive power is great enough to identify, and thus relieve, even the smallest degree of involuntary tension; this ultimately results in the subjects' ability to achieve voluntary and complete relaxation (electrical silence) in one muscle group after the other. Steinhaus and Norris (37), using Jacobson's methods on normal young subjects demonstrated a twenty-five to forty percent reduction in neuromuscular tension over a period of eight weeks. Control subjects showed no changes.

The ability to achieve voluntary control over the autonomic nervous system has long been claimed by practitioners of the ancient art of yoga, and objective evidence occasionally supports these claims. It has been reported that for a trained yogi the O_2 consumption during a live burial was depressed from a normal before-burial value of 19.5 liters per hour to 10.0 liters per hour, over several hours. Control subjects have been unable to depress their metabolic rate (3), and it is therefore obvious that such a depression of the metabolic rate could be accomplished only by a very great ability to achieve voluntary relaxation of the skeletal musculature. It would seem that such techniques as *shavasana*, the yogic technique for teaching relaxation, must also be effective.

Exercise and Relaxation. The earliest objective work relative to exercise and relaxation was done by Jacobson (22), who compared the ability of college athletes with normal subjects who were untrained in relaxation technique. He found that the athletes could relax more quickly and completely than the untrained controls; however, controls who were trained in the art of relaxation were superior to the athletes (as a group).

Obviously, this experiment does not tell us whether an athletic program contributes to relaxation ability or whether more relaxed persons take up athletics.

In the author's laboratory, twenty-nine young, healthy subjects were studied for EMG changes after five minutes of bench-stepping as standard exercise. Neuromuscular tension was decreased significantly in the experimental situation decreasing to a fifty-eight percent drop in electrical activity one hour after activity. No significant change was seen on the control day. A chronic effect of conditioning was also shown (11). More recent work in the laboratory was directed toward comparison of the exercise effect with that of a recognized tranquilizer drug, *meprobamate* (12). To make the experiment more sensitive, older people with complaints of nervous tension acted as subjects. EMG measurements were made before and after (immediately, thirty minutes, and sixty minutes after) each of the five following treatment conditions:

1. Meprobamate 400 mg (normal dosage)
2. Placebo, 400 mg lactose
3. Fifteen minutes of walking-type exercises at a heart rate of 100
4. Fifteen minutes of the same exercise at a heart rate of 120
5. Resting control

Conditions 1 and 2 were administered double blind. It was found that exercise at a heart rate of 100 lowered electrical activity in the musculature by twenty, twenty-three, and twenty percent at the first, second and third post-tests respectively. These changes were highly significant ($P < .01$). Neither meprobamate nor placebo treatments were significantly different from controls. Exercise at the higher heart rate was only slightly less effective, but the data were more variable and approached but did not achieve significance.

The data suggest that the exercise modality should not be overlooked when a tranquilizer effect is desired, since in single doses, at least, appropriate exercise has a significantly greater effect than does one of the most frequently prescribed tranquilizer drugs, meprobamate. It must be added that exercise has no undesirable side effects whereas tranquilizer drugs used in sufficient repeated dosage to bring about the same effect must also impair motor coordination, reaction time, etc., with subsequent hazards involved in driving an automobile and any other activity requiring normal reactions.

Relief of Neuromuscular Tension as an Important Part of Motor Learning. Physical education has pursued knowledge for developing more strength, more power, and more endurance in muscle tissue, but the future will demand emphasis in our curricula upon how to relax muscles, as well as how to tense them. Modern man, it seems likely, will have increasing problems in learning how to relax, and those who are most concerned with muscular activity, the physical educators, should provide the leadership. The need is well-defined, the methods are at hand, and we must proceed with the job.

SUMMARY

It is important to point out that although much evidence has been furnished that supports the value of exercise as a prophylactic and therapeutic measure, exercise is not a panacea. In none of the areas we have discussed in this chapter is the evidence final and conclusive, but we can confidently say that the evidence indicates the desirability of the vigorous life in maintaining optimum levels of health and well-being. Every physical educator should be dedicated to this principle, both in his personal and in his professional life. In no other way can the youth of this nation be led into the full life that only vigorous activity can bring about.

REFERENCES

1. Adams, A. 1966. Effect of exercise on ligament strength. *Research Quarterly* 37:163-67.
2. Anderson, J. J. B.; Milin, L.; and Crackel, W. C. 1971. Effect of exercise on mineral and organic bone turnover in swine. *Journal of Applied Physiology* 30:810-13.
3. Annotations. Yoga. 1962. *Journal of Sports Medicine and Physical Fitness* 2:50.
4. Bachman, J. C., and Horvath, S. M. 1968. Pulmonary function changes which accompany athletic conditioning programs. *Research Quarterly* 39:235-39.
5. Boyer, J. L., and Kasch, F. W. 1970. Exercise therapy in hypertensive men. *Journal of the American Medical Association* 211:1668-71.
6. Brunner, D. 1966. The influence of physical activity on incidence and prognosis of ischemic heart disease. In *Prevention of ischemic heart disease,* ed. W. Raab, pp. 236-43. Springfield: Charles C Thomas.
7. Cantone, A. 1964. Physical effort and its effect in reducing alimentary hyperlipemia. *Journal of Sports Medicine and Physical Fitness* 4:32-36.
8. Chapman, E. A.; deVries, H. A.; and Swezey, R. 1972. Joint stiffness: effects of exercise on young and old men. *Journal of Gerontology* 27:218-21.
9. Colacino, D., and Balke, B. 1972. Tumor reduction in endurance trained mice. Paper read at ACSM, May 1972, at Philadelphia.

10. deVries, H. A. 1962. Neuromuscular tension and its relief. *Journal of the Association for Physical and Mental Rehabilitation* 16:86-88.

11. ———. 1968. Immediate and long-term effects of exercise upon resting muscle action potential level. *Journal of Sports Medicine and Physical Fitness* 8:1-11.

12. deVries, H. A., and Adams, G. M. 1972. Electromyographic comparison of single doses of exercise and meprobamate as to effects on muscular relaxation. *American Journal of Physical Medicine* 51:130-41.

13. Eckstein, R. W. 1957. Effect of exercise on coronary artery narrowing and coronary collateral circulation. *Circulation Research* 5:230-35.

14. Fox, S. M., and Haskell, W. L. 1968. Physical activity and the prevention of coronary heart disease. *Bulletin New York Academy of Medicine* 44: 950-67.

15. Fox, S. M., and Boyer, J. L. 1972. Physical activity and coronary heart disease. In *Physical fitness research digest,* ed. H. H. Clarke. Washington, D. C.: The Presidents Council on Physical Fitness and Sports, series 2, no. 2.

16. Gollnick, P. D., and Taylor, A. W. 1969. Effect of exercise on hepatic cholesterol of rats fed diets high in saturated or unsaturated fats. *Internationale Zeitschrift für Angewandte Physiologie Einschliesslich Arbeitsphysiologie* 27:144-53.

17. Gottheiner, V. 1968. Long-range strenuous sports training for reconditioning and rehabilitation. *American Journal of Cardiology* 22:426-35.

18. Hellerstein, H. K. 1968. Exercise therapy in coronary disease. *Bulletin New York Academy of Medicine* 44:1028-47.

19. Heusner, W. W.; Van Huss, W. D.; Carrow, R. E.; Wells, R. L.; Anderson, D. J.; and Ruhling, R. O. 1972. Exercise, anxiety, and myocardial damage. Paper read at ACSM, 1 May 1972, at Philadelphia.

20. Holloszy, J. O.; Skinner, J. S.; Toro, G.; and Cureton, T. K. 1964. Effects of a 6-month program of endurance exercise on the serum lipids of middle-aged men. *American Journal of Cardiology* 14:748-55.

21. Holmgren, A. 1965. On the variation of DL_{co} with increasing oxygen uptake during exercise in healthy trained young men and women. *Acta Physiologica Scandinavica* 65:207-20.

22. Jacobson, E. 1936. The course of relaxation of muscles of athletes. *American Journal of Psychology* 48:98-108.

23. ———. 1938. *Progressive relaxation.* Chicago: University of Chicago Press.

24. ———. 1943. The cultivation of physiological relaxation. *Annals of Internal Medicine* 19:965-72.

25. Kannel, W. B.; Sorlie, P.; and McNamara, P. 1971. The relation of physical activity to risk of coronary heart disease: the Framingham study. In *Coronary heart disease and physical fitness,* eds. O. A. Larson and R. O. Malmborg, p. 256. Baltimore: University Park Press.

26. Malinow, M. R., and Perley, A. 1969. The effect of physical exercise on cholesterol degradation in man. *Journal of Atherosclerosis Research* 10: 107-11.

27. Montoye, H. J. 1962. Summary of research on the relationship of exercise to heart disease. *Journal of Sports Medicine and Physical Fitness* 2:35-43.
28. Morris, J. N.; Heady, J. A.; Raffle, P. A. B.; Roberts, C. G.; and Parks, J. W. Coronary herat disease and physical activity of work. *The Lancet* 2:1053-1111.
29. Nidever, J. E. 1959. A factor analytic study of general muscular tension. Doctoral dissertation (psychology), UCLA.
30. Oscai, L.; Williams, B. T.; and Hertig, B. A. 1968. Effect of exercise on blood volume. *Journal of Applied Physiology* 24:622-24.
31. Raab, W. 1960. Metabolic protection and reconditioning of the heart muscle through habitual physical exercise. *Annals of Internal Medicine* 53:87-105.
32. Raab, W.; van Lith, P.; Lepeschkin, E.; and Herrlich, H. C. 1962. Catecholamine-induced myocardial hypoxia in the presence of impaired coronary dilatibility independent of external cardiac work. *American Journal of Cardiology* 9:455.
33. Rigan, D. 1963. Exercise and cancer, a review. *Journal of the American Osteopathic Association* 62:596-99.
34. Rochelle, R. H. 1961. Blood plasma cholesterol changes during a physical training program. *Journal of Sports Medicine and Physical Fitness* 1:63-70.
35. Sainsbury, P., and Gibson, J. G. 1954. Symptoms of anxiety and tension and the accompanying physiological changes in the muscular system. *Journal of Neurology, Neurosurgery, and Psychiatry* 17:216-24.
36. Schneider, R. A., and Zangari, V. M. 1951. Variations in clotting time, relative viscosity and other physicochemical properties of the blood accompanying physical and emotional stress in the normotensive and hypertensive subject. *Psychosomatic Medicine* 13:289-303.
37. Steinhaus, A. H., and Norris, J. E. 1964. *Teaching neuromuscular relaxation.* Comparative Research Project 1529; Office of Education, U.S. Department of Health, Education and Welfare; Washington, D. C.
38. Stevenson, J. A. F.; Feleki, V.; Rechnitzer, P.; and Beaton, J. R. 1964. Effect of exercise on coronary tree size in the rat. *Circulation Research* 15:265-69.
39. Taylor, H. L. 1959. Relationship of physical activity to serum cholesterol concentration. In *Work and the Heart,* eds. F. F. Rosenbaum and E. L. Belknap, ch. 12. New York: Paul B. Hoeber, Inc.
40. Taylor, H. L.; Klepetar, E.; Keys, A.; Parlin, W.; Blackborn, H.; and Puchner, T. 1962. Death rates among physically active and sedentary employes of the railway industry. *American Journal of Public Health* 52:1697-1707.
41. Tepperman, J., and Pearlman, D. 1961. Effects of exercise and anemia on coronary arteries of small animals as revealed by the corosion-cast technique. *Circulation Research* 9:576-84.
42. Tipton, C. M.; James, S. L.; Mergner, W.; and Tcheng, T. K. 1970. Influence of exercise on strength of medial collateral knee ligaments of dogs. *American Journal of Physiology* 218:894-902.

43. Tipton, C. M.; Tcheng, T. K.; and Mergner, W. 1971. Ligamentous strength measurements from hypophysectomized rats. *American Journal of Physiology* 221:1144-50.

44. Zimkin, N. V. 1964. Stress during muscular exercise and the state of non-specifically increased resistance. In *International Research in Sport and Physical Education*, eds., E. Jokl and E. Simon. Springfield, Ill.: Charles C Thomas.

45. Zuckerman, J., and Stull, G. A. 1969. Effects of exercise on knee ligament separation force in rats. *Journal of Applied Physiology* 26:716-19.

14 Electromyography in Physiology of Exercise

Electromyography (EMG) has served the kinesiologist and neurologist well over several decades, but the exercise physiologist's needs have not been well satisfied by the instrumentation commercially available because it was designed for quite different purposes.

In physiology of exercise we have a major interest in the study of gross muscle function. Whereas the kinesiologist wants to identify the muscle involved in a given action, or its timing in the action, and the neurologist is interested in finding abnormal muscle function, we in physiology of exercise concern ourselves with the activation level of normal muscle tissue under various experimentally contrived conditions of exercise loading.

Consequently, the exercise physiologist is interested in "putting numbers on" the amount of muscle activation required for a given work load over a given period of time. His problems are basically needful of quantitative answers. It is the purpose of this chapter to point out some of the challenging uses to which EMG can be applied and also to suggest minimum requirements for instrumentation to serve those applications.

BASIC CONCEPTS OF ELECTRICAL PHENOMENA AND ELECTROMYOGRAPHY

It has been known, at least since the middle of the nineteenth century, that the contraction of muscle tissue is accompanied by an electrical change that can be recorded and measured. The electrical change is called a *muscle action potential*, and the recording of muscle action potentials (or their currents) is call *electromyography*. The muscle action potential arises at the muscle cell membrane (or sarcolemma) and passes lengthwise in wavelike form, as the fiber is stimulated to contract. The science of recording and analyzing muscle action potentials probably received its greatest impetus in the related science of *electrocardiography*, in which the events of the cardiac cycle are examined for abnormality. Physicians also use electromyography clinically, in the diagnosis of various types of muscular diseases (e.g., spasticity, paralysis, etc.).

Most EMG instrumentation and procedures have been developed for the use of physicians in diagnosing abnormal neuromuscular function and may be thought of as *qualitative* rather than *quantitative* in nature since the greatest concern is with the recording and analysis of the *wave form* of the *muscle action potential* (MAP) from single discrete motor units.

This is the area of greatest interest to physicians and medical researchers who investigate disease states in which changes in the activity of individual motor units can be observed (various paralytic and spastic conditions) as a means to diagnosis. Obviously, recording single motor units requires needle electrodes that contact only one motor unit or, at most, several motor units at a time. On the other hand, this type of electromyography does not require great sensitivity since the magnitude of the muscle action potential at the site of the fibers producing it is in the range of 100 to 3,000 microvolts (millionths of a volt).

Quantitative electromyography is the study of the amount of electrical activity that is present in a given muscle under varying conditions. Obviously, it is not electrical activity per se that is of interest here; rather, it is the fact that EMG recordings accurately reflect what the muscle is doing at a level of sensitivity at which palpation and other methods fail to produce evidence.

Investigators in exercise physiology and kinesiology (sometimes physical therapy and physical medicine) are mainly concerned with occurrences in the whole muscle rather than in isolated motor units. For this reason, surface electrodes on the skin over the belly or the motor point of the muscle are used. Thus the firing of many motor units is observed simultaneously, and a better statistical sampling is had than by the use of needle electrodes. This results, however, in a wave form that is a summation of the randomly organized activity of the many motor units observed, and it tells us nothing about any one motor unit. Also, the action potentials—in passing through the muscle tissue, fascia, subcutaneous fat, and skin—are severely attenuated (decreased in magnitude). Therefore, if we wish to know what is going on in a resting or relatively inactive muscle, we need extremely high sensitivity (the author has recorded meaningful differences in activity of resting muscles in which the difference between two conditions is less than one microvolt). The difference between recordings of individual motor units with needle electrodes and recordings of summated potentials from many motor units with surface electrodes is shown in figure 14.1.

It is important to realize that when many motor units fire randomly, some will by chance fire simultaneously, and the size of the wave form recorded at that point will be larger. Furthermore, as a muscle is required to produce more tension, recruitment of ever-greater numbers of motor units occurs; by the laws of chance, more will fire simultaneously, and the wave form will grow larger in amplitude as more tension is produced.

The information to be gained from the pattern of motor unit spikes shown in the right hand side of figure 14.1 is immediately obvious. We can count the spikes and measure the amplitude, but we have absolutely no quantitative knowledge of what the whole muscle is doing. Only what is going on in one motor unit. As it turns out, the physiological significance of the electrical activity in the total gross muscle rests on

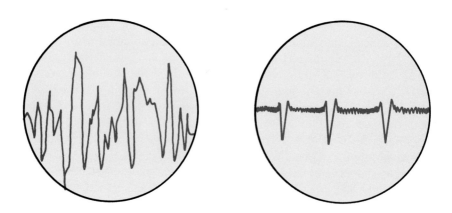

Figure 14-1. Differences between recordings of single motor-unit potentials with needle electrodes (right) and summated potentials from many motor units with surface electrodes (left).

the mean amplitude of the summated MAPs. The problem here is immediately recognized if we pose the question: what is the mean amplitude of the summated MAPs shown in the left side of figure 14.1? What do we measure to get a true mean value for a function which varies constantly and randomly over time as does the *interference pattern* (so called from electronics parlance) of figure 14.1? To do this requires integration (a procedure of the calculus). This concept of integration is depicted in figure 14.2. First, the integration process can be applied only to the electrically positive or negative halves of the spikes because otherwise the end result would be zero with the positive being balanced out by the negative aspects of the wave form. Thus, as the first step shown in figure 14.2(b) we have eliminated the negative swinging part of the spikes. Next, we must think of the spikes as having area as in figure 14.2(c). The dimensions of this area are: vertically, microvolts of electrical activity (uV) and horizontally, time in fractions of a second. The next step is to convert the area under the random spikes into a neat geometric figure such as a rectangle whose area equals height times length (or in this case uV times seconds). This conversion to the rectangle is accomplished by *planimetry* (tracing the curve with an engineering instrument which provides the area under any curve). Now we have the area of figure 14.2(d) in an approximate rectangle whose dimensions are a height of 1.0 uV and a time of 0.40 seconds thus

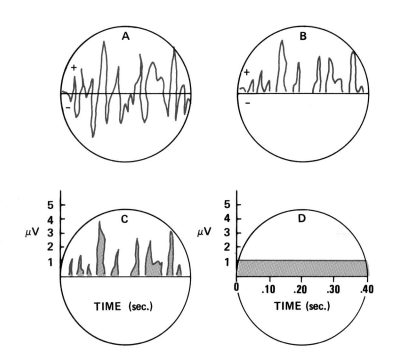

Figure 14-2. Integration of muscle action potentials to get true mean value of their amplitude.

providing an area of 1.0 times 0.40 or 0.40 uV seconds. This is the reading we would obtain from the planimeter. To get the mean uV level then we need only divide as follows.

$$\frac{uV \times sec}{sec} \text{ or } \frac{1.0 \text{ uV} \times 0.40 \text{ sec}}{0.40 \text{ sec}} = 1.0 \text{ uV}$$

So that we can now say that over the 0.40 second observation period the mean amplitude of the MAPs was 1.0 uV. Fortunately electronic integrators are available which accomplish the whole procedure without even the necessity for planimetry.

At this point it is imperative to recognize the need for integration because only through this procedure can accurate data regarding the physiological import of the electrical activity in the muscle be evaluated. It should be obvious by now that even such a tedious process as measuring spike amplitudes is of little value for precise data because the amplitude is constantly and randomly varying and to get a true mean one must know over what period of time the spike has acted. A fat spike is more important than a thin spike of equal amplitude in determining the true mean value.

Lippold (11) has found correlations of 0.93 to 0.99 between muscle tension and integrated EMG recordings from surface electrodes. Figure 14.3 shows the relationship between force of contraction and electrical activity when muscle tension is increased in the right elbow flexors.

The data in figure 14.3 have been corroborated by many investigators, and this issue is not in doubt; however, there is disagreement about the source of electrical activity that is recorded at the very low levels (0.0 to 10.0 uV) of resting muscle (which is also involved in the question of postural tonus). Hayes (10) regarded this as *tissue noise* and

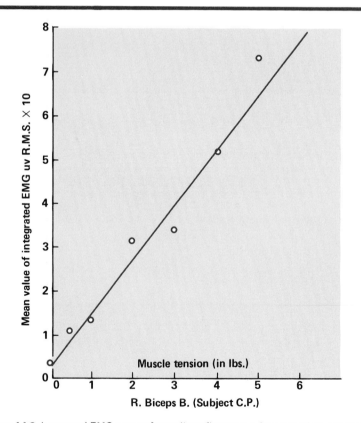

Figure 14-3. Integrated EMG output from elbow flexors as a function of muscle tension.

as separate and distinct from MAPs because he had no evidence that this low-level activity was related to muscular activity; but he also found differences that were related to the physiological state of the muscle. Other investigators appear to have recorded thermal noise (due to molecular activity) because they had not removed the horny layer of skin.

It seems, however, that much of the work at low levels has suffered from at least one of the following deficiencies:

1. Lack of sensitivity
2. Lack of integration (mathematical accumulation of data over a time period)
3. High source resistance that obscured or confounded the observed data
4. Lack of correction for the magnitude of the integrated signal due to noise factors.

For these reasons, equipment was developed for the author's laboratory (fig. 14.4) that simplifies the integration procedure and eliminates all four deficiencies. This equipment will record integrated EMG

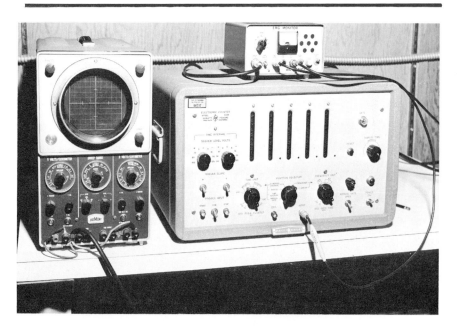

Figure 14-4. Equipment used in the author's laboratory to enable simple and precise evaluation of integrated muscle-action potentials. The basic noise level when the subject is in an electrically shielded room is considerably below one microvolt.

potentials with a sensitivity of 0.3 microvolts. Using this equipment, evidence has accumulated that the electrical activity from muscle tissue —even at the lowest levels—is indeed entirely similar to that at the higher levels. Figure 14.5 shows the high relationship between muscle tension in the elbow flexors and electrical output at the very lowest tension levels when all possible care has been taken to reduce electrode resistance to an essential minimum.

At our present state of knowledge, it is not possible to discriminate between electrical activity of the alpha motor neuron and its typical skeletal muscle fibers and the gamma efferent and its intrafusal fibers using surface electrodes, but evidence indicates that innervation of the intrafusal fibers contributes very little to the production of tension in mammalian muscle.

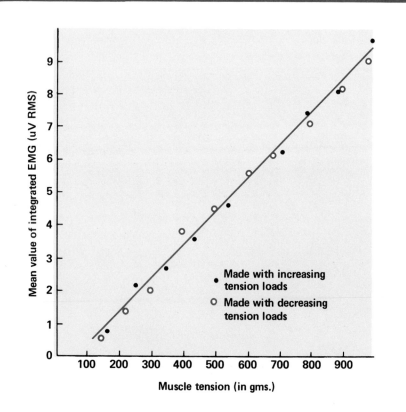

Figure 14-5. Integrated EMG output from elbow flexors as a function of muscle tension.

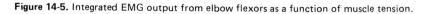

For these reasons the remainder of this chapter, and all further discussion of electromyographic data in this text, will rest upon the hypothesis that all electrical activity recorded over skeletal muscles is related to the total motor-unit activity in that muscle at any given time.

APPLICATIONS OF EMG TO PHYSIOLOGICAL PROBLEMS

Estimation of Tension Developed within a Muscle. Many situations arise in the physiology of exercise laboratory when it is desired to know the tension developed within a given muscle. It has been shown by Lippold and coworkers that the EMG voltage is proportional to the force of contraction in isometric contraction (11) and that in movements of constant velocity the electrical activity is proportional to the tension developed. In movements of constant tension the electrical activity is proportional to the velocity (constant velocity) (1). This work has been extended in our laboratory to include accelerated movements (2) and found that even here the electrical activity is proportional to the *effort impulse value*, a measurement of effort suggested by Starr (12). Thus we may conclude that in any kind of physical activity, a reasonably good estimate of the tension or effort developed within the muscle can be obtained through appropriate EMG instrumentation and techniques (integration is necessary of course). This would be difficult if not impossible to attain by any other means.

As an example of such use the reader is referred to chapter three in which the author presented EMG data to resolve the disagreement as to the involvement of the extensor muscles in the maintenance of the erect posture.

Estimation of Strength and Tonus. Where the musculature is relatively normal, measurement of maximal strength by cable tension, strain guage, or dynamometer provides one dimension which is unquestionably related to the functional state of the tissue. As a *physiological measurement,* however, maximal strength is notoriously contaminated by psychological factors such as motivation. Muscle tonus is another dimension for evaluating muscle function. Although this term is widely used by members of all the professions dealing with muscle tissue, a definition which satisfactorily encompasses all the experimental evidence available does not as yet exist.

A very interesting concept for evaluation of the functional state of muscle has been proposed (6, 9) in terms of the *Efficiency of Electrical Activity* (EEA). The concept is illustrated in figure 14.6. It is obvious that the stronger individual (flatter slope) needs less activation (electrical activity) for any given muscle loading. The author has shown

that this EMG slope or EEA as plotted in figure 14.6 is well related
(in young subjects) to measured strength ($r = -.75$ to $-.90$). The EEA
is also sensitive to hypertrophy and atrophy of muscle through use and
disuse as shown in figures 14.7 and 14.9. Figure 14.8 is of interest in
that is shows the cross-education strength effect clearly on the unexercised arm, while also showing that no hypertrophy (no change in EEA)
has occurred, thus suggesting that the cross-education effect is brought
about through neural changes, unaccompanied by any hypertrophy. This
requires further investigation.

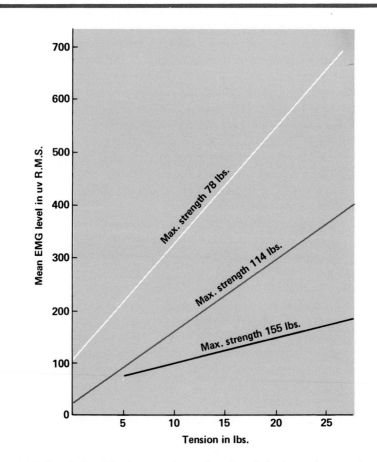

Figure 14-6. Electrical activity in a muscle as a function of the force of contraction. Note
the differences on the rate of increase in activity between subjects of varying levels of
strength.

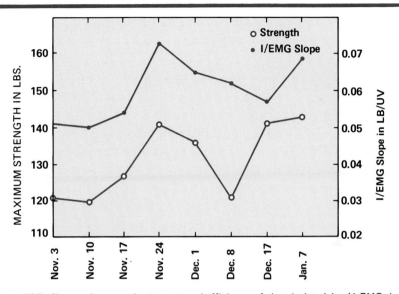

Figure 14-7. Changes in strength ⊙——⊙ and efficiency of electrical activity (1 EMG slope coefficient) ●——● as a result of intensive weight training of the right elbow flexors (subject D.Y.). (From deVries, H.A. *Am. J. Phy. Med.* 47:10, 1968.)

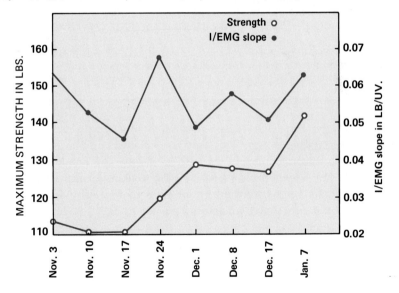

Figure 14-8. Changes in strength ⊙——⊙ and efficiency of electrical activity (1/EMG slope coefficient) ●——● in the left elbow flexors (untrained control) as a result of training the right elbow flexors (subject D.Y.). (From deVries, H.A. *Am. J. Phy. Med.* 47:10, 1968.)

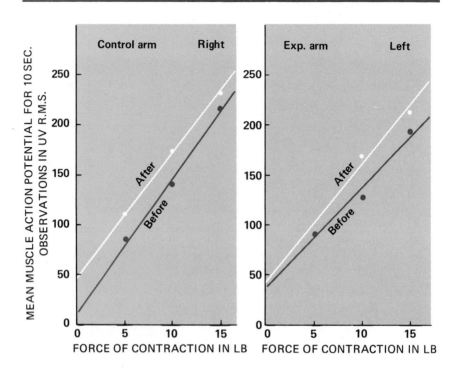

Figure 14-9. Changes in the experimental and control elbow flexors as the result of placing the left elbow flexors in a cast for four weeks. *Left:* right biceps (control arm). *Right:* left biceps (experimental arm). (From deVries, H.A. *Am. J. Phy. Med.* 47:10, 1968.)

Interestingly, the EEA is not predictive of strength in older men, aged fifty to eighty-six (8). This can be explained on the basis that in young people maximal muscle strength is largely the result of two determinants: (1) a *genotypic factor* related to muscle mass, and (2) a *phenotypic factor* related to the level of fiber hypertrophy. In older men it seems that the only muscular determinant of strength having predictive value is the genotypic factor of muscle mass, the factor of fiber hypertrophy no longer being involved in the more sedentary older population.

EMG Estimation of Endurance–Fatigue Parameters. When a muscle contracts isometrically against constant force, the electrical activity in that muscle increases with time as shown in figure 14.10. This phenomenon is thought to be the result of the fatigue process impairment of muscle fiber function so that recruitment must take place to compensate for the constantly decreasing force available per fiber. If the fatigue

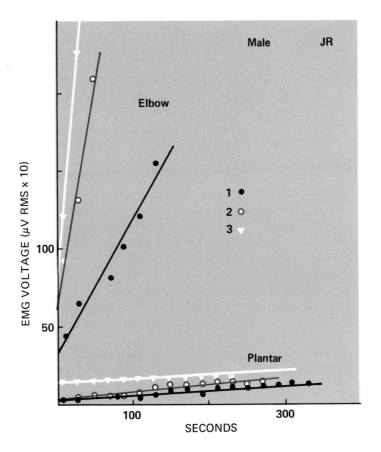

Figure 14-10. EMG fatigue curves in three test runs with increasing fatigue of elbow flexors and plantar flexors. (From deVries, H.A. *Am. J. Phy. Med.* 47:175, 1968.)

process is brought about quickly with loads of thirty to fifty percent MVC, the plot of EMG voltage as a function of time usually approximates linearity (later data in the laboratory show the curve to be an exponential with a considerable period of approximate linearity). The slope of this curve can be used under appropriate conditions for estimating the rate at which muscle fatigues (7). Test-retest reliability of such curves was found to be $r = .93$. The validity of this approach was evaluated by correlating the slope coefficient of the fatigue curve against measured maximal endurance time and the correlations were found to be $r = .79$ and $.82$ using isometric tensions of forty and fifty percent of MVC, respectively. The important point to remember here is that in plotting either the EEA curve or the fatigue curve only a few data points are required which can be obtained without the subject going beyond twenty-five to fifty percent of his maximum capacity in either case. Obviously, this eliminates the necessity for the usually invalid assumption that the investigator has obtained a true maximum effort from a subject under testing conditions since motivation and other psychological factors are no longer pertinent.

It is of interest to note in figure 14.10 the dramatic difference in the rate at which flexor muscles fatigue compared with the extensor muscles involved in posture.

EMG Estimation of the Level of Neuromuscular Tension (Relaxation). The nature of the author's work in this area has already been cited in the preceding chapter. At this point it is necessary only to describe the instrumentation requirements for accurate measurement of MAPs in resting muscle tissue for purposes of evaluation of the state of relaxation in the laboratory.

To begin, the instrumentation must be capable of a sensitivity of 1.0 uV per cm pen or scope deflection or its equivalent. This can only be achieved under rigorously controlled conditions which will usually require the services of a skilled electronics technician. The EMG amplifier must be of very high quality and the frequency spectrum must be closed down to about ten to 200 Hz. An electronic system for integration is an absolute *must*, and preferably by analog-digital conversion for reasons of both precision and simplicity of readout. The subject must be tested in an electronically shielded screen room sometimes called a *Faraday cage*. The electrodes should preferably be of the silver-silver chloride type to eliminate junction potential artifact, although if no movement is to occur the author has successfully used suction-cup electrodes of the type commonly used on infants for taking electrocardiograms. The electrode lead should be bipolar to take advantage of common-mode rejection factors built into the amplifier. Finally the electrode sites must be prepared with great care so that the source impedance is of the order of 1,000 to 2,000 ohms. Only under these conditions can precise measurements of resting MAPs be made. For more detail on suitable instrumentation the reader is referred to reference (4).

EMG Observation of Localized Muscle Spasm Related to Muscle Soreness. The requirements with respect to instrumentation are identical to those discussed above for measuring the state of relaxation, with the important exception that unipolar electrode leads should be used (5). This area is of sufficient concern to physical educators and coaches so that an entire chapter will be devoted to this subject (see chap. 15).

Observation of Other Physiological Phenomena by EMG. Many interesting physiological phenomena are mirrored in the electrical activity of the skeletal muscles. One of the more easily observed is that of the increase in electrical activity in irrelevant muscles when any one skeletal muscle is strained. Thus if we load the right elbow flexor group to fifty to seventy-five percent or more of MVC, one can detect measurable activity of at least five uV in the previously inactive left elbow flexors. The author has shown that even straining the eyes to read fine print raises the electrical activity in the elbow flexors by about 100 percent (3).

Another interesting demonstration which the author provides routinely for his students is the effect of hyperventilation upon the activity of irrelevant forearm muscles. The *blowing off* of CO_2 as discussed in chapter seven and eight results in a rising pH with concomitant greater irritability of muscle tissue which is displayed by increases of electrical activity of two to fivefold (best shown in the most peripheral flexor muscles). This, of course, is the reason for the commonly observed tendency of the fingers to curl (flex) toward a fist during moderate to severe hyperventilation.

Another use which has been made of this type of EMG is the observation of the onset of the *shivering response.* It must be noted, however, that all of these interesting phenomena alluded to in this section require an order of sensitivity beyond that which is ordinarily available in apparatus designed for the physician because he doesn't need it. Furthermore, without integration procedures, even a change in wave form which doubles the energy is not always easily discernible on the oscilloscope.

SUMMARY

1. Whenever a muscle is innervated, a *muscle action potential* (MAP) or potentials result which can be recorded and measured by *electromyography* (EMG).

2. By recording MAPs a quantitative measurement of muscle activation can be made. The author refers to this aspect of EMG as *quantitative EMG* in contradistinction to the methods and instrumentation commonly applied by the physician who is usually more concerned with the observation of the *wave form* of MAPs from single motor units.

3. When surface electrodes are used in EMG the *interference pattern* observed on the oscilloscope is the result of the summation of several or many different motor units firing randomly in time.

4. To make meaningful use of these data from the interference pattern requires integration procedures to calculate true mean amplitudes. Integration can be accomplished by *planimetry* or by electronic integrators which are discussed in the text.

5. That the integrals so achieved (or the true mean amplitude calculated from them) have physiological significance has been well verified in various laboratories.

6. The methods of quantitative electromyography have been applied to many aspects of exercise physiology:
   a. It has been shown that the tension developed within a muscle can be estimated (1) under isometric tension, (2) under constant velocity movement, and (3) under accelerated movements.
   b. Strength and functional quality of muscle tissue can be evaluated in young subjects by the slope of the EMG voltage regression upon force of contraction.
   c. The endurance (or fatigue rates) of muscles can be objectively evaluated by the slope of the EMG voltage regression upon time when the subject holds an isometric contraction of forty or fifty percent of maximal voluntary contraction.
   d. The only objective measurement of the state of neuromuscular tension (relaxation) presently available is that of measuring resting MAPs with EMG instrumentation of extremely high sensitivity.
   e. Highly sensitive EMG instrumentation also renders visible the reactions of muscle tissue to such homeostatic displacements as occur during hyperventilation.

REFERENCES

1. Bigland, B., and Lippold, O. C. J. 1954. The relation between force, velocity and integrated electrical activity in human muscles. *Journal of Physiology* 123:214-24.
2. Damon, E. L. An experimental investigation on the equating of isometric, concentric and eccentric muscular efforts. In preparation.
3. deVries, H. A. 1962. Neuromuscular tension and its relief. *Journal of Association for Physical and Mental Rehabilitation* 16:86-88.
4. ———. 1965. Muscle tonus in postural muscles. *American Journal of Physical Medicine* 44:275-91.

5. ———. 1966. Quantitative electromyographic investigation of the spasm theory of muscle pain. *American Journal of Physical Medicine* 45:119-34.

6. ———. 1968a. Efficiency of electrical activity as a physiological measure of the functional state of muscle tissue. *American Journal of Physical Medicine* 47:10-22.

7. ———. 1968b. Method for evaluation of muscle fatigue and endurance from electromyographic fatigue curves. *American Journal of Physical Medicine* 47:125-35.

8. deVries, H. A., and Lersten, K. C. 1970. Efficiency of electrical activity in the muscles of older men. *American Journal of Physical Medicine* 49: 107-11.

9. Fischer, A., and Merhautova, J. 1961. Electromyographic manifestations of individual stages of adapted sports technique. In *Health and fitness in the modern world,* ch. 13. Chicago: The Athletic Institute.

10. Hayes, Keith J. 1960. Wave analysis of tissue noise and muscle action potentials. *Journal of Applied Physiology* 15:749-52.

11. Lippold, O. C. J. 1952. The relation between integrated action potentials in a human muscle and its isometric tension. *Journal of Physiology* 117: 492-99.

12. Starr, I. 1951. New units for muscular work. *Journal of Applied Physiology* 4:21-29.

15 Physiology of Muscle Soreness — Cause and Relief

It is common experience that physical overexertion results in pain. In general, two types of pain are associated with severe muscular efforts: (1) pain during and immediately after exercise, which may persist for several hours, and (2) a localized soreness, which usually does not appear until twenty-four to forty-eight hours later.

The first type of pain is probably due to the diffusible end products of metabolism acting upon pain receptors (9). It is most likely that this pain is caused by either the potassium diffusion outward across the muscle cell membrane into the tissue spaces during contraction, or by the lactic acid formation from localized areas of ischemia. Both processes are known to occur, and each can produce the pain; but this is not a very serious problem because it is of short duration and is relieved by cessation of exercise or by short periods of rest.

The second type of pain can become chronic under certain conditions, and is at least annoying enough to constitute a deterrent to further exercise. The author has seen the *shin splint* problem develop to such a degree that an athlete has given up athletic activity rather than endure this nagging pain. This localized and delayed muscle soreness, or *lameness,* sometimes called a *myositis,* is often attributed to microscopic tears in muscle or connective tissues. It is this second type of pain that is important, and that concerns us in this chapter.

The hypothesis of torn muscle or connective tissues was probably first presented by Hough (11), at the turn of the century. It must be emphasized that he presented no direct evidence for this theory, nor has anyone since actually demonstrated the existence of torn tissue in relation to this type of soreness. While there is no question that violent trauma can result in the rupture of a muscle, most of the exercise that is known to result in soreness does not fall in this category. Furthermore, it is somewhat illogical to postulate that a tissue has been structurally damaged by the very function for which it is specifically differentiated.

A SPASM THEORY AS AN EXPLANATION OF DELAYED LOCALIZED SORENESS

A better hypothesis for the cause of soreness is suggested by observation of typical muscle fatigue curves in excised muscles (fig. 3.4, p. 41). It is readily seen that, in addition to the decrement in amplitude of contraction with increasing fatigue, an increasing inability to achieve complete relaxation is typical, and, significantly, this may end in contracture. Evidence (21) has shown the same phenomenon to occur in the intact human muscle. Petajan and Eagan interpreted their findings as showing the tendency of the untrained muscle after intense exercise to remain in the contracted condition since the increased intramuscular pressure of exercise limits the availability of factors important to the recovery process. For these reasons, the author has provided a more attractive hypothesis: the delayed localized soreness that occurs after unaccustomed exercise is caused by tonic, localized spasm of motor units.

Theoretical Basis for a Spasm Theory. A rationale based upon considerable physiological evidence can be constructed to support this hypothesis. First, it has been shown that exercise above a minimal level causes a degree of ischemia in the active muscles (9, 22). Second, ischemia can cause muscle pain, probably by transfer of *P substance* (15) across the muscle cell membrane into the tissue fluid, from which it gains access to pain nerve endings. Third, the pain brings about a reflex tonic muscle contraction, which prolongs the ischemia, and a vicious cycle is born. Evidence has been presented (20) that supports the concept of spasm caused by painful stimuli. This hypothesis agrees with the thinking of medical clinicians, who have suggested that many of the aches and pains of organic disease and anxiety states result from muscle spasm (10, p. 363).

From the standpoint of the physical educator and athletic coach, the spasm theory becomes even more attractive in that the vicious cycle hypothesized above has a vulnerable aspect that allows application of simple corrective measures for relief. Competitive swimmers and swimming coaches know that swimmer's cramp (gastrocnemius) is promptly relieved by gently forcing the cramped muscle into its longest possible state and holding it there for a moment, and this relief of cramp by stretching has also been demonstrated experimentally (20). It is very likely that the inverse myotatic reflex (see chapter four), which originates in the Golgi tendon organs, is the basis for this relief.

PHYSIOLOGY UNDERLYING STATIC STRETCHING

To test the spasm theory, several different lines of investigation have been pursued in the author's laboratory. First, it was hypothesized that, if the spasm theory had merit, the simple stretching technique that relieves a swimmer's cramp in the calf muscle should also be effective in providing prevention and relief for any sore muscle that can be put on stretch. Therefore a stretching technique was designed to take best possible advantage of the following neurophysiological concepts (see chapter four).

1. There are two components to the spindle reflex: phasic and static (14, 19).
2. The amount and rate of the phasic response in the spindle reflex are proportional to the amount and rate of stretching (19).

3. The Golgi tendon receptor organs have a relatively high threshold, but, when innervated, bring about inhibition not only of the muscle in which the receptors are situated but the entire functional muscle group (17).
4. Steady stretch depresses the monosynaptic response, even when the tendon organs are not active (12).
5. The amplitude of EMG in large human muscles characteristically diminishes when they are stretched (13).
6. Item five is related to tendon organ activity in human muscle (16).

The author's system of *static stretching* was developed around the six concepts outlined above: a body position is held that locks the joints around the sore muscle in a position of greatest possible muscle length and with as little concomitant muscle activity as possible. (Many yoga exercises have been found useful since they use the same principle.) This procedure results in the least possible reflex stimulation to the involved muscle. A *bouncing stretch,* on the other hand, would invoke stretch reflexes whose end result (contraction of the sore, stretched muscle) would be undesirable. The duration used in most cases has been two sets of two minutes with a one-minute rest intervening. Figure 15.1 illustrates the stretching principle for the gastrocnemius muscle.

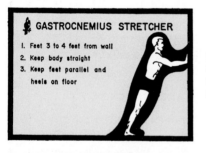

Figure 15-1. Illustration of the "static stretching" method as applied in the author's laboratory for relief of experimentally caused soreness (and also used for accidental soreness).

EXPERIMENTAL EVIDENCE SUPPORTING THE SPASM THEORY

The first experimental study to test the spasm theory (3) was done on seventeen college-age subjects, who did a four-minute standard exercise (designed to produce soreness) that consisted of wrist hyperextension against a resistance of 9½ pounds. Both arms were exercised simultaneously and immediately after exercise, and, at intervals thereafter, the wrist flexors and extensors of the nondominant arm were stretched by static methods. The dominant arm, which was not stretched, developed significantly greater levels of soreness for the group. The greatest soreness levels were found twenty-four and forty-eight hours after the exercise. The difference in soreness between stretched and unstretched arms was significant for both of these observations.

During the same period electromyographic equipment was designed to achieve very high sensitivity so that small differences in resting muscle tissue activity could be observed. Use of this instrumentation showed that static stretching markedly reduced resting EMG activity in six of seven subjects who had chronic muscular problems of the shin splint type (fig. 15.2). Symptomatic relief seemed to parallel lowered EMG values (4). The subject who was atypical showed a marked rise in electrical activity and increased levels of pain. It was hypothesized that in this case structural damage had indeed occurred—a truly ruptured muscle.

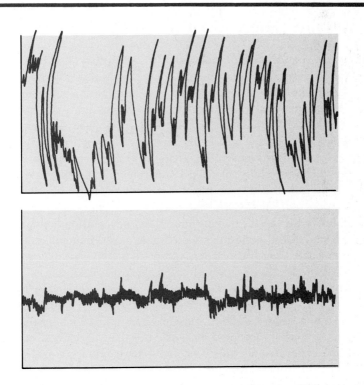

Figure 15-2. Effects of static stretching on muscle soreness of the "shin splint" type. Upper trace: electrical activity before stretching. Lower trace: electrical activity after stretching. Symptomatic relief accompanied the decrease in electrical activity.

This introduced the interesting possibility that ruptured muscle could be differentiated from those that are merely in spasm by applying static stretch and observing the EMG changes. To test this hypothesis, a series of eighteen subjects—three of whom had medically verified ruptured muscles—was recorded by the same technique. Of the fifteen subjects who showed no evidence of a torn muscle, thirteen had lowered levels of electrical activity after static stretching, and the three subjects with torn muscles showed higher levels (5).

In the most recent experiment (with more sophisticated EMG equipment, described in chapter fourteen), it has been possible to bring about muscular soreness experimentally and to relieve it by static stretching, with the entire series of physiological changes in electrical state of the muscle under electromyographic observation (8). Figure 15.3 illustrates the course of events in fifteen subjects (eleven male, four female) who did arm curls (ten sets with ten repetition maximum) with the right arm. The left arm was unexercised and thus furnished a control for comparison.

It can be seen from figure 15.3 that the electrical activity in both exercised and unexercised arms decreased as the result of the exercise. This is in agreement with previous data from the author's laboratory that demonstrated an improved ability to achieve voluntary relaxation after exercise (chapter thirteen). The relationship between the soreness that was present after forty-eight hours and the increased electrical activity (evidence of increased muscular activity or local spasm) is clearly shown. Over the biceps, activity increased ninety-eight percent, and over the brachialis (this included some biceps activity) by sixty-two percent, when soreness appeared. The relief of soreness by static stretching is also shown. Immediately after the forty-eight-hour EMG observation, both arms were stretched, and EMG recordings were again taken immediately after the stretching. Again, large decreases in electrical activity paralleled the symptomatic relief.

It would seem there is enough evidence that the Hough hypothesis for etiology of delayed local muscle soreness is untenable. It is unfortunate that this theory of "torn muscle fibers and/or connective tissues" has been so widely accepted because this has undoubtedly militated against any experimental work to achieve prevention or relief.

The rise in electrical activity in the exercised muscle and the relatively unchanged activity in the paired, unexercised muscle is difficult to explain on any other basis than a tonic local muscle spasm. The spasm could indeed accompany or result from torn tissues, however, if this were the case, relief from stretching would not occur because torn tissues would produce pain reflexes that would result in *higher*, not *lower*, muscle activity. Thus the spasm theory best fits all observed data. Most importantly, application of this theory allows us to assume a degree of control over the soreness phenomenon, in both prevention and relief.

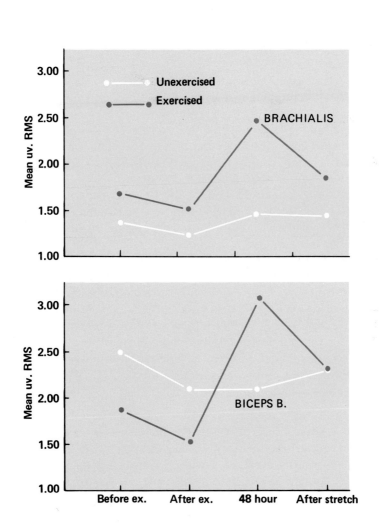

Figure 15-3. Effects of static stretching on experimentally induced soreness. Note that the electrical activity is virtually brought back to pre-soreness values by the static stretching. Symptomatic relief usually parallels the decreased electrical activity.

FACTORS IN THE PREVENTION OF SORENESS

Acceptance of the spasm theory allows us to bring theory and practice to bear on the problem of preventing this annoying phenomenon.

Warm-up. It has long been the popular opinion of coaches and athletes that *warm-up processes* serve to prevent muscle soreness. Experimental evidence is very meager, however, probably because no one cares to set up an experiment in which the subjects may be injured. All that is known of muscle physiology tends to support the need for warm-up as a protective measure.

In an experiment in which the author investigated the effects of flexibility upon O_2 consumption during 100-yard dashes, subjects ran under conditions of no warm-up, as a control situation, compared with a static stretching flexibility warm-up. In this experiment, two of the four subjects developed sore muscles as the result of running without warm-up. This would certainly seem to support prevailing opinion and theories of muscle physiology on the necessity for warm-up.

Progression in Training Programs. In the many experiments and pilot studies conducted in the author's laboratory, one factor especially stands out in regard to muscle soreness: soreness seems to occur only when large overloads of intensity or endurance are imposed upon an individual. In fact, one of the difficult problems to overcome in setting up systematic experimentation was development of standard exercises that would result in high levels of soreness in large percentages of the subjects. Thus if sore muscles are to be avoided, a *gradual increase* of work load should be planned, so that no one workout represents too great an overload for the physical condition of the musculature.

Types of Activity and Soreness. Some types of muscular activity are more likely to result in sore muscles than others. Activities most likely to result in soreness are:

1. Vigorous muscle contractions while a muscle is in a shortened condition, this often results in muscle cramp (20).
2. Muscle contractions that involve jerky movements. In this case, a muscle is temporarily overloaded when a full load is placed upon it before recruitment of sufficient motor units has occurred.
3. Muscle contractions that involve repetitions of the same movement over a long period of time (endurance imposed upon a limited number of muscle fibers). This repetitious movement causes even more soreness if a slight rest interval is allowed between repetitions because the bout can be disproportionately increased in length, and a greater total work load is demanded.
4. Bouncing-type stretching movements. At the end of a ballistic motion,

the movement is stopped by the muscle and connective tissues, which brings about reflex contraction at the time the muscle is being forcefully elongated.

Static Stretching. On many occasions it is impossible to avoid some of the conditions that predispose toward sore muscles, but in such situations a brief (ten-minute) period of static stretching after the workout can bring about a significant degree of prevention. (A well-rounded static stretching program for this purpose is described in the chapter on flexibility, p. 431.) In any event, application of the principles of kinesiology will enable a professionally trained coach or physical educator to design the exercise for a specific situation.

For example, in a running situation where shin splints may be expected, the muscles involved are the flexors of the ankle joint. Consequently, the athletes are put into a kneeling position, with the ankles extended (plantar flexed), and the full weight of the body is brought to bear—gently—by rocking back onto the ankles. This position is held a minimum of one minute, with *no bouncing*.

RELIEF OF MUSCULAR SORENESS

When a muscle becomes painful twenty-four to forty-eight hours (or more) after unaccustomed exercise, relief can usually be provided by the following procedure.

1. Determine (by palpation) which muscle or muscles are involved.
2. Determine the nature of the activity that brought about the situation.
3. Determine the muscular attachments of the involved muscle or muscles by consulting a textbook of anatomy or kinesiology.
4. Devise a simple position in which the attachments are held as far apart as possible with the least possible effort.
5. Have the subject hold this position for two-minute periods, with a one-minute rest period intervening. If the pain is severe, this should be repeated two or three times daily.

This procedure has proven effective even in chronic muscular problems (4).

SEVERE MUSCLE PROBLEMS

None of the foregoing discussion should be construed as suggesting that all painful muscles are due to muscle spasm; nor is it suggested that muscles cannot, under certain conditions, be torn (ruptured). It is obvious that a muscle can be put under such great, sudden strain that some of the tissue exceeds its elastic limits and rupture may occur, but this probably occurs much less often than athletes and coaches seem to think.

In any event, muscular pain that is severe, or that persists longer than a few days, should be diagnosed by a physician as should any muscle injury in which deformation, swelling, or inflammation occurs.

SUMMARY

1. Two types of muscle pain result from overexertion: (1) pain during and immediately after exercise, which is probably due to diffusion of metabolites into the tissue spaces, and (2) a localized, delayed soreness that appears in twenty-four to forty-eight hours.
2. The spasm theory explains the localized delayed soreness as follows: (1) exercise causes localized ischemia; (2) ischemia causes pain; (3) pain brings about greater reflex motor activity; (4) greater motor activity creates greater local muscle tension, which causes ischemia; (5) a vicious cycle is born.
3. The spasm theory is supported by the following evidence: (1) static stretching procedures, which are effective in relieving a cramp, also furnish a degree of prevention against soreness; (2) where muscle soreness exists, electromyography shows markedly higher electrical activity; (3) when a muscle is stretched, as for relief of cramp, symptomatic relief is usually seen, along with decreased electrical activity; (4) muscular soreness has been produced, and relieved, under experimentally controlled conditions. EMG observations showed the predicted rise with soreness and decline with relief.
4. Several factors are important in the prevention of sore muscles: (1) proper *warm-up* is essential; (2) workouts should be designed with *progressive* increases in work load; (3) activity that involves vigorous muscle contraction with the muscle in a shortened condition, jerky movements, long-term repetition of a movement, or bouncing-type stretching is most likely to produce muscular soreness.
5. *Static stretching* has been found to be effective in providing both prevention and relief of muscular soreness.

REFERENCES

1. Barcroft, H., and Millen, J. L. E. 1939. The blood flow through muscle during sustained contraction. *Journal of Physiology* 97:17-31.
2. Davis, J. F. 1959. *Manual of surface Electromyography*. W.A.D.C. Technical Report 59-184, project 7184, task 71580; McGill University, Allen Memorial Institute of Psychiatry, Montreal, Canada.

3. deVries, H. A. 1961a. Electromyographic observations of the effects of static stretching upon muscular distress. *Research Quarterly AAHPER* 32: 468-79.

4. ———. 1961b. Prevention of muscular distress after exercise. *Research Quarterly of AAHPER* 32:177-85.

5. ———. 1961c. Treatment of muscular distress in athletes. *Proceedings of the 65th Annual College Physical Education Association*, Kansas City, 28 December 1961.

6. ———. 1962. Evaluation of static stretching procedures for improvement of flexibility. *Research Quarterly of AAHPER* 33:222-29.

7. ———. 1965. Muscle tonus in postural muscles. *American Journal of Physical Medicine* 44:275-91.

8. ———. 1966. Quantitative electromyographic investigation of the spasm theory of muscle pain. *American Journal of Physical Medicine* 45:119-34.

9. Dorpat, T. L., and Holmes, T. H. 1955. Mechanisms of skeletal muscle pain and fatigue. *Archives of Neurology and Psychiatry* 74:628-40.

10. Fulton, J. F. 1955. *A textbook of physiology.* Philadelphia: W. B. Saunders Co.

11. Hough, T. 1902. Erogographic studies on muscular soreness. *American Journal of Physiology* 7:76-81.

12. Hunt, C. C. 1952. The effect of stretch receptors from muscle on the discharge of motoneurons. *Journal of Physiology* 117:359-79.

13. Inman, V. T.; Ralston, H. J.; Saunders, J. B.; Feinstein, B.; and Wright, E. W., Jr. 1952. Relation of human electromyogram to muscular tension. *EEG and Clinical Neurophysiology* 4:187-94.

14. Katz, B. 1950. Depolarization of sensory terminals and the initiation of impulses in the muscle spindle. *Journal of Physiology* 111:261-82.

15. Lewis, T. 1942. *Pain.* New York: The Macmillan Co.

16. Libet, B.; Feinstein, B.; and Wright, E. W., Jr. 1955. Tendon afferents in autogenetic inhibition. *Federation Proceedings* 14:92.

17. McCouch, G. P.; Deering, I. D.; and Stewart, W. B. 1950. Inhibition of knee jerk from tendon spindles of crureus. *Journal of Neurophysiology* 13: 343-50.

18. Morehouse, L. E., and Miller, A. T. 1963. *Physiology of exercise.* St. Louis: C. V. Mosby Co.

19. Mountcastle, V. B. 1961. Reflex activity of the spinal cord. In *Medical physiology*, ed. P. Bard, ch. 60. St. Louis: C. V. Mosby Co.

20. Norris, F. H., Jr.; Gasteiger, E. L.; and Chatfield, P. O. 1957. An electromyographic study of induced and spontaneous muscle cramps. *Electroencephalography and Clinical Neurophysiology* 9:139-47.

21. Petajan, J. H., and Eagan, C. J. 1968. Effect of temperature and physical fitness on the triceps surae reflex. *Journal of Applied Physiology* 25:16-20.

22. Rohter, F. D., and Hyman, C. 1962. Blood flow in arm and finger during muscle contraction and joint position changes. *Journal of applied physiology* 17:819-23.

16 Environment and Exercise

The efficiency of the human organism in various forms of work or exercise may vary between fifteen and thirty percent. This means that, of the energy consumed, only fifteen to thirty percent is converted into useful work, and that the remaining energy (seventy to eighty-five percent) is wasted as heat energy. This wasted heat energy must be dissipated; otherwise the body temperature will rise unduly. Furthermore, in a hot climate the body also absorbs heat from its environment. These two factors tend to increase the body heat stores and thus increase body temperature.

PHYSIOLOGY OF ADAPTATION TO HEAT AND COLD

There are four means by which the body can maintain thermal balance by losing heat to the environment.

Conduction. This is the process by which heat exchange is accomplished through contact with another substance. The rate of exchange is determined by the temperature difference between the two substances and by their thermal conductivities. For example, the body loses heat in this manner when submerged in cold water.

Convection. This is the process by which heat is transferred by a moving fluid (liquid or gas). Thus in the example of a man submerged in cold water, the heat that is transferred from the body to the water by conduction is carried away from the body by convection (the water that has been warmed rises, making way for new molecules to be heated by conduction, etc.).

Radiation. This is the process of heat transfer by way of electromagnetic waves. These waves can pass through air without imparting much heat to it; however, when they strike a body their energy is largely transformed into heat. This is the means by which the sun heats the earth, which also explains why a man can be perfectly comfortable in air that is below the freezing point if he receives enough solar radiation. (Skiing in high mountains in subtropical latitudes is an example; the air may be cold due to the altitude, yet the sun's declination is such as to transfer much radiant heat.)

Evaporation. Changing a liquid into a gas is called evaporation, or vaporization, and requires large amounts of heat energy. Thus while one kilocalorie can raise the temperature of one liter of water one degree centigrade, it takes 580 kilocalories to evaporate one liter of water at body temperature. These 580 kilocalories are taken from the surroundings, and this of course is the principle that underlies the operation of a kitchen refrigerator. Human beings function much as refrigerators when they leave a swimming pool and allow the atmosphere to absorb the water on their skin.

Thus it seems that man's problems in adjusting to his thermal environment are twofold: (1) heat dissipation in hot climates and (2) heat conservation in cold climates. He can gain heat from two sources: environment and metabolism; and he can lose heat from one, or a combination, of four factors: conduction, convection, radiation, and evaporation.

Under normal indoor atmospheric conditions, a resting individual maintains body temperature equilibrium within narrow limits. In this situation his heat gain is entirely due to metabolism, and his heat loss is estimated to occur approximately forty percent by convection, forty percent by radiation, and twenty percent by evaporation (insensible perspiration); conduction is usually negligible. His input is balanced by his output, and his body temperature remains constant—at, or close to, 98.6° F. In fact, within the range of about 30° to 170° F environmental temperature, the body temperature of a nude man is maintained at a constant temperature within about 1° F of his normal resting temperature. This very precise regulatory function is brought about by nervous feedback mechanisms operating through the temperature regulatory center (*thermostat*) in the hypothalmas. The temperature receptors which feed into this thermostat sense the body temperature (1) at the preoptic area of the anterior hypothalmus, (2) in the skin, and (3) probably in some of the internal organs.

When the body temperature is too high the thermostat in the hypothalamus having received the error signals from the temperature sensors, increases the rate of heat loss from the body in two principal ways: (1) by stimulating the sweat glands to secrete, which results in evaporative heat losses from the body, and (2) by inhibiting the sympathetic centers in the posterior hypothalamus, thus reducing the vasoconstrictor tone of the arterioles and microcirculation in the skin. This allows vasodilation of the skin vessels and thus better transport of metabolic heat to the periphery for cooling.

When the body temperature is too low mechanisms are brought into play to (1) produce more metabolic heat and (2) conserve the heat produced within the body. Heat production is increased by hypothalamic stimulation of (1) shivering which can increase metabolic rate by two to fourfold, (2) catecholamine release which increases the rate of cellular oxidation processes, and (3) the thyroid gland which results in considerably higher metabolic rates.

Heat conservation is brought about by vasoconstriction of the skin vessels and abolition of the sweating response.

EXERCISE IN THE COLD

Some sports and athletic activities are of necessity carried on in cold environments. Skiing and ice skating depend upon snow and ice, and many other sports, such as football and soccer, are occasionally played in very cold weather. A cold environment ordinarily poses few problems for an athlete because increased metabolic heat due to the activity soon warms him to a normal *operating temperature,* and heat dissipation to the atmosphere occurs easily by radiation, convection, and when he starts sweating, by evaporation.

The chief problem in this situation is to prevent sudden changes in temperature (chilling), and athletic dress is extremely important, especially when there are intermittent periods of activity and rest (as in football). The athlete must be dressed in attire that (1) keeps him comfortably warm while waiting for his event and while warming up, and (2) can be removed (in part) after warm-up has been accomplished.

It is possible for metabolic rates to increase by as much as twenty-five or thirty times basal values in very vigorous activity. This means that even in the coldest weather (no wind) an athlete has large heat loads to dissipate if a sport is extremely vigorous. Many athletes sweat profusely even in cold environments, and the important consideration is that the clothing worn during actual participation (and after warm-up) be as light as possible in weight and provide as little barrier to passage of water vapor (sweat) as possible. Sweat will otherwise accumulate on the skin or in soaked jerseys, etc., thus providing a chilling problem in the interim between the end of exercise and showering.

Cold Acclimatization. It is well known that continued exposure to cold environments results in greater ability to withstand cold; however, the physiological adjustments are not yet well-defined. The most important factor is the maintenance of *core temperature* (rectal temperature, which reflects the temperature of the central nervous system and deep viscera). Core temperature is maintained at a fairly constant 99° F even though skin temperature may fall from its normal average temperature of 92° F to as low as 60° F.

On the basis of the earlier discussion it is seen that the body can react to cold (1) by reduction of heat loss and (2) by increased metabolism. When a resting and naked man is cooled from a comfortable environment of 85° F to approximately 72° F, no increase in metabolism occurs, and heat is conserved by vasoconstriction of cutaneous blood vessels that prevents loss of the heat carried by the blood from the core. Below 72° F increased metabolism results from shivering; the involuntary contraction of the muscles in shivering may raise the metabolic rate from two to four times the resting rate.

For these reasons investigators have looked for changes in basal metabolic rates, peripheral circulation, and skin temperature as indicators of acclimatization. The results are controversial. An increased basal metabolic rate (BMR) of thirty-five percent in Korean women who dive for commercial purposes in winter water (temperature 50° F) has been observed (Kang et al. 1963), and Eskimos have been found to have a higher BMR than Caucasians; forty-six kilocalories per M² per hour compared to thirty-seven kilcalories per M² per hour (Milan, Hannon, and Evonuk 1962). However, experiments during expeditions into antarctic regions have failed to find significant BMR changes in their personnel.

Local adaptation to cold has been shown in the fishermen of Gaspé Bay, Canada, who gave lower pressor responses to immersion of hands and feet in ice water than did controls (13). It is interesting to note that hypnosis suppressed shivering, lowered the heart rate, and improved vigilance-task performance significantly over the controls during cold exposure at 40° F (12).

It seems likely that adaptation to cold is comprised of physiological and psychological factors, and it may well be that the interaction between the two—as well as the type of physiological changes—can vary from individual to individual.

Human Limitations in Cold Environments. Ability to withstand cold environments varies widely with individuals. Truly remarkable resistance to cold has been claimed by some of the adherents of religions that practice religious pilgrimages (Yoga, etc.). In one such pilgrimage, which was observed under scientific conditions (18), a Nepali pilgrim was uninjured by four days of exposure at 15,000 to 17,000 feet altitudes, with temperatures ranging between 5 and 9° F at night, although he wore only light clothing and no shoes or gloves. It was found that his resistance to cold depended upon elevated metabolism.

Body build and tissue proportions are important factors in determining an individual's ability to withstand cold. Other things being equal, the more rotund (*endomorphic*) a person, the less surface area he has in relation to volume (mass of tissues); consequently, heat loss occurs at a slower rate than in a person of angular (*ectomorphic*) build. Furthermore, fat tissue is an excellent insulator against heat loss. These two factors make the round fat man better able to withstand cold; conversely, the tall thin man is better able to dissipate heat (and remain cool) in a hot climate.

Effect of Ice-cold Showers. A shower of ice-cold water (32 to 35° F) over the chest causes large increases in systolic and diastolic arterial pressures (11); it also causes increased pulse pressure, heart rate, and cardiac output. These changes are not necessarily dangerous in themselves for healthy individuals, but they would almost certainly be hazardous for anyone with impaired cardiac performance or in the presence of circulatory overload. Whether the same experimentally observed cardiovascular changes can be extrapolated to a mildly cold shower (60 to 70° F) is not yet known.

EXERCISE IN THE HEAT

Exercise in hot climates is a more serious problem than exercise in the cold. Whereas in a cold climate the increased metabolic heat production combats the increased heat loss to the environment, in a hot climate metabolism and environment combine to increase heat gain in body tissues. The problem is further complicated by the fact that when environmental temperature approaches skin temperature (approximately 92° F), heat loss through convection and radiation gradually comes to an end, so that at temperatures above skin temperature the *only* means for heat loss is *evaporation of sweat*. Radiation and convection reverse their direction and add heat to the body.

Sweating, then, is the only avenue for heat loss at temperatures above skin temperature, and it is the most important avenue at temperatures that approach skin temperature. At this point it is most important to understand that the mere process of sweating is not in itself effective in dissipating heat; *liquid sweat must be converted to a gas by evaporation before any heat loss occurs.* Sweat that merely roles off is virtually ineffective, but large heat losses can result when the weather is so dry that the liquid is evaporated from the skin so rapidly that sweating is imperceptible. For these reasons, this topic will be discussed as two separate and distinct environmental problems: hot and dry environment, and hot and humid environment.

Hot, Dry Environment. When a man works or plays in a hot and dry environment, cooling of the skin is brought about by evaporation of sweat; there is no problem for the evaporative processes because the air can absorb considerable moisture before becoming saturated (but not in humid climates). Cooling the skin is not the desired end result, however; it is the *internal environment* that must be cooled at all costs. To retain a normal core temperature, heat must be transported from the core to the skin, and this requires adjustments from the normal, resting circulatory state. As we discussed earlier (chapter six), the arteriovenous anastomoses of the microcirculation open up along with precapillary sphincters, to increase flow through the skin and subcutaneous tissues. This results in greater volumes of slower-moving blood in and close to the skin for better transfer of heat to the evaporative surfaces, and thus in better cooling.

Along with the improved cooling, however, it must be noted that the volume of the circulatory system has increased by a considerable amount. Under these conditions, venous return to the heart is somewhat impaired, and this results in a decreased stroke volume (in accord with Starling's law). To maintain a constant cardiac output for the demands of both exercising muscles and skin circulation, the heart rate must increase (19, 23). Because increases in rate depress cardiac efficiency, exercise at temperature close to or above skin temperature can impose very severe loads upon the cardiovascular system, even when the air is relatively dry.

Since the entire process of heat dissipation now depends upon elimination of water in perspiration, it is obvious that dehydration is a distinct possibility. How important this factor may be has been pointed out by Adolph and his associates (1), who note that a man walking in the desert (temperature 100° F) will lose approximately one quart of water per hour. Furthermore, their extensive desert experimentation indicates that voluntary thirst results in adequate water replacement during rest but *not* during work or exercise.

Hot, Humid Environment. When the air surrounding an individual is not only hot but is also loaded with moisture, evaporative cooling is impaired because evaporation cannot take place unless volumes of air are available to take up the water vapor given off. To illustrate this, let us take the extreme example where the air is completely saturated (100 percent relative humidity) and the air temperature is higher than the skin temperature. Under these conditions no heat dissipation can occur; consequently, the metabolic heat accumulates and raises body temperature, until death ensues (108 to 110° F).

It may therefore be concluded that the problems in a hot, dry atmosphere are related to increased cardiovascular loads and dehydration if water intake is insufficient. In a hot, humid climate the same problems exist, and are aggravated by a lessened ability to unload water vapor into an already-loaded ambient atmosphere. These facts are illustrated in figure 16.1, where the hot, wet environment is 90° F and eighty-five percent relative humidity; the hot, dry environment is 100° F and twenty-five percent relative humidity compared with a normal or control environment (room temperature) of 72° F and forty-two percent relative humidity. It is clearly seen that although the temperature is lower in the hot, wet situation, it is considerably more stressful in terms of heart rate response than the hot, dry climate.

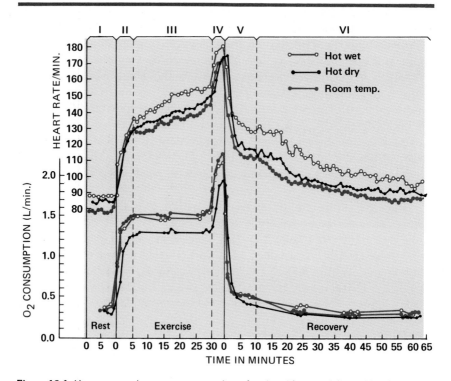

Figure 16-1. Heart rate and oxygen consumption of male subjects pedaling a bicycle ergometer at 540 Kg.m./min. during phases II and III, and at 720 Kg.m./min. during phase IV, under the different environments. (From Brouha. "Effect of Work on the Heart," ch. 21 in *Work and the Heart,* Rosenbaum and Belknap, eds., 1959. Courtesy of Harper & Row, Publishers, New York.)

HUMAN LIMITATIONS IN THE HEAT

The combination of hot weather and strenuous physical activity resulted in almost 200 deaths from heatstroke in recruits at training centers in the US during World War II. In just one summer (1952) there were approximately 600 heat casualties at one Marine Corps Recruit training center (16). From August 1959 to October 1962, twelve heatstroke deaths were reported in football players, seven in high school and five in college (8). These statistics show the need for greater familiarization among physical educators and coaches with the physiological effects of combinations of heat stress and physical activity.

First, we need to define the problem. Unfortunately, we cannot evaluate the heat stress of any given situation by simply reading the thermometer because, as has been pointed out earlier, the transfer of heat into or out of the body is dependent upon the balance of heat gain from metabolism plus environment against the heat lost to the environment. Thus we need information regarding not only the temperature, but also humidity, air movement, and heat gain from solar radiation. What is really needed is one index which is sensitive to all of the above factors, to give us an *effective temperature* which tells the whole story of heat stress. Such an index was developed by Yaglou (25) in 1927 and has gained wide usage in industry and in the military. His effective temperature or ET was defined as that temperature with 100 percent relative humidity and still air that brings about an equivalent physiological response to the environment under observation. It was later corrected for radiation effect and was then called *Corrected Effective Temperature* or CET. Estimation of CET requires the reading of three instruments, *dry bulb, wet bulb* and *globe* temperatures plus the necessary calculations to arrive at CET. Botsford developed a new instrument (4) the *wet globe thermometer* (WGT) which exchanges heat with the surroundings by conduction, convection, evaporation, and radiation essentially as a perspiring man does (see fig. 16.2); so the one reading, temperature of

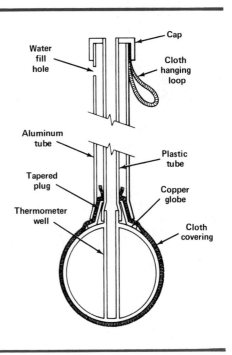

Water fill hole

Cap

Cloth hanging loop

Aluminum tube

Plastic tube

Tapered plug

Copper globe

Thermometer well

Cloth covering

Figure 16-2. Sectional sketch showing construction of the Wet Globe Thermometer (not to scale). (From Botsford, J.H. *Am. Ind. Hyg. J.* 32:9, 1971.)

the globe without further calculation, provides a comprehensive measure of the cooling capacity of the work environment.[1] This instrument provides a simple readout and consequently should be placed in every institution where heat stress can conceivably become a problem in the conduct of physical education or athletics. Figure 16.3 shows Botsfords compilation of data for maximal allowable WGT at various metabolic rates with the author's extrapolations to caloric value of various athletic activities.

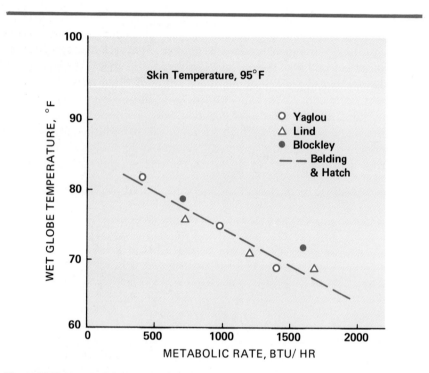

Figure 16-3. Maximum Wet Globe Temperatures for continuous work according to various authorities. 500 BTU or 125 Kcal/hour would be the approximate metabolic rate for standing at ease, 1000 BTU or 250 Kcal about that of light calisthenics, 1500 or 375 Kcal that of playing singles tennis, and 2000 BTU or 500 Kcal that of heavy activity in football, basketball or handball. (From Botsford, J.H. *Am. Ind. Hyg. J.* 32:1, 1971.)

One note of caution is advisable in the use of such an approach. All of the data on which figure 16.3 is based was taken on subjects where

1. This instrument is now commercially available from: Howard Engineering Co., P. O. Box 3164, Bethlehem, Pa. 18017

no artificial barriers were imposed to vapor loss during sweating. The "suit of armor" worn by our football players creates a greater load by virtue of its weight and more importantly cuts off about fifty percent of the players evaporative surface area. This was shown to increase the sweat loss by seventy-eight percent. Thus the uniform both adds to the metabolic heat load and also simultaneously prevents transfer of the heat away from the body (8).

To emphasize this point the author has used the temperature and humidity data relating to the football heat stroke deaths of Fox et al. to estimate the WGT at the time of each football fatality. Since only temperature and humidity were available, the estimates were based on an 8 mph breeze blowing and no radiant effect.

Figure 16.3 suggests a maximal WGT of about 64° for a metabolic rate of 2000 BTU/hr which probably is a good approximation of the metabolic rate during football. But table 16.1 shows that only two of the nine fatalities occurred above that level of heat stress. This suggests (1) that the heat stress was considerably greater for uniformed football players than for equivalent metabolic levels of lightly clothed individuals on whom the data were taken, and (2) that the data of figure 16.3 must be used very conservatively with respect to football players.

The feasability of reducing heat stress casualties through enlightened control of activity when heat loads are hazardous has been shown in

TABLE 16.1

Estimations of the ET and WGT at the Time of Each Football Fatality

Football Fatality	Dry Bulb Temp °F	Wet Bulb Temp °F	Relative Humidity	Effective Temp (ET)	Wet Globe Temp (WGT)
1	64	64	100%	52	52
2	90	75	50	77	67
3	85	76	62	74	64
4	75	67	75	63	59
5	82	73	68	71	62
6	85	71	50	72	63
7	83	72	60	71	62
8	93	76	45	79	68
9	81	75	78	71	62

From Fox et al. *Research Quarterly* 37:333, 1966.

the Marine Corps recruit training program (16). They reduced the weekly heat casualty rate from 12.4 to 4.7 per 10,000 recruits by instituting a program involving:

1. Curtailed activity when heat loads were high
2. Gradual breaking in period for the first week or two
3. Increased emphasis on physical fitness
4. Allowing water ad libitum
5. Replacement of salt
6. Loosening of uniform regulations to allow T-shirts, etc.

We can certainly make no less effort on behalf of our athletes.

Results of Overexposure

Heat Cramps. This problem is common in athletes in hot environments; the cause is loss of salt in perspiration. Prevention, as well as the cure, lies in taking additional salt in the diet. It has been found that, even under extreme conditions, thirteen to seventeen grams of salt per day will maintain normal electrolyte balance (21). If more than this is taken, the superfluous amount is merely excreted, but may cause nausea in many individuals.

This special salt requirement, which represents about one-half ounce, can best be taken by more liberal salting of food at mealtime. If we can assume that the average diet includes about half the salt necessary for severely dehydrating conditions, the balance can be taken by adding one-half teaspoon of salt to each of four glasses of drinking water each day. This amount of salt in water is not found to be disagreeable if a need exists (one level teaspoon equals approximately four grams of salt). Sweetening the solution with glucose or sugar also has physiological benefit if the exercise is of long duration.

Heat Exhaustion. This condition occurs when the limitations of the cardiovascular system are exceeded. The symptoms are weak, rapid pulse, and cold skin, and the inadequate circulation usually results in dizziness or syncope (fainting). A victim of heat exhaustion must be rested and given adequate fluid.

Heat Stroke. This condition occurs as the result of failure of the heat regulatory system, and is serious enough to demand medical attention. The symptoms are a hot, flushed skin (usually dry), high body temperature, and possibly delirium.

ACCLIMATIZATION TO HOT ENVIRONMENTS

In these days of rapid transportation, individual athletes and whole teams frequently travel far enough for their competitions to encounter a severe climatic change. If an athlete goes from a cold to a hot climate, this will entail a considerable decrement in performance if the event involves heavy demands upon the cardiovascular system.

It has been shown that complete acclimatization can be brought about artificially by workout sessions in hot rooms in four to five days (20), and will last at least three weeks during cold weather (9). Acclimatization results in lower work-pulse rates, lower rectal temperatures, and more stable blood pressures for any given level of work. There is also a possibility that sweat rates are increased, but the evidence is not clear.

Evidence has been presented that even persons who live in hot climates are only partially acclimatized (fifty percent) when compared with subjects who have been systematically exercised under artificial hot-room conditions (24). Buskirk, Iampetro, and Bass (5) have shown that mere exposure to heat is not as effective as a combination of conditioning and heat exposure in resisting the effects of dehydration.

Thus the evidence seems clear cut. When competition is scheduled for a different, hot climate, artificial acclimatization is a must for preventing serious decrements in performance.

Even after full acclimatization has been brought about, two other precautions should be followed for maintaining optimum health and performance in hot climates. First, and most importantly, athletes must maintain adequate intakes of water and salt. The simplest way to check this is by recording weight records under consistent conditions. Dehydration shows up quickly as a loss in weight, and any weight loss more than two or three pounds should be corrected by adding salt and water to the diet. Second, athletes should be encouraged to decrease the protein in their diet because the specific dynamic action of protein digestion causes more heat formation than the other foodstuffs. Inclusion of more foods with high water content, such as fruits and salads, is also advisable.

WATER REPLACEMENT SCHEDULE TO IMPROVE PERFORMANCE

The need for water replacement during exercise under conditions of heat and humidity has already been discussed but the *schedule of replacement* is also important. It has been shown that taking more water than is expected to be lost during the athletic activity (overhydration) and taking it prior to participation in addition to during the activity results in the best physiological conditions for maximum performance (14, 17). Under conditions of heavy heat stress such as early season football in hot climates, one may estimate a loss of one to two liters per hour. As much of the replacement as can be managed easily should be taken pregame and most of the balance in the first and second quarters. The ideal replacement fluid is a hypotonic salt solution to which glucose or sugar has been added as suggested earlier. Taking salt without water, a practice which is common among athletes is undesirable because it has been shown that plasma sodium concentration becomes elevated during exercise in the heat due to loss of hypotonic sweat (6).

EXERCISE AT HIGH ALTITUDES

Man's travels to find athletic competition often involve not only changes in temperature and humidity but large changes in altitude as well. It has been known since the turn of the century, and the advent of aviation, that whenever man ascends to higher altitudes he encounters lower atmospheric pressures. Because oxygen maintains a constant 20.93 percent of decreasing total pressure regardless of altitude, a gradually decreasing partial pressure drives oxygen into the blood. This decreasing availability of oxygen to the tissues would be expected to hamper physical performance, and indeed it does.

The O_2 saturation of arterial blood at sea level approaches 100 percent, even under conditions of exercise, but at 19,000 feet saturation is only sixty-seven percent at rest; and exercise at this altitude may drop the value below fifty percent (22). We do not have to go to this extreme altitude, however, to find changes that may be of great importance in athletic competition. At 3,000 feet even acclimatized subjects have lost five percent of their aerobic capacity, and fifteen percent at 6,500 feet (2).

This decreased aerobic capacity (maximum O_2 consumption) is brought about by a combination of factors, probably most importantly by reduction in O_2 saturation of arterial blood, decreased cardiac output, and the higher cost of lung ventilation. The impaired lung diffusion is the result of the lowered O_2 pressure gradient. The decreased cardiac output is undoubtedly due to the hypoxic myocardium. The lung ventilation is increased progressively with altitude. All this results from the necessity of breathing more air to attempt to get the same number of molecules of O_2. The increased effort of the respiratory muscles results in greater O_2 consumption by the respiratory muscles and in lowered efficiency.

Limitations in Performance at High Altitudes. Not all athletic performances suffer because of the hypoxia of higher altitudes. Obviously, *one maximal effort* activities, such as the shot put, broad jump, high jump, etc., do not suffer because they do not depend upon O_2 transport. Furthermore, events of less than one minute duration, such as the 100-

and 220-yard dashes, are also performed (very largely) anaerobically, and consequently they are unimpaired, but recovery times are longer (see fig. 16.4).

In any event that lasts one minute or more, aerobic capacity is more important, and this importance increases as duration increases. Considerable losses in performance may be expected in such events unless athletes have had adequate time for acclimatization.

Acclimatization. The need for artificially increasing the available oxygen at higher altitudes has been recognized by the US Air Force. In aircraft that are not pressurized, regulations require breathing *aviator's oxygen* at altitudes above 10,000 feet. Experiments in low-pressure chambers (to simulate high altitude) have shown that without additional oxygen the average individual may remain conscious *at rest* (with varying degrees of impairment) for about thirty minutes at 18,000 feet, but for one minute or less at 30,000 feet. Exercise would obviously shorten these times greatly.

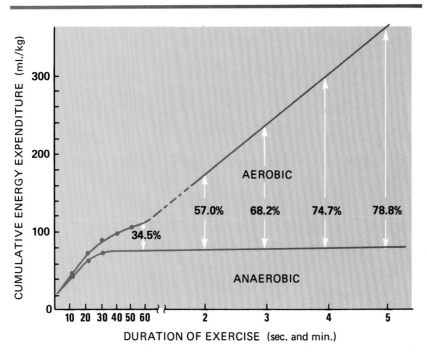

Figure 16-4. The relative importance of oxygen debt and steady oxygen intake during maximum exercise of varying duration. (From Shephard, R.J. *J. Spt. Med.* 10:73, 1970.)

On the other hand, man's ability to adjust to higher environments over a period of time is truly phenomenal. It has been reported (3) that a member of the 1924 British Mt. Everest expedition reached an altitude of 28,126 feet without oxygen equipment.

The acclimatizing process can be accomplished by various systems of physical conditioning, and at progressively higher altitudes if possible. If altitude cannot be increased systematically, a progressive conditioning program at the *game altitude* is undertaken in which cardiorespiratory endurance is gradually improved by progressively increasing demands.

Altitudes below 3,000 feet probably require no acclimatization, the problem is slight up to about 5,000 feet, and the problem of altitude is only academic above 10,000 feet since no serious competition occurs above that level so that the area of concern for physical education and athletics in the USA is really for altitudes between 5,000 and 10,000 feet.

D. B. Dill (1968) has provided evidence which suggests that the physiological adaptation to altitude occurs in four phases:

1. The *acute phase*: in the first thirty minutes of exposure to the altitudes of concern here, the loss in maximal O_2 consumption and, consequently, in performances which depend upon aerobic capacity is less than ten percent.
2. In the *second phase* the decrements may be from twenty to thirty percent (in one to three days) and this requires a matter of weeks for adaptation, to achieve the *third phase*.
3. In the *fourth phase*, adaptation depends upon the increase of red blood cell volume which reaches a maximum in about a year or more.

Over a period of years it is eventually possible to achieve sea level performance up to as high as 13,200 feet. Above 17,500 feet there is only deterioration, no adaptation seems to occur. This represents a schema (fig. 16.5) which is widely variable from individual to individual with respect to both rate and capacity for adaptation to altitude.

Thus, the coach faced with the prospect of competition at a site such as Mexico City at an altitude of 7,350 feet is faced with the choice of timing his trip to compete within minutes of arrival (impossible) or to arrive several weeks early to allow time for acclimatization (also usually impossible, except for the fortunate few in Olympic competition). Possibly, the only real solution is for the flatlanders to limit their interscholastic competitions to other flatlanders or to accept the alternative of a predictable loss of performance in aerobic events gracefully.

The physiological mechanisms that bring about the acclimatization process have been well demonstrated, at least in part. Increases of ten

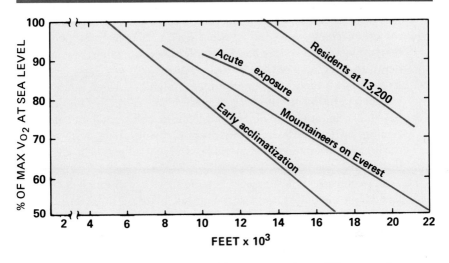

Figure 16-5. Decrement in capacity for supplying oxygen to tissues, VO_2 max, at four stages of acclimatization. (From Dill, D.B. *J.A.M.A.* 205:753, 1968.)

to fifty percent in the number of erythrocytes and in the hemoglobin content of the blood have been reported. Ability to increase the maximum ventilation rate has also been demonstrated, and there is a possibility that vascularization of lung and muscle tissue is also improved.

Administration of Oxygen to Improve Performance. There seems to be no evidence that breathing enriched mixtures of O_2 *before* an athletic event has a significant effect upon the subsequent performance. Use of O_2 *during* work at high altitudes, however, is not only advantageous but absolutely necessary—at 18,000 to 20,000 feet—for most people without a long acclimatization period. (This, of course, is of no practical value for athletics.)

One use of O_2 for athletes that rests on sound theoretical and experimental bases is for shortening recovery times at altitude. In sports that involve rest periods between heavy, endurance work bouts, such as basketball and soccer, repayment of the O_2 debt can be hastened in the unacclimatized athlete who has competed at an altitude substantially higher than the altitude he is used to.

SUMMARY

1. Human thermal balance is maintained by striking a balance between heat gain and heat loss. Heat gain is due to metabolism, and also

to gains from radiation and convection when environmental temperatures are above skin temperature (92° F). Heat loss occurs by *radiation, convection,* and *evaporation* at temperatures below skin temperature; and by *evaporation* only when the environmental temperature is greater than skin temperature.

2. In vigorous athletic events an athlete's metabolic heat maintains his *core temperature* in all but the most severe cold.

3. The most serious problem for athletes in cold environments is obtaining sufficient flexibility in dress to bring about heat retention during warm-up and rest periods, and yet allow heat dissipation during the competitive periods.

4. Cold acclimatization is probably brought about through a combination of physiological and psychological factors. The most important physiological factors seem to be an increased metabolic rate and a greater temperature gradient between core and skin temperatures.

5. In hot, dry environments the ability to adjust to the severely increased cardiovascular load is most critically limited by *dehydration.*

6. In hot, wet environments the ability to adjust to the severely increased cardiovascular load is most critically limited by rising body-core temperature due to inability to dissipate heat by evaporation.

7. For both hot, dry and hot, wet environments, acclimatization can be brought about by progressively increasing work bouts in an artificial hot room over four or five days. This acclimatization will persist at least three weeks in cold weather.

8. Water replacement schedules should be set up to achieve both early replacement and overhydration to maintain performance at its highest level.

9. Exercise or competitive sport performance at altitudes higher, by 3,000 feet or more, than the home environment will be noticeably impaired by hypoxia if the activity depends largely upon aerobic energy (one minute or greater duration).

10. Physiological adaptation to altitude appears to follow a time course of four phases: (1) *acute phase*: up to thirty minutes in which performance is not greatly affected (up to ten percent at 10,000 feet), (2) in one to three days performance falls off more severely, (3) over several weeks acclimatization brings performance back to that of phase one, and (4) red blood cell volume increases over a period of months reaching its maximum after a year or more with commensurate improvement in performance, and eventual return to sea level performance at altitudes up to 13,200 feet.

11. Administration of oxygen to athletes at high altitudes should result

in faster recovery times, but its use before an event cannot be expected to bring about large changes in performance.

REFERENCES

1. Adolph, E. F. 1947. *Physiology of man in the desert*. New York: Interscience Publishers.
2. Astrand, P. O. 1963. Physiological aspects on cross-country skiing at the high altitudes. *Journal of Sports Medicine and Physical Fitness* 3:51-52.
3. Balke, B. 1960. Work capacity at altitude. In *Science and Medicine of Exercise and Sports*, ed. W. R. Johnson, ch. 18. New York: Harper & Row.
4. Botsford, J. H. 1971. A wet globe thermometer for environmental heat measurement. *American Industrial Hygiene Association Journal* 32:1-10.
5. Buskirk, E. R.; Iampetro, P. F.; and Bass, D. E. 1958. Work performance after dehydration: effects of physical conditioning and heat acclimatization. *Journal of Applied Physiology* 12:189-94.
6. Cade, J. R.; Free, H. J.; De Quasada; A. M.; Shires, D. L.; and Roby, L. 1971. Changes in body fluid and volume during vigorous exercise by athletes. *Journal of Sports Medicine* 11:172-78.
7. Dill, D. B. 1968. Physiological adjustments to altitude changes. *Journal of American Medical Association* 205:123-30.
8. Fox, E. L.; Mathews, D. K.; Kaufman, W. S.; and Bowers, R. W. 1966. Effects of football equipment on thermal balance and energy cost during exercise. *Research Quarterly* 37:332-39.
9. Henschel, A.; Taylor, H. L.; and Keys, A. 1943. The persistence of heat acclimatization in man. *American Journal of Physiology* 140:321-25.
10. Kang, B. S.; Song, S. H.; Suh, C. S.; and Hong, S. K. 1963. Changes in body temperature and basal metabolic rate of the ama. *Journal of Applied Physiology* 18:483-88.
11. Keatinge, W. R.; McIlroy, M. B.; and Goldfien, A. 1964. Cardiovascular responses to ice-cold showers. *Journal of Applied Physiology* 19:1145-50.
12. Kissen, A. T., Reifler, C. B.; and Thaler, V. H. 1964. Modification of thermoregulatory responses to cold by hypnosis. *Journal of Applied Physiology* 19:1043-50.
13. LeBlanc, J. 1962. Local adaptation to cold of Gaspé fishermen. *Journal of Applied Physiology* 17:950-52.
14. Londeree, B. R.; Updyke, W. F.; and Burt, J. J. 1969. Water replacement schedules in heat stress. *Research Quarterly* 40:725-32.
15. Milan, F. A.; Hannon, J. P.; and Evonuk, E. 1962. Temperature regulation of Eskimos, Indians, and Caucasians in a bath calorimeter. *Journal of Applied Physiology* 18:378-82.
16. Minard, D. 1961. Prevention of heat casualties in marine corps recruits. *Military Medicine* 126:261-72.
17. Moroff, S. V., and Bass, D. E. 1965. Effects of overhydration on man's physiological responses to work in the heat. *Journal of Applied Physiology* 20:267-70.

18. Pugh, L. G. C. E. 1963. Tolerance to extreme cold at altitude in a nepalese pilgrim. *Journal of Applied Physiology* 18:1234-38.
19. Saltin, B. 1964. Circulatory response to submaximal and maximal exercise after thermal dehydration. *Journal of Applied Physiology* 19:1125-32.
20. Taylor, H. L.; Henschel, A. F.; and Keys, A. 1943. Cardiovascular adjustments of man in rest and work during exposure to dry heat. *American Journal of Physiology* 139:583-91.
21. Taylor, H. L.; Henschel, A.; Mickelson, O.; and Keys, A. 1943. The effect of the sodium chloride intake on the work performance of man during exposure to dry heat and experimental heat exhaustion. *American Journal of Physiology* 140:439-51.
22. West, J. B.; Lahiri, S.; Gill, M. B.; Milledge, J. S.; Pugh, L. G. C. E.; and Ward, M. P. 1962. Arterial oxygen saturation during exercise at high altitude. *Journal of Applied Physiology* 17:617-21.
23. Williams, C. G.; Bredell, G. A. G.; Wyndham, C. H.; Strydom, N. B.; Morrison, J. F.; Peter, J.; Fleming, P. W.; and Ward, J. S. 1962. Circulatory and metabolic reactions to work in the heat. *Journal of Applied Physiology* 17:625-38.
24. Wyndham, C. H. 1964. Heat reactions of caucasions in temperate, in hot dry, and hot humid climates. *Journal of Applied Physiology* 19:607-12.
25. Yaglou, C. P. 1927. Temperature, humidity and air movement in industries: the effective temperature index. *Journal of Industrial Hygiene* 9:297-309.

17 Age and Exercise

If we consider the human lifespan in terms of the biblical concept of three score and ten, we have a lifetime of seventy years; however, if we judge the interest of the physical education profession by the nature of the curricula offered in teacher training institutions, it would seem that virtually all of our efforts are directed to ten years of that lifespan, the years involved in secondary and college education. Should physical education start in junior high school and end after two or four years of college? This seeming preoccupation of physical education with only fourteen percent of the total lifespan is certainly undesirable.

That the need for physical education exists at all ages is amply demonstrated by the success of various athletic programs for children (Little League, Pop Warner League, and age-group swimming) and by weight training and conditioning gyms for adults. It seems inevitable that the scope of physical education must somehow grow to include programs that are organized and administered by professional people for *all ages* and not just for high school and college students who need the exercise least. It behooves us, then, to consider the physiological changes that occur as a function of the aging process.

With respect to the entire age range of human life, physical performance measures in general improve rapidly from early childhood to a maximum somewhere between the late teens and about thirty years of age. In most cases a slow decline occurs during maturity and becomes more rapid with increasing age. The decline in physical performance with age deserves a great deal more emphasis by scientific investigators than it has been accorded in the past.

Indeed the entire body of knowledge regarding the loss of function with increasing age must be viewed with caution since in very few cases has the effect of habitual physical activity been controlled or ruled out. Wessel and Van Huss (48) have shown that physical activity decreases significantly with increasing age. This is not surprising news but does provide scientific validation of the need for consideration of this variable in all investigations directed toward aging changes in performance. To further support this contention they showed that agewise losses in physiological variables important to human performance were more highly related to the *decreased habitual activity* level than they were to *age itself.*

Statistics on population trends for the United States indicate that we are rapidly becoming a nation of older people. The absolute number, as well as the proportion of our older population segments, is increasing rapidly. In evaluation of the effects of the aging process on human performance, several problems arise. First, it is difficult to separate the effects of aging per se from those of concomitant disease processes (particularly cardiovascular problems) that become more numerous as age progresses. Second, the sedentary nature of adult life in the United States makes it very difficult to find *old* populations for comparisons with *young* populations at equal activity levels. Third, very little work has been done on longitudinal studies of the same population over a period of time. Conclusions drawn from cross-sectional studies in which various age groups are compared must be accepted with reservations because the weaker biological specimens are not likely to be represented in as great numbers in the older populations tested as in the younger (due to a higher mortality rate).

Just as various individuals age at different rates, various physiological functions seem to have their own rates of decline with increasing age (see fig. 17.1). Indeed, some functions do not seem to degenerate with age (41), under resting conditions, there seem to be no changes in blood sugar, blood pH, or total blood volume. In general, the functions that involve the coordinated activity of more than one organ system decline most with age, and, as might be expected, changes due to the aging process are most readily observed when the organism is stressed. Homeostatic readjustment is considerably slower with increasing age.

AGE CHANGES IN MUSCLE FUNCTION

All investigators have found that rapid improvement in strength accompanies the growth of children, and maximal strength is found to occur for most muscle groups between the ages of twenty-five and thirty (26). Rodahl et al. (39) have shown that this increase in strength is almost entirely accounted for by the increased size of the muscle. Even sex differences in muscle quality are not very large. When strength is expressed per unit of cross-sectional area (kg per cm²), differences due to age and sex are very small.

Strength decreases very slowly during maturity. After the fifth decade, strength decreases at a greater rate, but even at age sixty the loss does not usually exceed ten to twenty percent of the maximum, with women's losses being somewhat greater than those of men (fig. 17.1).

Damon (13) has extended the older work to show that these age decrements exist whether measured in isometric, concentric, or eccentric muscle contraction and also whether measured as maximal instantaneous force achieved, or as a mean value over a finite time period. However, his work showed isotonic strength to be affected to a greater extent than isometric. The maximum velocity produced against any given mass is

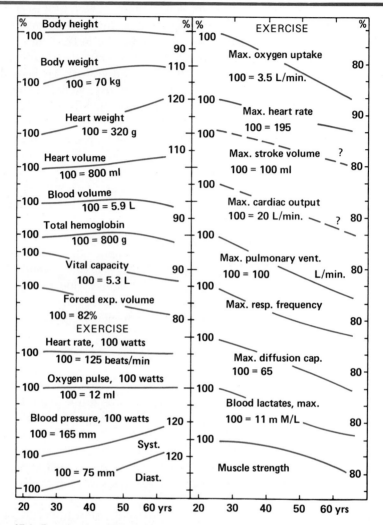

Figure 17-1. Functional variables with age. Data have been collected from various subjects, including healthy men. For data on the same function, only one study has been consulted. The values for the twenty-five-year-old subjects = 100 percent; for the older ages the mean values are expressed in percentage of the twenty-five-year-old individuals' values. The values should not be considered "normal values," but they illustrate the effect of aging. Note that heart rate and oxygen pulse at a given work load (100 watts or 600 kpm/min, oxygen uptake about 1.5 liters/min) are identical throughout the age range covered, but the maximal oxygen uptake, heart rate, cardiac output, etc., decline with age. The data on cardiac output and stroke volume are based on few observations and are therefore uncertain. (From I. Astrand. *Measurement in Exercise Electrocardiography* 1969. Courtesy of Charles C. Thomas, Publisher, Springfield, Illinois.)

less for the old than the young although the shape of the force velocity curve is similar (see fig. 17.2). Thus loss of strength with age consists of two components: (1) a decrease in ability to maintain maximum force statically, and (2) a decrease in ability to accelerate mass.

With respect to muscular endurance, or fatigue rate, Evans (25) has shown, with the EMG fatigue curve techniques described in chapter fourteen, that fatigue rate is significantly greater in the old than the young when holding isometric contractions of twenty, twenty-five, thirty, thirty-five, forty or forty-five percent of MVC.

AGE AND THE CARDIOVASCULAR SYSTEM

The effects of a lifetime of vigorous exercise upon the cardiovascular system have not yet been investigated extensively by scientific methods. Evidence, however, has been presented from observations on isolated individuals who have trained very hard into old age. Clarence De Mar, the famous marathon runner, made it a habit to run twelve miles every

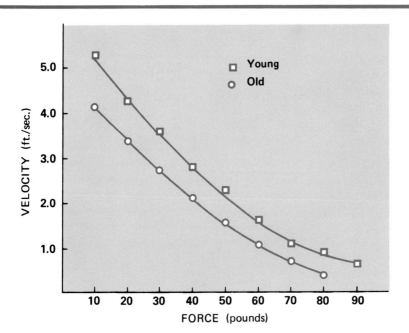

Figure 17-2. Comparison of young and old groups on force-velocity relationship. (From Damon, E.L. *An Experimental Investigation of the Relationship of Age to Various Parameters of Muscle Strength,* Doctoral dissertation, Physical Education U.S.C. 1971.)

day, and this level of training was maintained throughout his lifetime. He was still competing in twenty-five- and twenty-six-mile marathons at age sixty-five, and he ran his last fifteen-kilometer race at sixty-eight— two years before his death (from cancer). At the autopsy it was found that this unusually strenuous exercise had not only *not* hurt his heart, but that the myocardium was unusually well developed, the valves were normal, and the coronary arteries were estimated to be two or three times normal size (8).

Maximum Heart Rate.   As was discussed in chapter five, the maximum heart rate attainable during exercise decreases with age. Maximum heart rate for young adults is usually between 190 and 200 beats per minute; in old age this value decreases gradually. The maximum heart rate in older adults can be estimated as follows: MAX HR = 220 − age.

Cardiac Output.   No data are available for cardiac output under conditions of heavy exercise in aging populations; however, the at-rest cardiac output declines approximately one percent per year after maturity (10). This evidence is supported by the fact that the strength of the myocardium measured by ballistocardiography also declines at a similar rate (44). It is very likely that the maximal cardiac output declines at a rate no less than the rate for the resting values.

Coronary Artery Changes.   Simonson has shown (43) that in normal hearts the cross-sectional area of the lumen of coronary arteries is reduced with age. The percentage of the total arterial cross-section that is open to blood flow is twenty-nine percent less in age group forty to fifty-nine than in the group ten to twenty-nine.

Circulatory Changes.   One method for assessing vasomotor responsiveness to stress is strapping a subject to a tilt board so that his orientation in space can be changed quickly from the supine to the vertical posture, as well as to intermediate postures, thus bringing about quick changes in hydrostatic pressures within the circulatory system. After a tilt to forty-five degrees, older subjects showed larger decreases and slower recovery of systolic blood pressure than the younger group. When tilted to standing, the older group had larger decreases and slower recovery of diastolic blood pressure. In both cases the younger group had a greater increase in heart rate (a desirable response) to increase the blood pressure available to compensate for the increased hydrostatic pressure (29).

There appear to be no significant differences in the blood flow to the extremities at rest nor in the vasomotor reflex responses to warming and cooling between healthy young and old adults. However, the response of blood flow to the stimulus of exercise is markedly less in the old than in young subjects (35).

Circulation time from arm to thigh was measured in 237 normal subjects and found to be slowed by thirty to forty percent in older subjects (over sixty) compared with the values for the young (9).

Capillary density does not appear to change with age, but the ratio of capillary to muscle fibers decreases because of the greater number of fibers per unit cross section due to atrophic processes (32).

A more hopeful note is sounded by Russian workers who have reported that the hardening of the arteries associated with aging may be reversible through systematic physical conditioning. They found a fourteen percent slowing of pulse wave velocity after six to seven months of training in a group whose age averaged fifty-four years (46). A slower pulse wave propagation is associated with better elasticity in the arterial wall.

CHANGES IN PULMONARY FUNCTION

Lung Volumes and Capacities. It has been firmly established that vital capacity declines with age (30, 31, 33). There appears to be no very good evidence for any change in total lung capacity and consequently residual volume increases with age (30, 31). Aging increases the ratio of RV/TLC and anatomic dead space also increases with age (12).

Thoracic Wall Compliance. Some tissues of the lungs and chest wall have the property of elasticity. Thus in inspiration the muscles must work against this elasticity which then aids the expiration phase through elastic recoil. This relationship between force required (elastic force) per unit stretch of the thorax is called *compliance*. It is measured by the size of the ratio of volume change per unit pressure change. It may be thought of as the elastic resistance to breathing. That is to say, the less compliant the tissues the more elastic force must be overcome in breathing. There are two tissues which offer elastic resistance to breathing, the lung tissue itself and the wall of the thoracic cage. The evidence suggests that lung compliance increases with age (45) but more important, thoracic wall compliance decreases (28, 37, 45). Thus the older individual may do as much as twenty percent more elastic work at a given level of ventilation than the young and most of the additional work would be performed in moving the chest wall (45).

It seems entirely likely that the agewise differences in lung volumes and capacities noted above can be explained largely on the basis of this lessening mobility of the chest wall with age.

Pulmonary Diffusion. There is a significant decrease in the capacity for pulmonary diffusion both at rest and at any given work load which accompanies the aging process (24).

Ventilatory Mechanics in Exercise. In view of the changes in pulmonary function already cited, it is not surprising to find that the process of breathing becomes less efficient with age. Figure 17.3 shows work

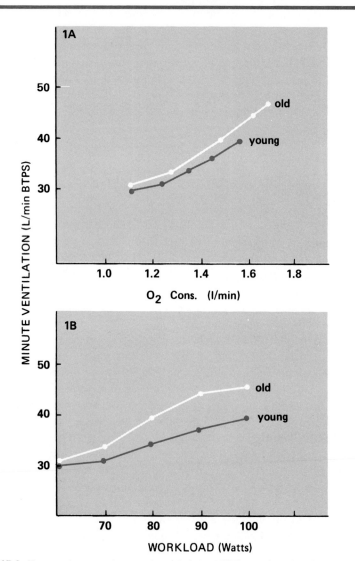

Figure 17-3. *Top:* expiratory minute volume (L/min BTPS) as a function O_2 consumption (L/min STPD). *Bottom:* expiratory minute volume as a function of work load in watts. (From deVries, H.A., and Adams, G.M. *J. Geront.* 27:350, 1972.)

from the author's laboratory which shows clearly the need for greater ventilation in older men compared with young men at any given level of work or O_2 consumption (19). Interestingly, the right side of figure 17.3 shows also that there is a difference in the mechanics by which the old subjects met the increased ventilatory demand. While the young first increased breathing frequency, the older men increased their tidal volume (the more efficient mechanism) thus reaching their maximal TV early at work loads where the young still had large reserves of TV for work at higher loads.

AGE AND PHYSICAL WORKING CAPACITY (PWC)

Maximal O_2 Consumption. As was mentioned earlier, the best single measure of physical working capacity (PWC) is *maximal oxygen consumption*, and two excellent studies have related this variable to age. Robinson (38) tested a total of seventy-nine male subjects, ranging in age from six to seventy-five years; the results are shown in table 17.1. Astrand (3) tested forty-four women, ranging in age from twenty to sixty-five, and these results are tabulated in table 11.2, page 235.

For boys, it is seen (table 17.1) that, in terms of absolute quantities, maximal O_2 consumption increases rapidly with age. When the results are

TABLE 17.1

Highest Oxygen Intake Attained in Maximal Work as Related to Body Weight and Age

Age Group	No. of Subjects	Age in Years (Mean)	Weight in kg (Mean)	Maximal O_2 Intake*			
				L per min		Ml per kg per min	
				(Mean)	(Extremes)	(Mean)	(Extremes)
I	4	6.1	21.0	0.98	0.80—1.30	46.7	42.8—49.5
II	9	10.4	30.0	1.56	1.24—2.00	52.1	49.0—56.1
III	9	14.1	55.8	2.63	1.89—3.41	47.1	36.4—55.4
IV	11	17.4	68.5	3.61	2.96—4.20	52.8	44.6—62.5
V	11	24.5	72.5	3.53	2.56—4.50	48.7	41.9—55.6
VI	10	35.1	79.3	3.42	2.76—3.97	43.1	37.6—52.8
VII	9	44.3	74.1	2.92	2.30—3.62	39.5	33.7—46.5
VIII	7	51.0	68.7	2.63	2.24—3.35	38.4	33.7—43.2
IX	8	63.1	67.4	2.35	1.64—3.15	34.5	30.2—41.7
X	3	75.0	67.4	1.71	1.43—1.90	25.5	21.8—29.6

After S. Robinson, *Arbeitsphysiologie* Vol. 10, p. 279 (1938). Verlag Julius Springer, Berlin.
*Dry gas at O° C. and 760 mm. Hg.

stated in terms of O_2 consumption per unit of body weight, however, there are only very small changes with age, which may not be significant. Thus the mean maximal O_2 consumption for boys of 6.1 years is 0.98 liters per minute, compared to 2.63 liters per minute for boys of mean age 14.1. But when growth (or body size) is canceled out, the six-year-olds can achieve 46.7 milliliters per kilogram of body weight, which is virtually as good as the 47.1 milliliters per kilogram for fourteen-year-olds and not very far from the best value for all ages, which is achieved at mean age 17.4 years. Thus the working capacity of young boys is probably not limited by ability to transport and consume oxygen. (Equivalent data for girls are lacking.)

For adults, there is a gradual decline in maximal O_2 consumption with age, for both sexes. For men, the maximal values were found at mean age 17.4 years, and they declined to less than half those values at mean age seventy-five. For women, the maximal values were found in the age group twenty to twenty-nine, and they fell off by twenty-nine percent in the age group fifty to sixty-five.

It is of interest to consider the physiological functions whose decline, with increasing age, might contribute to this loss of ability to transport and utilize O_2. The following functions are probably the most important in achieving maximal O_2 consumption: (1) lung ventilation, (2) lung diffusion capacity for O_2, (3) heart rate, (4) stroke volume, and (5) O_2 utilization by the tissues. The implication of direct or indirect evidence is that all of these functions decline with age.

Muscular Efficiency.   According to the data of Robinson (38), adults tended to be more economical in their adjustment to work than boys. He found no clear-cut differences with increasing age during maturity. Astrand found significant decreases in efficiency with age in women (3). These differences were very small, however: 21.9 percent for the twenty to twenty-nine age group, and 19.6 percent for the fifty to sixty-five age group.

The only longitudinal data available were done on D. B. Dill (21). It was found that his efficiency in running on a treadmill declined greatly between age forty-one and age sixty-six; however, two confounding factors operated in this comparison. First, he had gained sixteen and one-half pounds in the interim; secondly, although the same work load was used in both instances, it represented his maximum effort at sixty-six but only some sixty-six percent of his maximal effort at forty-one. Consequently, considerably more energy utilized at age sixty-six came from anaerobic sources, which are less efficient. In summarizing these data it would appear that muscular efficiency decreases with age, but probably to a very slight degree.

TABLE 17.2

Maximal Oxygen Intake and Heart Rate
as Related to Age in Subject DBD

Age Year	Maximum O$_2$ Intake L/min	Maximum Heart Rate	Age Year	Maximum O$_2$ Intake L/min	Maximum Heart Rate
37	3.28	172	45	3.17	
39	3.26		46	2.90	163
40	3.35		48	2.98	
42	3.23		50	2.87	162
44	3.26		66	2.80	160

From D. B. Dill, S. M. Horvath, and F. N. Craig, "Responses to Exercise as Related to Age," *Journal of Applied Physiology* 12:195, 1958.

Longitudinal Studies of PWC. Longitudinal data taken over a period of years on the same individuals provide information that is only implicit in data from cross-sectional studies. Very few data of this type are available, and it seems only fitting that two of these investigations should have been made on two of the pioneers in the relatively new science of exercise physiology: Percy M. Dawson and David B. Dill, who have contributed much to our fund of knowledge in this area. Table 17.2 shows the changes in maximal O$_2$ consumption over a period of twenty-nine years. It is seen that, even in a physically active, vigorous man such as Dr. Dill, aging results in decreased work capacity. More important, however, is the fact that the rate of decrease has been slowed down. Robinson's data on men of a size and age similar to Dill's (table 17.1) show a mean maximal O$_2$ consumption of 2.35 liters per minute compared to 2.80 liters per minute for Dill.

Asmussen and Mathiasen (2) were able to persuade thirty-six of their former physical education students to return to the laboratory to repeat measurements that had been made on them twenty-six to twenty-eight years earlier. The results are shown in table 17.3.

PWC under Environmental Stress. In another longitudinal study, two subjects repeated the same work loads after a twenty-nine-year interval under environmental temperatures that varied from 32° to 124° F. Although the PWC had decreased because of aging, the response to the added stress of high temperatures was relatively unchanged (22).

TABLE 17.3

Values for Various Physiologic Functions Expressed as
Percentages of Values Recorded 25 Years Previously
in Male and Female Physical Education Students

Subjects	Height	Weight	Resting Pulse	Systolic BP	Metabolism (resting O_2 uptake)	Vital Capacity	Hand-grip Strength (Right)	Metabolism during Work (at 617 mkg/min)	Maximum Aerobic Capacity
25 Males	100	107	103	112.5	100	96	81	94	78
11 Females	100	103	96	113.0	98	94	73	99	64

From E. Asmussen and P. Mathiasen, "Some Physiologic Functions in Physical Education Students Reinvestigated after 25 Years," *Journal of the American Geriatrics
Society* 10:379, 1962.

Data on altitude acclimatization seem to indicate that individual differences (both innate qualities and acquired physical fitness) are far
more important in withstanding high altitude than the factor of age per
se (23).

AGE AND THE NERVOUS SYSTEM

Age changes (slowing) in reaction time and speed of movement have
been verified. Birren and his co-workers (6, 7), who have done extensive
investigation in this area, have reached the conclusion that this psycho-
motor slowing is probably an effect of the aging of the central nervous
system because the slowing is common to several sensory modalities and
to several motor pathways. The decreases in conduction time, both afferent and efferent, are insufficient to account for the total slowing.

Cerebral function is much more vulnerable to circulatory deficits than
most tissues, it must have a constant source of O_2, and it cannot function
anaerobically (as can muscle tissue, for instance). For this reason there
is a temptation to associate the effects of aging with a decreased cerebral
blood flow and with the resulting hypoxia; however, when the effects
of aging per se have been separated from the effects of arteriosclerosis,
which frequently accompanies the aging process, it appears that it is
the arteriosclerosis that is at fault. Aging per se, in the absence of arteriosclerotic changes, probably does not result in circulatory or metabolic changes in cerebral function (6, 7).

The German neurophysiologists, C. and O. Vogt, have made the extremely interesting observation that the degree of activity of a particular type of nerve cell has a great effect on its aging process. They have found that involution (part of the aging process) "is delayed not only by normal but also by such excessive activity of nerve cells as results in their hypertrophy (47)." This suggests that physical activity involving overuse of neural pathways of the central nervous system may have beneficial effects, such as we know occur in the case of muscle tissue. Their work has received support from the work of Retzlaff and Fontaine (36) who also found improved spinal motor neuron function as the result of conditioning in rats. Much more scientific research into the possible benefits of vigorous exercise for aging populations is needed.

AGE AND BODY COMPOSITION

As has been discussed in earlier chapters, it is typical for aging humans to increase their weight, and Brozek (11) has provided interesting data on th ecomposition of the human body as it ages (table 17.4). It is clearly seen that this weight gain represents a mean increase in Brozek's sample of 12.24 kilograms (twenty-seven pounds) of fat while the fat-free body weight has actually decreased from age twenty to

TABLE 17.4

Average Estimated Changes in Body Composition during Maturity (20-55 Years) (Standard Weights Refer to Men 176 Cm Tall)

Age	Standard Weight (kg)	Standard Fat %	Fat (kg)	Fat-free Weight (kg)
20	67.6	10.30	6.96	60.6
25	69.9	13.42	9.38	60.5
30	71.3	16.20	11.55	59.8
35	72.9	18.64	13.59	59.3
40	74.1	20.74	15.37	58.7
45	75.5	22.50	16.99	58.5
50	76.0	23.92	18.18	57.8
55	76.8	25.01	19.20	57.6

From J. Brozek, "Changes of Body Composition in Man during Maturity and Their Nutritional Implications," *Federation Proceedings* 11:787, 1952.

fifty-five. It is obvious that, to maintain a constant proportion of body fat as one ages, weight must not merely be maintained at a constant level, it must be decreased. It is conceivable, however, that the loss in fat-free weight represents disuse atrophy of muscle tissue and may not be a necessary component of the aging changes if vigorous exercise is maintained.

Shock and his co-workers (42) have furnished compelling evidence that this loss of active tissue is the cause of the well-known decline in the basal metabolic rate (BMR) with age. When they computed BMR on the basis of body water (which reflects the amount of active tissue cells in the body), no significant changes were observed in relation to age. The customary method of calculating BMR (per unit of surface area) does not differentiate between fat and active tissue; thus we find that the aging body contains fewer and fewer cells, although the activity of individual cells probably does not change significantly. Again, we should like to know the effects vigorous exercise programs might have on this process.

Stature.   It has been shown that, on the average, we also grow shorter as we grow older and fatter. De Queker, Baeyens, and Claessens showed the loss rate to average about one-half inch per decade after age thirty (14).

EFFECTS OF PHYSICAL CONDITIONING ON AGEWISE LOSSES IN FUNCTIONAL CAPACITIES

It must be emphasized at this point that all of the agewise changes described thus far can only be said to *accompany* the aging process. *Causal relationships* have not been established. We may infer that observations of changes in these various functional capacities made upon different groups of subjects at increasing age levels, may be the resultant of a combination of at least three factors: (1) true aging phenomena, (2) unrecognized disease processes whose incidence and severity increase with age, and (3) *disuse phenomena* or the increasing sedentariness of our life style as we grow older. Since we can do little to modify the first two factors, and since the third factor offers potential for modification by the methods of conditioning and training already well known to our profession the author and other investigators have addressed themselves to the question of "How trainable is the older human organism?"

The capacity for improvement of performance by training in children and young adults has long been established. For middle-aged adults the results of investigations over the last two decades which demonstrate the beneficial effects of physical conditioning are also too numerous to cite. However only recently have we turned our attention to the problem of maintaining and improving physical fitness and associated functional capacities in the elderly male and female, arbitrarily defined here as the age bracket over 60. Table 17.5 shows the results of recent research in this direction.

There seems little doubt that the physical working capacity of the older individual can be improved by very significant increments. It should be pointed out that while this improved PWC may have no effect in adding years to our life, it most certainly does add "life to our years." The improvement of PWC is tantamount to increasing the *vigor* of the older individual and this can make a very important contribution to the later years of life, certainly in terms of life syle and possibly even in terms of *health*.

The physiological basis for the improvement in PWC is still very much in question. All of the data reported seem to agree on the fact of potential for trainability in the older organism and the capacity for improvement percentagewise is probably not greatly different from that of the young. The capacity for maximum achievement is of course severely compromised since the older subject starts from a lower level. As to the mechanism by which improved PWC is brought about, the results reported by Saltin et al. (40) and Hartley et al. (27) suggest a difference in the mechanisms of adaptation from young to middle age (thirty-four to fifty-five years) in that the young respond with increases of (1) cardiovascular dimensions (heart size), (2) better redistribution of blood flow to the active tissues, and (3) increased cardiac output and other functional improvements. In the middle-aged men the third factor alone seems to account for the improvement of aerobic capacity. Whether this is also true for the older population (sixty and over) remains unanswered at this time. The data of table 17.5 suggest that improvement of respiratory function may be another important factor in improvement of PWC in the older male.

PRINCIPLES FOR CONDUCT OF CONDITIONING PROGRAMS FOR OLDER MEN AND WOMEN (OVER SIXTY)

Although the principles set forth in this section have been developed around programs for the elderly they would hold in general also for the middle-aged (thirty to sixty). Indeed they would provide a measure of conservatism for this age group.

Medical Examination. It is absolutely essential that every individual over thirty who has a history of sedentary life style be examined and approved by his physician before entry into any physical conditioning program. In recent years, many cardiologists have added stress-tests to

TABLE 17.5

Effects of Physical Conditioning on the Functional Capacities of Older Men and Women (Mean Age over 60)

Measurement	Sex	N	% Improvement	Source
Cardiovascular system				
1. Decrease in HR at submax work	M	5	19	Barry et al. (1966)
	F	3		
2. O$_2$ pulse	M	13	11	Benestad (1965)
	M	48	4 (6 weeks)	deVries (1970)
	M	5	29 (42 weeks)	deVries (1970)
	F	17	7 (12 weeks)	Adams and deVries (1973)
3. Increased blood Vol.	M	13	9	Benestad (1965)
4. Increased total Hb.	M	13	7	Benestad (1965)
5. Cardiac output at 75 watts	M	34	0	deVries (1970)
6. Stroke volume at 75 watts	M	34	6	deVries (1970)
7. Resting systolic BP	M	5	13	Barry et al. (1966)
	F	3		
	M	66	2	deVries (1970)
	F	17	0	Adams and deVries (1973)
8. Resting diastolic BP	M	5	6	Barry et al. (1966)
	F	3		
	M	66	4	deVries (1970)
	F	17	0	Adams and deVries (1973)
9. Regression of EKG abnormalities	M	5	50 percent of abnorm. showed definite improvement	Barry et al. (1966)
	F	3		
Respiratory system				
1. Vital capacity	M	5	0	Barry et al. (1966)
	F	3		
	M	66	5 (6 weeks)	deVries (1970)
	M	8	20 (42 weeks)	deVries (1970)
	F	17	0	Adams and deVries (1970)
2. Max ventilation during exercise	M	47	12 (6 weeks)	deVries (1970)
	M	7	35 (42 weeks)	deVries (1970)
	M	5	50	Barry et al. (1966)
	F	3		
	M	13	0	Benestad (1965)
	F	17	0	Adams and deVries (1973)
Physical work capacity	M	61	9 (6 weeks)	deVries (1970)
	M	8	16 (42 weeks)	deVries (1970)
	F	17	37	Adams and deVries (1973)
	M	5	76	Barry et al. (1966)
	F	3		
Muscular strength	M	68	6 (6 weeks)	deVries (1970)
	M	8	12 (42 weeks)	deVries (1970)
	M	5	50	Perkins and Kaiser (1962)
	F	15		

their examination in which the individual's EKG is monitored *during* the stress of progressively increasing exercise work loads. Such data are invaluable in the conduct of conditioning programs for middle-aged and older people.

Physiological Monitoring (in the Laboratory). Ideally, the individual's initial condition and progress in the program would be evaluated in depth including his responses with respect to O_2 consumption, cardiovascular function (blood pressure, cardiac output, EKG, etc.), respiratory function, muscular status, and anthropometric measurements. This is seldom feasible and it is fortunate that simple measures can provide considerable insight into the individual's status (assuming prior medical clearance). At a minimum expense of money, time, and effort, at least the following parameters can and should be measured: (1) HR and blood pressure response to submaximal exercise (Astrand test), (2) resting blood pressure, (3) strength of selected muscle groups, (4) body weight, and (5) percentage of body fat estimated from skinfolds. Such measurements form the basis for a scientific approach to the use of exercise in conditioning older people in that they (1) allow prescription of exercise on a dose-response basis, and (2) provide considerable motivation for the participants who can thus see their own progress with respect to health benefits they can understand.

Physiological Monitoring (Gym or Field). Every participant should be taught to take his own heart rate, usually at the radial or carotid artery. He should be taught to find the artery quickly (in five to ten seconds) and to count pulse beats accurately over a fifteen second period immediately following exercise. While such a count immediately after exercise in the young may involve considerable error because of the very rapid exponential decline in rate, the rate of decline in older people is much slower, and the rate thus counted is a very valuable criterion of the adequacy of response to any given exercise workout in the middle age and elderly.

Prescription of Exercise (Dose-Response Data). Figure 17.4 shows that the threshold for a training effect in older people requires that they work above that percentage of their heart rate range (% HRR) which is represented by their Astrand score for estimated maximal O_2 consumption in ml/kg/min. For example an estimated maximal O_2 of 30 ml/kg/min would require exercising at levels which would bring HR at least thirty percent of the way from resting toward maximal (16). Thus a man seventy-five years old with a resting rate of seventy and a maximum rate of 152 (taken from table 17.6) would need to work above

$$70 + .30 \ (152\text{-}70) = 70 + 25 = 95$$

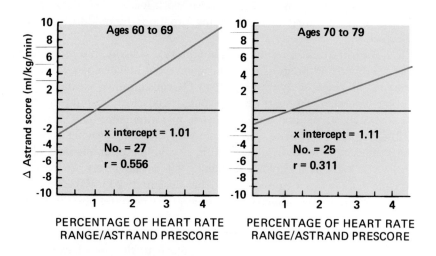

Figure 17-4. Change in Astrand test score after six weeks of training as a function of percentage of heart rate range/Astrand prescore. (From deVries, H.A. *Geriatrics* 26:94, 1971.)

TABLE 17.6

Maximal Heart Rates in Older Men

Age	Heart Rate	Age	Heart Rate	Age	Heart Rate	Age	Heart Rate
50	174	60	166	70	156	80	147
51	173	61	165	71	155	81	146
52	172	62	164	72	154	82	145
53	172	63	163	73	153	83	145
54	171	64	162	74	152	84	144
55	170	65	161	75	152	85	143
56	169	66	160	76	151	86	143
57	168	67	159	77	150	87	142
58	168	68	158	78	149	88	141
59	167	69	157	79	148	89	141

From *Arbeitsphysiologie* 10:251-323, 1938.

Since ninety-five represents the *threshold* for a training effect and since there are errors in our calculations one might raise that value by fifteen to twenty percent and estimate the desirable working heart rate as approximately 109 to 114 which would be a safe load for the healthy normotensive older individual.

Now, using that figure for a target heart rate we may enter the nomogram of figure 17.5 (17) to find what combination of jog-walk would furnish the appropriate challenge to achieve HR 109 to 114. For a maximum O_2 consumption of 30 ml/kg/min even the fifty steps jog-fifty steps walk would raise HR to 118 after five sets of 50-50 and therefore the subject would be recommended to start with only two to three sets of fifty jog-fifty walk and advised to monitor his HR carefully.

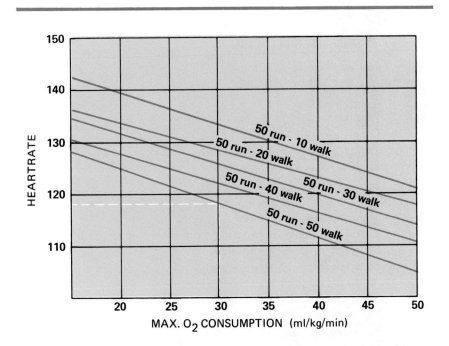

Figure 17-5. Nomogram for the estimation of heart rate response to a given "dose" of jogging for men aged 60-79. Example: for a man in this age bracket with a measured (or estimated from Astrand test) maximal oxygen consumption of 30 milliliters per kilogram per minute, go vertically from 30 on the horizontal axis to the intersection with the 50 run-50 walk regression line. Now go horizontally to the heart rate axis to read 118 which represents the mean response to this dose. The standard error for the 5 regression lines is 8 to 10 beats. (From deVries, H.A. *Geriatrics* 26:110, 1971.)

Progression.   The system of gradual progression of exercise work load used in the author's laboratory and geriatric exercise program is shown in table 17.7. The warm-up is accomplished by calisthenics, the cardio-vascular-respiratory challenge is provided by the run-walk program, and static stretching is used to improve joint mobility and to prevent muscular problems (15). The run or jog phase of the run-walk is done at the cadence and stride length normal and comfortable to the individual with no attempt at regulation for time, etc., in this age level. This program has been shown to be both safe and effective (on a three times per week basis) for a normal population of older men (15) and women (1) in the presence of medical and physiological monitoring.

TABLE 17.7

Exercise Regimen (3 Times/Week)

A. Calisthenics (15-20 minutes)
   1. 5BX
   2. President's Council & Administration on Aging Series (1968)
   3. Others

B. Run-Walk program (15-20 minutes)
   1. 50 steps run, 50 steps walk
      a. 5 sets the first day
      b. Each day increase the number of sets by one until 10 sets have been completed
      c. Use the same set procedure for each new series of run-walk
   2. 50 steps run, 40 steps walk
   3. 50 steps run, 30 steps walk
   4. 50 steps run, 20 steps walk
   5. 50 steps run, 10 steps walk
   6. 75 steps run, 10 steps walk
   7. 100 steps run, 10 steps walk
   8. 125 steps run, 10 steps walk
   9. 150 steps run, 10 steps walk
   10. 175 steps run, 10 steps walk
   11. 200 steps run, 10 steps walk
   12. Individual program

C. Static stretching to prevent soreness and to improve joint mobility (15-20 minutes)

Type of Exercise as a Determinant of Heart Stress in Older People.
deVries and Adams conducted an experiment on twelve older men (mean
age—sixty-nine) in which the work of the heart relationship to total body
work was explored for exercises involving (1) heavy but rhythmic arm
and leg work (crawling), (2) heavy rhythmic leg work with moderate
static contraction of the upper limbs (cycling), and (3) heavy rhythmic
leg work without any static muscular activity (walking). The data indicated that the cardiac effort rises more slowly in walking (rhythmic)
type exercise with increasing loads of total body work than it does for
either cycling or crawling type effort due to the static muscular contractions. It is important in exercising older people to reduce the sympathetic adrenergic vasoconstrictor reflex to a minimum, by maximizing
the rhythmic activity of large muscle masses and by minimizing (1) high
activation levels of small muscles and (2) static muscle contraction of
any kind. The natural activities of walking and running (jogging) are
well suited to this purpose.

IMPLICATIONS FOR PHYSICAL EDUCATION AND ATHLETICS

After the foregoing review of the effects of aging upon physical performance and related physiological functions, the future for the college-
age student using this text must seem unattractive indeed. However, two
very important mitigating factors must be considered.

First, each of the performance measures discussed has wide variability
in its measurement. Since all of the discussion has centered about comparisons of *means* for various age groups, it is extremely important to
recognize that, in all of the measurements, it is possible for a superior
individual in an older age bracket to surpass the performance of an inferior young individual (superior or inferior in respect to his age group).

Second, for many of the measurements discussed in this chapter we
have no way of knowing how much of the age decrement can be attributed to aging per se and how much to increasingly sedentary habits or
increasing degrees of unrecognized disease processes (such as arteriosclerosis).

That some decline in physical performance must occur with advanced
age is certainly undeniable, but that the ravages of old age can be slowed
down by a sensibly vigorous regimen of physical exercise is supported
by the available scientific evidence. Let us now consider the implications
the foregoing information may have for the philosophy and curricula of
physical education in regard to four arbitrarily defined age groups: (1)
childhood, six to twelve years; (2) adolescence, thirteen to twenty years;
(3) maturity, twenty-one to sixty years; and (4) old age, sixty-one and
over.

Childhood.   There seems to be no physiological disadvantage for this age group in respect to energy supply. In relation to their mass, children can transport and utilize oxygen at rates comparable to young adults.

In regard to strength, it is well known (e.g., observation of norms for motor performance tests) that strength per unit of weight increases with age. Or one might say that the younger the child the less able he is to handle his body weight.

In regard to the nervous system and coordination, all evidence indicates that reaction time and speed of movement are at a low level in early childhood and improve rapidly to their maximal values in young adulthood.

According to the evidence cited, it would seem that childhood is a time for games and activities that are vigorous enough to bring about maximal physical development. Such activities as gymnastics (at least apparatus events), where strength per unit of body weight is at a premium, would be most successfully accomplished during the adolescent years. Activities that test, and possibly develop, speed of reactions and movements are challenging and are well-received by this age group. Baseball, basketball, and soccer are ideal activities.

Adolescence.   During these years an individual achieves or closely approaches the maximum in all performance and physiological measurements. There are two considerations for physical education for this age range: (1) supplying the immediate needs for exercises that will provide the greatest physical development, and (2) forming the foundation for exercise habits in later years.

The first consideration requires the inclusion of vigorous strength and endurance activities, and there are no limitations for a healthy individual in this age bracket. Every individual should be exposed to and challenged by heavy-resistance activities for developing strength, and to activities of sufficient intensity and duration of effort to build muscular and cardio-respiratory endurance. Examples of the first category are such activities as gymnastics, wrestling, and weight training. The second category includes such activities as swimming and distance running (against time, at least occasionally), and all of the vigorous sports activities, football, soccer, handball, tennis, badminton, etc.

The second consideration, forming the foundation for exercise in later years, requires a good instructional program that is geared to the needs of adults and that is readily provided by the physical recreational opportunities of a particular geographic area. Primary consideration must be given to the fact that adults cannot always count on even one available partner or opponent much less seventeen for baseball or nine for basketball. Individual and dual sports must be introduced and skills must be taught so that future *participation* is encouraged rather than *spectatoritis*.

Maturity. It is the author's conviction that limitations on exercise in the adult years are self-imposed by a lack of consistency and continuity in an individual's exercise habits. Probably every activity that is mastered during adolescence or young adulthood can be continued by a healthy individual well into old age. This is true, however, only if participation occurs a minimum of three times weekly. If occupational obligations prevent this degree of participation, calisthenics or weight training programs can be designed to provide the mid-week conditioning necessary to prevent the weekend's activity from becoming a strain instead of an exhilarating experience.

For example, skiing, especially cross-country skiing, can be one of the most demanding of all sports; few adults can ski every weekend, let alone three times per week, but it is a simple matter for a trained physical educator to provide mid-week exercise programs for maintaining the physical capacities needed for successful weekend skiing. Suitable calisthenic or weight training exercises can maintain the muscular strength and range of movement needed, while simple application of interval training principles to bench-stepping or stair climbing can maintain the requisite cardiorespiratory fitness.

From the standpoint of *preventive medicine*, it is most important that every healthy adult possess skill in one or several sports that are vigorous enough to maintain optimum levels of cardiorespiratory fitness. Such activity will also provide benefits in maintaining body weight and relieving nervous tension (chapter 13). Ideally, this activity should be so enjoyable and challenging that it is self-motivating. Activities that are interpreted as drudgery are not likely to be long continued, no matter how rewarding. Excellent activities that meet the above criteria are tennis, handball, volley ball (if played correctly), badminton, skiing, surf boarding, etc. It will be noted that some excellent activities, from a fun standpoint have been omitted; golf, for instance, is not vigorous enough for young adults (nor is swimming, as ordinarily performed) to form the *only* physical recreation if maximum benefits in physical condition are desired.

It should also be emphasized at this point that any layoff from vigorous activities must be followed by a period of progressive rebuilding to the former level of competency. In general, the older the individual, the lower the first work load should be, and the longer the period of progressive rebuilding of condition.

Old Age. Depending upon the health of the individual, a greater or lesser reduction in work load (both intensity and duration) is indicated. Most activities allow for such adjustment without complete cessation. In tennis and badminton one plays doubles instead of singles; in skiing one skis for shorter periods of time with increasing lengths of rest intervals, etc. Obviously, in all competitive dual sports, one modification exists simply in playing opponents of roughly equivalent age.

There is no evidence that vigorous exercise can in any way injure a *healthy* individual in the older age brackets; however, frequent physical examinations, at least yearly, are necessary to protect the individual from overstrain during an incipient illness.

Indeed, there is a growing body of experimental evidence to show that the healthy older individual improves his functional capacities through physical conditioning much as does the young person. Percentagewise his improvement is comparable to that in the young, although he starts at and progresses to lower achievement levels and probably requires less training stimulus to bring about the desired response. In general, it may be said that the effects of physical conditioning upon the middle-aged and older individual are opposite in direction to those commonly associated with the aging process.

REFERENCES

1. Adams, G. M., and deVries, H. A. Physiological effects of an exercise training regimen upon women aged 52-79. *Journal of Gerontology* 28:50-55, 1973.
2. Asmussen, E., and Mathiasen, P. 1962. Some physiologic functions in physical education students reinvestigated after 25 years. *Journal of the American Geriatrics Society* 10:379-87.
3. Astrand, I. 1960. Aerobic work capacity in men and women with special reference to age. *Acta Physiologica Scandinavica* 49 suppl. 169.
4. Barry, A. J.; Daly, J. W.; Pruett, E. D. R.; Steinmetz, J. R.; Page, H. F.; Birkhead, N. C.; and Rodahl, K. 1966. The effects of physical conditioning on older individuals. *Journal of Gerontology* 21:182-91.
5. Benestad, A. M. 1965. Trainability of old men. *Acta Medica Scandinavica* 178:321-27.
6. Birren, J. E.; Imus, H. A.; and Windle, W. F., eds. 1959. *The process of aging in the nervous system.* Springfield, Ill.: Charles C Thomas.
7. Birren, J. E.; Butler, R. N.; Greenhouse, S. W.; Sokoloff, L.; and Yarrow, M. R. eds. 1963. *Human aging, a biological behavioral study.* Washington, D. C.: Public Health Service Publication no. 986.
8. Bock, A. V. 1963. The circulation of a marathoner. *Journal of Sports Medicine and Physical Fitness* 3:80-86.
9. Borner, W.; Moll, E.; Schroder, J.; and Rau, F. P. 1964. Abhängigkeit der Kreislaufzeit von Alter Geschlecht und Körperlänge. *Archiv für Kreislaufforschung* 43:221-35.

10. Brandfonbrener, M.; Landowne, M.; and Shock, N. W. 1955. Changes in cardiac output with age. *Circulation* 12:557-66.
11. Brozek, J. 1952. Changes of body composition in man during maturity and their nutritional implications. *Federation Proceedings* 11:784-93.
12. Comroe, J. H.; Forster, R. E.; Dubois, A. B.; Briscoe, W. A.; and Carlsen, E. 1962. *The lung*. Chicago: The Yearbook Publishers, Inc.
13. Damon, E. L. 1971. An experimental investigation of the relationship of age to various parameters of muscle strength. Doctoral dissertation, USC (physical education).
14. Dequeker, J. V.; Baeyens, J. P.; and Claessens, J. 1969. The significance of stature as a clinical measurement of aging. *Journal of the American Geriatrics Society* 17:169-79.
15. deVries, H. A. 1970. Physiological effects of an exercise training regimen upon men aged 52-88. *Journal of Gerontology* 25:325-36.
16. ———. 1971a. Exercise intensity threshold for improvement of cardiovascular-respiratory function in older men. *Geriatrics* 26:94-101.
17. ———. 1971b. Prescription of exercise for older men from telemetered exercise heart rate data. *Geriatrics* 26:102-11.
18. deVries, H. A., and Adams, G. M. 1972a. Comparison of exercise responses in old and young men: I. The cardiac effort/total body effort relationship. *Journal of Gerontology* 27:344-48.
19. ———. 1972b. Comparison of exercise responses in old and young men: II. ventilatory mechanics. *Journal of Gerontology* 27:349-52.
20. ———. Effect of the type of exercise upon the work of the heart in older men. In preparation.
21. Dill, D. B.; Horvath, S. M.; and Craig, F. N. 1958. Responses to exercise as related to age. *Journal of Applied Physiology* 12:195-96.
22. Dill, D. B., and Consolazio, C. F. 1962. Responses to exercise as related to age and environmental temperature. *Journal of Applied Physiology* 17:645-49.
23. Dill, D. B.; Robinson, S.; Balke, B.; and Newton, J. L. 1964. Work tolerance: age and altitude. *Journal of Applied Physiology* 19:483-88.
24. Donevan, R. E.; Palmer, W. H.; Varvis, C. J.; and Bates, D. V. 1959. Influence of age on pulmonary diffusing capacity. *Journal of Applied Physiology* 14:483-92.
25. Evans, S. J. 1971. An electromyographic analysis of skeletal neuromuscular fatigue with special reference to age. Doctoral dissertation, USC (physical education).
26. Fisher, M. B., and Birren, J. E. 1947. Age and strength. *Journal of Applied Psychology* 31:490-97.
27. Hartley, L. H.; Grimby, G.; Kilbom, A.; Nilsson, N. J.; Astrand, I.; Bjure, J.; Ekblom, B.; and Saltin, B. 1969. Physical training in sedentary middle aged and older men: III. Cardiac output and gas exchange at submaximal and maximal exercise. *Scandinavian Journal of Clinical and Laboratory Investigation* 24:335-49.

28. Mittman, C.; Edelman, N. H.; Norris, A. H.; and Shock, N. W. 1965. Relationship between chest wall and pulmonary compliance and age. *Journal of Applied Physiology* 20:1211-16.

29. Norris, A. H.; Shock, N. W.; and Yiengst, M. J. 1953. Age changes in heart rate and blood pressure responses to tilting and standardized exercise. *Circulation* 8:521-26.

30. Norris, A. H.; Shock, N. W.; Landowne, M.; and Falzone, J. A. 1956. Pulmonary function studies: age differences in lung volume and bellows function. *Journal of Gerontology* 11:379-87.

31. Norris, A. H.; Shock, N. W.; and Falzone, J. A. 1962. Relation of lung volumes and maximal breathing capacity to age and socio-economic status. In *Medical and Clinical Aspects of Aging*, ed. H. T. Blumenthal, pp. 163-71. New York: Columbia University Press.

32. Pariskova, J.; Eiselt, E.; Sprynarova, S.; and Wachtlova, M. 1971. Body composition, aerobic capacity and density of muscle capillaries in young and old men. *Journal of Applied Physiology* 31:323-25.

33. Pemberton, J., and Flanagan, E. G. 1956. Vital capacity and timed vital capacity in normal men over forty. *Journal of Applied Physiology* 9:291-96.

34. Perkins, L. C., and Kaiser, H. L. 1962. Results of short term isotonic and isometric exercise programs in persons over sixty. *Physical Therapy Reviews* 41:633-35.

35. Redisch, W.; Meckeler, K.; and Steele, J. M. 1962. Changes in peripheral blood flow and vascular responses with age. In *Medical and Clinical Aspects of Aging*, ed. H. T. Blumenthal, pp. 453-59. New York: Columbia University Press.

36. Retzlaff, E., and Fontaine, J. 1965. Functional and structural changes in motor neurons with age. In *Behavior Aging and the Nervous System*, ed. A. T. Welford and J. E. Birren. Springfield: Charles C Thomas.

37. Rizzato, G., and Marazzini, L. 1970. Thoracoabdominal mechanics in elderly men. *Journal of Applied Physiology* 28:457-60.

38. Robinson, S. 1938. Experimental studies of physical fitness in relation to age. *Arbeitsphysiologie* 10:251-323.

39. Rodahl, K. 1961. Physical work capacity. *AMA Archives of Environmental Health* 2:499-510.

40. Saltin, B.; Hartley, H.; Kilbom, A.; and Astrand, I. 1969. II. Physical training in sedentary middle aged and older men. *Scandinavian Journal of Clinical and Laboratory Investigation* 24:323-34.

41. Shock, N. W. 1961. Current concepts of the aging process. *Journal of the American Medical Association* 175:654-56.

42. Shock, N. W.; Watkin, D. M.; Yiengst, M. J.; Norris, A. H.; Gaffney, G. W.; Gregerman, R. I.; and Falzone, J. A. 1963. Age differences in the water content of the body as related to basal oxygen consumption in males. *Journal of Gerontology* 18:1-8.

43. Simonson, E. 1957. Changes of physical fitness and cardiovascular functions with age. *Geriatrics* 12:28-39.

44. Starr, I. 1964. An essay on the strength of the heart and on the effect of aging upon it. *American Journal of Cardiology* 14:771-83.
45. Turner, J. M.; Mead, J.; and Wohl, M. E. 1968. Elasticity of human lungs in relation to age. *Journal of Applied Physiology* 25:664-71.
46. Vasiliyva, V. Y. 1962. The effect of physical exercise on the cardiovascular system of elderly persons. *Excerpta Medica Gerontology and Geriatrics* 5: 5, no. 641. From Papers presented at 2nd conference on Gerontology and Geriatrics at Moscow, 1960.
47. Vogt, C., and Vogt, O. 1946. Aging of nerve cells. *Nature* 158:304.
48. Wessel, J. A., and Van Huss, W. D. 1969. The influence of physical activity and age on exercise adaptation of women aged 20-69 years. *Journal of Sports Medicine* 9:173-80.

Part Three

PHYSIOLOGY APPLIED
TO THE TRAINING
AND CONDITIONING
OF ATHLETES

18 Physiology of Muscular Strength

The desirability of a *minimum quantity* of strength has long beer. recognized in athletics; however, the advantages of maximum levels of strength for all sports in which power is a factor were not recognized by physical educators, athletes, or coaches until quite recently. This strange neglect of the strength factor in athletes was the result of an unscientific acceptance, by virtually everyone concerned, of an old wives' tale that claimed that the development of large amounts of strength in the musculature (through weight training, etc.) inevitably resulted in a condition known as *muscle bound*. Being muscle bound was supposed to limit both range and speed of movement in those who participated in weight training, and therefore was anathema to all but the most heretical coaches. This belief persisted until shortly after World War II.

At the end of World War II the need for rehabilitation procedures to restore strength to various body segments of injured veterans was acute. This need brought about a scientific evaluation of weight training procedures, and the pioneering work of De Lorme and Watkins brought about acceptance of weight training for rehabilitation purposes (13). Acceptance of weight training by the medical profession apparently stimulated the research-oriented members of the physical education profession to put the muscle bound hypothesis to the test by the scientific method. The results are now history, for many well-controlled investigations laid the ghost of the muscle bound myth. It is now generally accepted that properly conceived weight training programs not only do not slow or restrict joint motion but may even (in some cases) improve these factors while providing very substantial gains in strength.

The importance of strength in athletics is not always obvious, although in such an activity as shot putting the need for maximum power is readily apparent. It would be well to recall earlier discussion at this point and to note that power is the rate of doing work (producing force). We may therefore think of power as the result of two factors: (1) strength to produce the force and (2) speed to increase the rate at which the force can be applied. In other words, we can improve an athlete's power in three different ways: (1) increase his speed, strength remaining constant, (2) increase his strength, speed remaining constant, and (3) improve speed and strength.

It is a matter of practical experience in coaching that speed of movement improves rapidly in the training program to a plateau, from which it can be increased only with great difficulty. On the other hand, very few athletes have even begun to approach their maximum strength levels, and thus large gains in power are possible by improving strength while simply maintaining speed.

That power is a factor in almost all athletic activities is best demonstrated by the onslaught on the record books in all sports where strength training has been pursued as part of the conditioning regimen. Even such a seemingly unlikely sport as swimming has borne witness to the beneficial effects of strength training. Prior to World War II, swimming coaches were loathe to have their stars even walk unduly lest they develop bunchy muscles; the few heroic and heretical coaches who used weight training in those days were cause for much grave "head shaking."

This chapter will discuss the physiological bases of strength and its improvement; it will culminate in a set of principles, based upon our present knowledge, for the formulation of programs designed to improve the strength (and power) factor in athletes.

PHYSIOLOGY OF STRENGTH

Strength and Hypertrophy. One of the outward manifestations of great strength is large muscles of firm texture; however, the relationship between size and strength is not absolute. We have all seen the skinny fellow who possesses greater strength than his build would warrant believing. When this relationship is described mathematically, positive correlations are found between strength and muscle girth. It has been the author's experience that this correlation is very high when the group examined is composed of well-conditioned, nonobese young men. The relationship grows smaller as interfering factors, such as fatty tissue and differing levels of training, appear in the group tested.

In any event, it is known that the development of strength in any one individual is the result of increasing the size of the muscle fibers involved not by increasing the number of fibers in the muscle. This increase in fiber size is called *hypertrophy*. Hypertrophy and strength are brought about only by subjecting a muscle to greater loads than those to which it is accustomed. This is known as the *overload principle*.

Disuse and Atrophy. Anyone who has had a limb in a cast can attest to the basic fact of muscular atrophy (shrinking of a muscle). Scientific evidence has been presented (15, 21) to show that immobilization of a limb (whether mechanically—as by cast—or by denervation) results in decreased fiber size and (at least over a short period of time) in no loss in number of fibers. Thus we may say that all of the changes in muscle tissue brought about by training programs are impermanent, and that training must be carried on systematically throughout a lifetime, or a degree of atrophy from disuse will set in.

Strength and Usable Force. If strength development and muscle hypertrophy proceed together, we might expect to find no change in the ratio of strength per unit of cross-section as training proceeds. Indeed, Hettinger and Muller (19) found this to be true in their work with isometric training. Furthermore, it has been suggested that this ratio remains very constant regardless of age or sex (32). Uncertainty exists, however, in that one investigator found differences between the sexes in this regard, and differences from muscle to muscle in the same individual (27).

In any event, strength per unit of cross-section is a theoretical concept, and it tells us little about the forces that can be produced at the ends of the bony lever systems. It will be recalled from earlier discussions that two factors interact to determine the force available at the end of a bony lever: (1) the length at which the muscle is working and (2) the angle of pull. Figure 18.1 illustrates this in respect to the third-class lever that works at the elbow during elbow flexion. At full extension (180 degrees) where the muscle length is greatest, the angle of pull is poor. At full flexion (forty degrees), the muscle is doubly at a disadvantage because it is short and because it works at a poor angle. The best combination of the two factors seems to be at approximately 115 degrees (11).

When a muscle works directly in pulling upon a bone (without going through a mechanical lever, as in pulling a rope over a pulley), the curve approximates a length-tension diagram in which the muscle length is the dominant factor in determining the force available (fig. 18.2). In figure 18.2 it is seen that the best force of contraction results when the hip is fully flexed at 50° because this position has the hip extensors fully stretched. Thus it can be seen that the strength available for doing use-

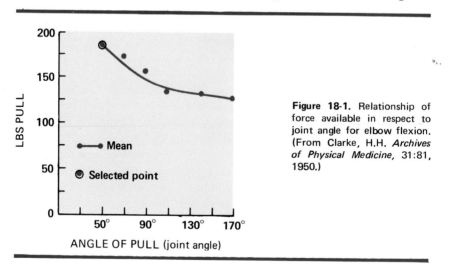

Figure 18-1. Relationship of force available in respect to joint angle for elbow flexion. (From Clarke, H.H. *Archives of Physical Medicine,* 31:81, 1950.)

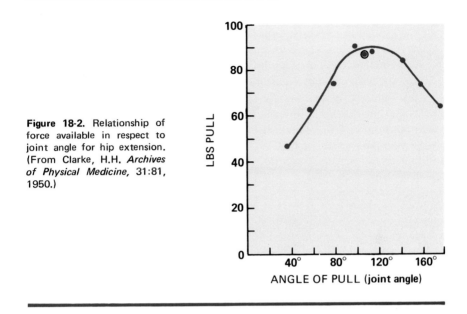

Figure 18-2. Relationship of force available in respect to joint angle for hip extension. (From Clarke, H.H. *Archives of Physical Medicine,* 31:81, 1950.)

ful work varies from joint to joint and also with the angle of each joint. This is a very important point to bear in mind when one considers the effects of an exercise. It will be discussed in greater detail in a following section.

The Training Stimulus for Strength. Our training procedures for the development of strength could undoubtedly be greatly improved if we knew precisely what quantity and quality of stimulus are required to bring about a training effect. The early work of Hettinger and Muller (19), which formed the basis for the current popularity of isometrics, indicated that the threshold value of the resistance necessary to bring about gains is approximately one-third the maximal contraction strength of the muscle under consideration. It was their opinion that the training stimulus for strength gain was the occurrence of an oxygen deficit in the tissue involved. Below a contraction strength of one-third maximum, no O_2 deficit occurred. Analysis of isometric fatigue curves (34) supports their contention in that the ability to replenish energy meets its upper limit at about one-third of the maximum contraction strength, probably due to mechanical occlusion of the muscle.

However, more recent studies have failed to verify hypoxia (oxygen deficit) as the necessary stimulus (18, 26). In fact, Morehouse and his associates at UCLA have been unable to find evidence in favor of any of the following postulated factors as stimuli for strength gain: (1) temperature change, (2) hypoxia, (3) stretching, or (4) cerebration (22). They suggest the interesting possibility that the training stimulus resides in the central nervous system and that training effects are brought about by reduction of the normal inhibitory effects of the extrapyramidal system upon the lower motorneuron.

It is interesting to note that two investigations have independently demonstrated the feasibility of developing strength in muscles by involuntary contractions initiated by electrical stimulation (25, 29); but in both experiments the results were considerably inferior to those of normal, voluntary contraction. Since the motor pathways are probably minimally involved in electrical training, this constitutes evidence for a training stimulus that resides in the muscle tissue itself; but the fact that the training effect was quantitatively inferior to voluntary contraction indicates that some of the training effect resides in the nervous system. Until more conclusive evidence is available, it seems logical to hypothesize the existence of training effects in the nervous system and in the muscle tissue itself.

SPECIFICITY OF STRENGTH GAIN TO ANGLE OF EXERCISE

Since there is so much interest in isometric training for strength, we must ask how specific muscle training may be to the angle at which the training takes place. This question is also important for such isotonic methods as weight training because the *net effect* of the weight changes with the angle of the joint.

Logan demonstrated that the strength training effect is specific to the angle at which the greatest resistance is applied (24). Of his three experimental groups (fifteen in each), one used weight resistance and one used spring resistance to strengthen the knee extensors, while the third group was a control. Using weight resistance the greatest resistance was encountered from about 155 degrees to full extension, and in spring resistance (on this particular device) the greatest resistance was offered at 115 degrees. The weight training group made significantly greater gains than the spring resistance group when tested at 155 degrees, and the spring resistance group showed significantly greater gains when tested at 115 degrees.

It should be noted that these differences existed despite the fact that both groups exercised isotonically throughout the whole range of motion, the only real difference in resistance at various angles being that of degree. These results implied that even greater differences in training due to joint angle specificity would be found as the result of isometric training, and this has indeed been the case. Two independent investigations (3, 16) have shown that strength tested at angles other than that at which isometric training took place may show gains less than fifty percent of that at the exercised angle. This difference in gains appeared when the test angle was as little as twenty degrees removed from the exercise angle. The lesser specificity for isotonic training has also been demonstrated (12).

It has also been shown that the rate of strength gain is greater when a muscle is trained isometrically at a short length compared with a long length. This was found to be true for all muscles tested, elbow flexor and extensor and the wrist pronators and supinators (33).

ISOTONIC VERSUS ISOMETRIC STRENGTH TRAINING METHODS

Until quite recently, when man wanted to increase his strength he usually used some form of weight lifting in application of the overload principle. In 1953 Hettinger and Müller (of Germany) published their work on isometric training (19), and their findings indicated that a maximum training effect could be obtained from one daily six-second isometric contraction against two-thirds of an individual's maximal contraction strength. Greater force, duration, or number of repetitions did not seem to increase the rate of strength gain, which they found averaged five percent per week when training was performed five times per week. Strength improved in various muscles from thirty-three to 181 percent.

Coaches and athletes have trampled each other ever since in getting on the isometric bandwagon, and an evaluation of the comparative merits of isotonic (classic) and isometric training methods seems to be in order. Comparison is difficult, however, for at least two reasons: (1) it is extremely difficult to compare equal work loads of isometric and isotonic training sessions, and (2) most investigators have used isometric methods (cable tensiometer, strain gauge, dynamometer, etc.) for testing results from both types of training; and both reasons probably preclude a valid comparison.

Advantages of Isotonic Methods. Both isometric and isotonic methods have been shown to bring about significant gains in strength in short periods of time, but in investigations where direct comparisons have been made, the differences—although not large—favor the isotonic method.

Probably the greatest advantage in isotonic methods is that strength gains are specific to the angle at which the resistance is encountered.

Thus isotonic exercises can be designed to work the entire range of motion in one contraction, but several contractions would be needed at different angles to work the whole range of motion with isometric methods.

Another advantage for isotonic methods may be that the individual sees work being done, and this appears to be a psychological advantage for those who find a static contraction boring.

Muscular hypertrophy appears to be somewhat greater in isotonic exercise (31), and greater endurance effects have also been noted (14). There is also reason to believe that dynamic strength is better related to motor ability since motor ability correlated 0.76 with dynamic strength and only 0.45 with static strength (7).

Advantages of Isometric Methods.   The chief advantages here are administrative in nature. If only one contraction per day is used (as in the original work of Hettinger and Müller), great savings in time are possible. Furthermore, a little ingenuity can reduce the equipment needed to pieces of apparatus that are already available in the gym or on the practice field. The elimination of the need for barbells, dumbbells, etc., also makes it possible to work out larger groups in shorter periods of time.

However, recent work from the same German laboratory (28) has modified the original work of Hettinger and Muller, and it now appears that the rate of strength gain approximately doubles when maximal contraction strength is used instead of two-thirds of the maximum. Also, a higher end strength can be reached by increasing the number of six-second repetitions to between five and ten.

If these changes are made in the procedure, plus working each joint at three to four angles to eliminate the specificity problem, isometric results may well match isotonic results, but making these changes would nullify the advantage in time. It is also important to recall the discussion of chapter six in which the well-defined effect of isometric tension in raising the arterial blood pressure was pointed out. Isometric exercises must be considered potentially hazardous for people in cardiac rehabilitation or adult exercise programs because of the greater rise in blood pressure.

TRAINING METHODOLOGY

Isometric Contraction.   The work of Müller and Rohmert (28) seems to be definitive, so there are few choices to be made as to frequency, intensity, etc. Best results appear to be obtained by using maximal contraction strength, held for five seconds, and repeated five to ten times daily. It would be desirable to apply these contractions at varying points in the range of motion if a well-rounded workout is desired, or, if the activity that is trained for demands strength or power, throughout the entire range of motion. In some cases, as in ballistic movements, analysis may indicate the need for maximal power at the beginning of the motion; and exercises should be designed accordingly.

Isotonic Contraction. Many combinations of resistance, repetitions, and number of sets are possible here, but let us first define our terms. *Repetitions* (although used incorrectly, it is firmly entrenched in the literature) means the total number of executions. *Execution maximum* and *repetition maximum* can be used interchangeably, and they indicate the maximum weight that can be lifted for the indicated number of repetitions; that is, 10 EM (RM) is the greatest weight that can be lifted ten times. *One set* is the number of repetitions done consecutively, without resting.

The investigations that have been performed in this area are not in close agreement, but a general picture seems to emerge. The classic work of De Lorme and Watkins (13) recommended the following program:

> 1 set of 10 repetitions, with ½ 10 RM
> 1 set of 10 repetitions, with ¾ 10 RM
> 1 set of 10 repetitions, with   10 RM

Other investigators have furnished support for the effectiveness of this method of weight training (2); however, systematic investigations of the value of varying numbers of repetitions seem to indicate that fewer repetitions may be even more effective: four, five, or six. Berger's data (5) are provided in figure 18.3, and they provide rather good evidence that

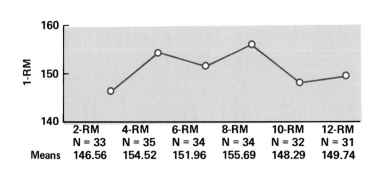

	2-RM	4-RM	6-RM	8-RM	10-RM	12-RM
	N = 33	N = 35	N = 34	N = 34	N = 32	N = 31
Means	146.56	154.52	151.96	155.69	148.29	149.74

Figure 18-3. Mean strength resulting from weight training programs involving six different methods. (From Berger. *Research Quarterly,* 33:334, 1962.)

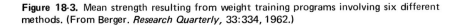

between four and eight repetitions provide maximal results in terms of strength gain. Another approach which has been validated under laboratory conditions as being very effective is that of doing ten repetitions in which each repetition is done against the maximum possible for that particular execution (8). Thus the individual starts with his 1 RM and uses as large a weight as possible for each successive lift. In comparison with the use of one set of ten repetitions with the 10 RM it was shown that significantly greater gain in strength was achieved although the total work in foot-pounds was greater in the 10 RM groups. Muscle hypertrophy seems to be best brought about by the De Lorme and Watkins procedure (2).

The optimal number of workouts per week is probably between three and five, depending upon the amount of other vigorous activity a given individual may be indulging in (work or play) beyond the weight training program.

RATE OF STRENGTH GAIN AND RETENTION OF STRENGTH

Hettinger and Müller, in their original study on isometric strength training, reported mean gains for their subjects of about five percent per week (19), but many subsequent investigators have been unable to demonstrate this rapid a gain with isometric methods. On the other hand, forearm pronation has been reported to increase by as much as seventy-three percent in one week (12) by isometric methods. The same investigators found that isotonic training improved the same movement by as much as 168 percent in one week.

Such divergent results require explanation, and Muller and Rohmert (28) have furnished the logical explanation. Their work has shown that strength gain does not proceed at a constant rate: gain is very rapid when a muscle's beginning strength is a small proportion of its maximal possible end strength, and, as the muscle approaches its maximum possible end strength, the gain is very much slower. Thus the high rates of gain have occurred in such muscles as the pronators of the hand, which would not be expected to be in a high state of training. Muscles that are heavily used have usually shown more modest gains, of from one to ten percent per week in isotonic training and of one to five percent in isometric training.

Retention of Strength Training Effects. After a strength training program is terminated, the gains persist for a considerable period of time. Unfortunately, no data are available on the effects of immobilization after a rigorous training program, but data have been presented on subjects who have simply ceased their training. In one case, observations repeated twelve months after the end of training showed retention of strength in an amount double the pretraining value, although it had declined from the post-training level (12). This does not appear to be unusual; indeed similar observations show the same result. It would seem that long-lasting changes of this type can be attributed to changes brought about in the nervous system by the training regimen.

METHODS OF MEASURING STRENGTH

Isotonic Versus Isometric Methods. As with many other physiological parameters, accurate and objective measurement of strength is a problem. To begin with, measuring strength by isotonic methods degenerates into a trial-and-error situation. For example, if we wish to determine the maximal weight that can be lifted by a muscle group, we may start with a weight that is estimated to be less than maximal and work up to the maximal in small increments; however, the number of trials needed to establish the maximum will vary from subject to subject (according to our "guessing" ability) and varying levels of fatigue will influence the maximum attained. This is hardly objective measurement, and consequently it is not often used for scientific purposes. Also, this method is too time-consuming for classwork.

On the other hand, measurement of isometric tension is done easily and quickly, and it can be fairly precise, but does this measure the same capacity that is developed by isotonic exercise? A well-controlled study showed that no significant correlation exists between isotonic and isometric measurements of strength gains (4). Even absolute strength, when measured by isotonic and isometric methods, yielded a correlation of only 0.622- 0.800 (1, 4). The result of isotonic programs should therefore be measured isotonically and the results of isometric programs should be measured isometrically.

Cable Tension Strength Tests. Of all the methods for measuring isometric strength, probably the simplest and most widely used is the cable tension testing method of Clarke. Figure 18.4 illustrates the cable tensiometer instrument used in the testing, and figure 18.5 shows the application of the method in testing elbow flexion strength. Objectivity coefficients of 0.90 and above were obtained when the tests were administered by experienced testers. Thirty-eight such tests have been devised and validated for testing the various muscle groups of the body (10).

Isokinetic Strength Measurement. In recent years measurement of strength under conditions of constant velocity muscular contractions has become popular. This is called *isokinetic strength* measurement and prob-

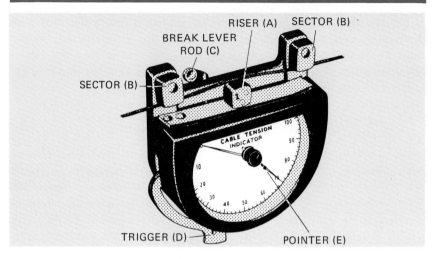

Figure 18-4. The cable tensiometer used for evaluation of muscular strength. (From Clarke and Clarke. *Developmental and Adapted Physical Education,* Copyright © 1963, Prentice Hall, Inc., Englewood Cliffs, N.J.)

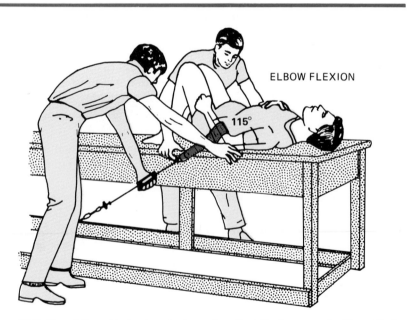

Figure 18-5. Use of the cable tensiometer in testing elbow flexion strength. (From Clarke and Clarke. *Developmental and Adapted Physical Education,* Copyright © 1963, Prentice Hall, Inc., Englewood Cliffs, N.J.)

ably got its impetus from the work of Asmussen, et al. (1) who designed a device using strain gauges with which the force of contraction could be measured and recorded during movement, but limited to constant velocity conditions. Figure 18.6 shows the results of their work in which it can be seen that at all velocities eccentric contraction can develop more and concentric contraction less force than isometric contraction. They also showed that the correlation between maximum isometric and dynamic contraction was 0.80 at a velocity of fifteen percent of arm length per second.

While this approach represents a distinct improvement over isometric tests and those using repeated measures of ability to lift weight, it still does not measure the quality of muscle which is really most important to athletic ability i.e., the ability to produce force in accelerated movement which is typical of almost all skilled muscle action in sports. Interestingly, the basis for such measurement of force (strength) in accel-

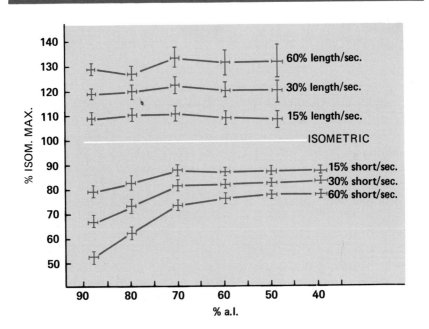

Figure 18-6. Concentric force (lower three curves), and excentric force (upper three curves) at three different velocities of movement, expressed as percentages of isometric force in the different positions. Extended arm to the left. Horizontal and vertical bars denote ± 1 s.e. (From Asmussen, Hansen, and Lammert. *Communications from Testing and Observation Institute of The Danish National Association for Infantile Paralysis* 1965.)

erated movement was provided in the early 1920s by A. V. Hill (22). It hardly seems too early to rejuvenate the methods of Hill to study the production of force by muscles under game conditions which are really not isometric or isokinetic but in fact necessitate the production of force in accelerating-decelerating movements.

Individual Variability. Strength may be expected to vary somewhat in an individual from day to day. The amount of this variability has been found to range from 1.5 to 11.6 percent for women, and from 5.3 to 9.3 percent for men (calculated as the standard deviation from the mean) (36).

Generality Versus Specificity. We often speak of a strong man or a weak man, and imply that strength is a general quality, that all muscles are strong or weak to the same degree. Obviously, the relationships of strength among the various muscles of any individual are not perfect, but there is a high degree of generality. When the strength of single muscle groups was correlated against the total of twenty-two representative muscle groups, all correlations were positive and were significant at better than 0.01 the level of confidence. Muscle groups that correlated highest (most representative of general strength) were leg extensors, 0.89; hip flexors, 0.72; knee extensors, 0.70; hand grip, 0.69; and elbow flexors, 0.64 (35). Thus strength tests that use several of these muscle groups can estimate the general strength quite accurately.

Quantity and Quality of Muscle Tissue. It is apparent that *quantity* and *quality* enter into the determination of the ultimate strength of a muscle. When we relate strength and size of the same muscle group in different subjects, substantial correlations are found. The author has found this relationship to be between $r = 0.80$ to 0.90 for well-trained, nonobese young men in the elbow flexor group.

The quality (or absolute muscle force) varies from muscle to muscle within an individual, however, and the quality of muscle tissue is best measured as strength per unit of physiological cross-section. Physiological cross-section is the same as anatomic cross-section only when the muscle fibers are parallel to the tendon of the muscle; otherwise it is obtained by dividing the volume of the muscle by the length (30). The mean strength per unit of cross-section has been estimated for various muscle groups, and it varies from 4.36 kilograms per square centimeter for the rectus femoris (female) to 14.76 kilograms per square centimeter for the triceps muscle (male) (27).

The available evidence indicates that in strength training programs the strength and size of muscles increase proportionately; consequently, it is the quantity (volume, not number of fibers) that increases, not the quality (19).

EFFECT OF VARIOUS FACTORS UPON STRENGTH

Age. As a child grows from infancy to adulthood, strength grows commensurately with the growth in the size of the muscles. Changes in the quality of muscle tissue seem to be small in magnitude since almost all the gain in strength can be accounted for by the increased size (32). Although experimental data are not available for the older segments of the population, it is quite probable that the decline in strength beyond age thirty can be attributed to decreased quantity of muscle tissue rather than to qualitative changes.

Sex. Most of the difference in strength between the sexes can be accounted for by the difference in muscle size (32); however, evidence has been presented that also shows differences of quality (27). It is possible that differences in motivation (culturally inspired) may be responsible for the observed qualitative differences, and that in a histological sense no difference exists.

Diurnal Variation. A clear-cut picture of variation in grip strength with time of day has been presented. Figure 18.7 shows the diurnal vari-

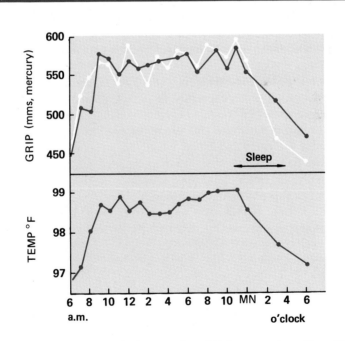

Figure 18-7. Diurnal variation of grip strength and body temperature. (From Wright. *Research Quarterly*, 30:114, 1959.)

ation and its close relationship to the diurnal variation in oral body-temperature readings (37). The closeness of the relationship does not establish a cause-effect relationship, but other evidence (in relationship to athletic warm-up) tempts one to relate the two factors causally.

Another investigator, working with other muscles, including the elbow flexor and knee extensor groups, was unable to show a systematic variability in strength that was related to time of day in these muscles (35). It is possible there are differences from muscle to muscle.

Seasonal Effects on Strength Gain. Experiments in Germany on twenty-one subjects, who were observed for strength gains as a result of isometric training, indicated seasonal variations. A minimum strength gain was found to occur in January and February, and a tenfold higher gain rate was observed in September and October. The investigators attributed this to changes in the diet: availability of fresh fruit and vegetables (20). This finding is interesting, but it requires verification by other investigators.

Effects of Heat and Cold on Strength. Immersion of the arm in hot water (120° F) for eight minutes resulted in small but significant gains in grip strength in eight of twelve subjects. With the same subjects, immersion in cold water (50° F) resulted in a mean decrease in grip strength of eleven percent, which was highly significant (17). It would be of interest to extend these observations to varying temperatures and to other muscle groups.

Psychological Factors in Strength. It has long been known, on empirical bases, that strength as expressed by voluntary maximal contractions is limited by psychological factors before physiological limits are reached; and many examples illustrate this point. In one instance, a young man working under his car was pinned when the jack failed; his mother, a woman of less-than-average size, lifted a corner of the car to release him. Unquestionably, her usual inhibitory processes were inhibited, allowing her to exert her full physiological strength.

Some interesting experiments support this view. It was shown that forearm flexor strength can be significantly increased by the following factors:

1. A pistol shot from two to ten seconds before strength effort, +7.4 percent.
2. A subject shouting at application of force, +12.2 percent.
3. Hypnosis that suggests a greater strength, + 26.5 percent; hypnosis that suggested weakness brought about a significant decline in strength, 31.7 percent (23).

SUMMARY

1. Strength is a very important factor in any physical activity in which muscular forces move the body or extraneous sports implements that possess appreciable mass.
2. Athletic power is the rate of producing force. Power can usually be improved to the greatest extent by increasing the available force (strength).
3. The overload principle means that gains in muscular strength and hypertrophy are brought about only when a muscle works against considerably greater resistance than that to which it is accustomed. For isometric training, a minimum resistance of one-third maximum contraction is required to furnish a training stimulus.
4. Strength gains are specific to the angle in the range of motion at which the resistance is met in training.
5. The rate of strength gain is most rapid when a muscle has achieved only a small proportion of its possible maximal end strength. The rate of gain slows down as muscle strength approaches its maximal end strength.
6. The rate of strength loss after training ends is a very much slower process than strength gain. Retention of strength can probably be brought about by as little as one maximal contraction per week.
7. The strength of any muscle is the result of both the quantity and quality of the muscle tissue. Quality (strength per unit of cross-section area) varies considerably from muscle to muscle within an individual, but strength gains appear to be brought about largely by quantitative increases in fiber size.
8. Strength testing, to achieve maximal accuracy, should be applied under conditions that are constant in (1) time of day, (2) ambient temperature, and (3) psychological factors.

Training Methodology and Isometric Training

1. Maximal contraction produces the fastest gains.
2. Duration of five seconds is optimal.
3. Higher end strength values can be attained by increasing repetitions from one to between five and ten daily.
4. If contraction strength less than the maximum is used, it should be based on a maximum that is measured weekly.
5. Workouts four or five times per week appear to be optimal.

Training Methodology and Isotonic Training

1. All contractions should be made through the full range of motion.
2. For the development of *strength*, a program based on two or three

sets of four to ten repetitions each, using maximum resistance for the number of repetitions, seems to rest on sound experimental bases.

3. For the development of *hypertrophy*, the De Lorme technique is probably most effective.

> 1st set: 10 repetitions with ½ 10 RM.
> 2d set: 10 repetitions with ¾ 10 RM.
> 3d set: 10 repetitions with full 10 RM.

4. Workouts should be scheduled no less than three and no more than four times weekly for optimal results.

5. The total exercise program should be scheduled so that no more than one workout per week approaches exhaustion.

REFERENCES

1. Asmussen, E.; Hansen, O.; and Lammert, O. 1965. The relation between isometric and dynamic muscle strength in man. *Communications* from the Danish National Association for Infantile Paralysis 20:1-11.

2. Barney, V. S., and Bangerter, B. L. 1961. Comparison of three programs of progressive resistance exercise. *Research Quarterly* 32:138-46.

3. Bender, J. A., and Kaplan, H. M. 1963. The multiple angle testing method for the evaluation of muscle strength. *Journal of Bone and Joint Surgery* 45A:135-40.

4. Berger, R. A. 1962a. Comparison of static and dynamic strength increases. *Research Quarterly* 33:329-33.

5. ———. 1962b. Optimum repetitions for the development of strength. *Research Quarterly* 33:334-38.

6. ———. 1963. Comparison between static training and various dynamic training programs. *Research Quarterly* 34:131-35.

7. Berger, R. A., and Blaschke, L. A. 1967. Comparison of relationships between motor ability and static and dynamic strength. *Research Quarterly* 38:144-46.

8. Berger, R. A., and Hardage, B. 1967. Effect of maximum loads for each of ten repetitions on strength improvement. *Research Quarterly* 38:715-18.

9. Capen, E. K. 1956. Study of four programs of heavy resistance exercises for development of muscular strength. *Research Quarterly* 27:132-42.

10. Clarke, H. H., and Clarke, D. H. 1963. *Developmental and adapted physical education*. Englewood Cliffs: Prentice-Hall, Inc.

11. Clarke, H. H.; Elkins, E. C.; Martin, G. M.; and Wakim, K. G. 1950. Relationship between body position and the application of muscle power to movements of the joints. *Archives of Physical Medicine* 31:81-89.

12. Darcus, H. D., and Salter, N. 1955. The effect of repeated muscular exertion on muscle strength. *Journal of Physiology* 129:325-36.

13. De Lorme, T. L., and Watkins, A. L. 1951. *Progressive resistance exercise*. New York: Appleton-Century-Crofts.

14. Dennison, J. D.; Howell, M. L.; and Morford, W. R. 1961. Effect of iso-metric and isotonic exercise programs upon muscular endurance. *Research Quarterly* 32:348-52.

15. Eichelberger, L.; Roma, M.; and Moulder, P. V. 1963. Tissue studies during recovery from immobilization atrophy. *Journal of Applied Physiology* 18:623-28.

16. Gardner, G. W. 1963. Specificity of strength changes of the exercised and nonexercised limb following isometric training. *Research Quarterly* 34:98-101.

17. Grose, J. E. 1958. Depression of muscle fatigue curves by heat and cold. *Research Quarterly* 29:19-31.

18. Hettinger, T. 1955. Der Einfluss der Muskeldurchblutung beim Muskel-training auf den Training-erfolg. *Arbeitsphysiologie* 16:95-98.

19. Hettinger, T., and Müller, E. A. 1953. Muskelleistung und Muskeltraining. *Arbeitsphysiologie* 16:90-94.

20. Hettinger, T., and Müller, E. A. 1955. Die Trainierbarkeit der Muskulatur. *Arbeitsphysiologie* 16:90-94.

21. Hettinger, T., and Muller-Wecker, H. 1954. Histologische und Chemische Veranderungen der Skeletmuskulatur bei Atrophie. *Arbeitsphysiologie* 15:459-65.

22. Hill, A. V. 1922. The maximum work and mechanical efficiency of human muscles and their most economical speed. *Journal of Physiology* 56:19-41.

23. Ikai, M., and Steinhaus, A. H. 1961. Some factors modifying the expression of human strength. *Journal of Applied Physiology* 16:157-63.

24. Logan, G. A. 1960. Differential applications of resistance and resulting strength measured at varying degrees of knee flexion. Doctoral dissertation, USC.

25. Massey, B. H. 1964. The effect of involuntary training with high frequency electrical stimulation upon strength and muscle size. Paper read at 11th Annual Meeting of the American College of Sports Medicine, March 1964, at Hollywood, Calif.

26. Morehouse, L. E. 1960. Physiological basis of strength development. In *Exercise and Fitness*. New York: The Athletic Institute.

27. Morris, C. B. 1948. The measurement of the strength of muscle relative to the cross-section. *Research Quarterly* 19:295-303.

28. Muller, E. A., and Rohmert, W. 1963. Die Geschwindigkeit der Muskel-kraft Zunahme bei Isometrischen Training. *Internationale Zeitschrift fur Angewandte Physiologie* 19:403-19.

29. Nowakowska, A. 1962. Influence of experimental training by electric current stimulation of skeletal muscle. *Acta Physiologica Polonica* 12:32-38.

30. Ralston, H. J.; Polissar, M. J.; Inman, V. J.; Close, J. R.; and Feinstein, B. 1949. Dynamic features of human isolated voluntary muscle in isometric and free contractions. *Journal of Applied Physiology* 1:526-33.

31. Rasch, P. J., and Morehouse, L. E. 1957. Effect of static and dynamic exercises on muscular strength and hypertrophy. *Journal of Applied Physiology* 11:29-34.

32. Rodahl, K. 1961. Physical work capacity. *AMA Archives of Environmental Health* 2:499-510.
33. Rohmert, W., and Neuhaus, H. 1965. Der Einfluss Verschiedener Ruhelänge des Muskels auf die Geschwindichkeit der Kraftzunahme durch Isometrisches Training. *Internationale Zeitschrift für Angewandte Physiologie Einschliesslich Arbeitsphysiologie* 20:498-514.
34. Royce, J. 1958. Isometric fatigue curves in human muscle with normal and occluded circulation. *Research Quarterly* 29:204-12.
35. Tornvall, G. 1963. Assessment of physical capabilities. *Acta Physiologica Scandinavica* 53:suppl. 201:1-102.
36. Wakim, K. G.; Gersten, J. W.; Elkins, E. C., and Martin, G. M. 1950. Objective recording of muscle strength. *Archives of Physical Medicine* 31: 90-100.
37. Wright, V. 1959. Factors influencing diurnal variation of strength of grip. *Research Quarterly* 30:110-16.

19 Development of Endurance

The ability to persist in physical activity, to resist muscular fatigue, is referred to as endurance. If there is any one most important factor in human performance, it is endurance. It is probably the most important component of physical fitness in that it reflects the state of some of the physiological systems that are most important to the general health of an individual. In athletics, there are few sports in which endurance is not a factor, and in many sports the entire training and conditioning programs are directed toward this end.

The concept of endurance is not altogether simple. Analysis of this factor into its component parts is apt to mislead a student into a concept of discrete elements when in fact the elements are interwoven and interrelated, and basically inseparable. Realizing that analysis of endurance into its several components is essentially artificial, we shall nevertheless make the analysis to aid in achieving better understanding of the physiology involved.

I. **Analysis of Endurance as a Factor in Human Performance**
    A. Psychological elements
        1. Motivation
        2. Willingness to take pain
    B. Physiological elements
        1. Local endurance: involvement of only one, or several, localized muscle groups
            a. Strength of a particular muscle group
            b. Energy stores
            c. Peripheral circulatory factor
        2. General endurance: whole body activity
            a. Strength of general musculature
            b. Energy stores
            c. Systemic circulatory factor
                (1) Aerobic activity: limited by maximal O_2 consumption
                    (a) Respiratory function
                    (b) Cardiac output
                    (c) O_2-carrying-capacity of blood
                    (d) Vascularization of muscle tissues
                (2) Anaerobic activity
                    (a) Muscle glycogen
                    (b) ATP and CP stores
                    (c) Alkaline reserve: blood buffers
            d. Efficiency of heat regulatory mechanisms
            e. Effectiveness of the nervous system in maintaining high levels of skill and coordination

    3. Muscular efficiency: energy input required to bring about de-
      sired level of muscular performance

We shall dismiss the psychological elements (although they are very
important) as beyond the scope of this text; and muscular efficiency,
warrants a chapter by itself. Thus the remainder of this chapter will be
concerned with the physiology of endurance considered with respect to
its two major components: (1) local or muscular, endurance, and (2)
general, or systemic, endurance.

LOCAL OR MUSCULAR ENDURANCE

Strength and Endurance. Let us consider for a moment the simplest
possible illustration of muscular endurance. Let us concern ourselves with
the maintenance of an isometric contraction of the elbow flexors against a
load that is at least sixty percent of the *maximal* voluntary contraction
(MVC). A load of this magnitude results in virtually complete occlusion
of the blood vessels that supply the muscle tissue because the pressure
of the contracted muscle exceeds systolic arterial pressure (26).

Under these conditions the duration of the isometric contraction may
be limited by a finite energy supply or by the buildup of acid metabolic
end products. Thus the contracting muscle group utilizes its only available sources of direct energy, the breakdown of ATP and creatine phosphate, and, subsequently, the energy available from the breakdown of
glycogen. Neither of these energy sources can be replenished because the
circulation is occluded; consequently, the duration of this isometric contraction becomes a function of the amount of energy stored and the rate
of energy depletion and the concomitant drop in tissue pH that decreases
the contractility of the muscle. The exact factor which actually sets the
limit for duration of this isometric contraction is still in question. Recent
work (1) suggests that depletion of muscle glycogen does not set the limit
for isometric contraction but the depletion of high energy phosphates
has not been ruled out. Lowering blood pH due to acid metabolites can
probably also be ruled out, but decreases in pH *within the muscle cell*
are such as to offer a possible explanation for rapid fatigue from very
heavy work (18). Such pH decreases in the muscle cell may reduce the
binding capacity for calcium ion through an inactivation of the fibrillar
protein, troponin (see chapter two).

Figure 19.1 illustrates the relationship of muscular endurance to the
magnitude of the load imposed upon the muscle. It will be noted that
load is designated in terms of the percentage of MVC; this is necessary
because strength is such a large factor in local muscular endurance. It
is obvious that if a load of fifty pounds were used for subjects of widely

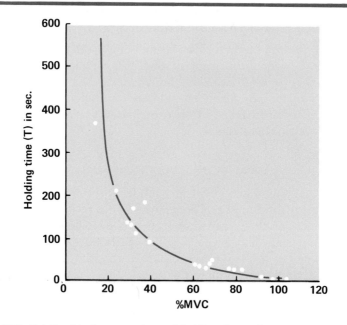

Figure 19-1. Relationship between observed holding times of contractions sustained to fatigue vs. % MVC. (From Ahlborg, B., et al. *J. Appl. Physiol.* 33:224, 1972.)

varying strength, a weak subject would find it required close to a maximal contraction, and his duration would be only a few seconds. For a very strong subject, the load would be light and the duration might be several minutes (even longer if the contraction is below that which causes occlusion). Thus the test results would be more closely related to strength than to muscular endurance.

To further illustrate this fact, many investigators have found the relationship between strength and *absolute endurance* to be high, from $r = 0.75$ to $r = 0.97$, while the relationship between strength and *relative endurance* is practically nil (4, 29). Absolute endurance is measured by using the same load for everyone, whereas the relative endurance is measured by using a given percentage of each individual's MVC (thus ruling out strength as a factor).

Measurement of Muscular Endurance

Maintenance of Isometric Tension. The simplest and most direct method has already been described, but another method that involves isometric tension is illustrated by figure 19.2. The subject holds a *maximal contraction* and the effects of energy depletion upon his maximum strength are observed over time. It is also of interest to note that the effects of the circulatory factor do not become apparent (there are no differences between open circulation and circulation occluded by a pressure cuff) until the contraction strength falls below (approximately) sixty percent of MVC (this value is also supported by data for the arm musculature). However, the percentage of MVC at which occlusion occurs undoubtedly varies from muscle to muscle (it is probably very much lower in such muscles as the gastrocnemius, with bipennate fiber orientation). The plotting of these "fatigue curves" is a laboratory procedure however, and does not lend itself readily to practical situations.

Isotonic Testing by Ergographic Methods. F. A. Hellebrandt and her colleagues (16) have modified the classic Mosso ergograph into a very

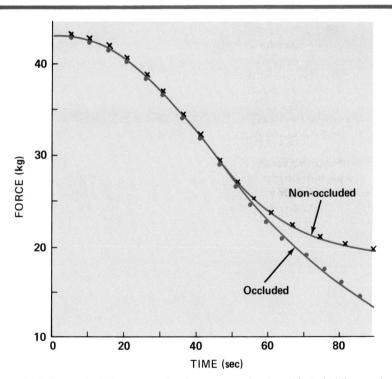

Figure 19-2. Isometric fatigue curves for forearm muscles. In subjects holding maximum voluntary contraction, the decrement in MVC is a function of fatigue. (From Royce. *Research Quarterly,* 29:204, 1958.)

useful instrument for muscle endurance testing by isotonic methods (see fig. 19.3). The main advantage in the use of this instrument is that the applied force is constant throughout the range of motion, and consequently the range of contraction decreases with increasing fatigue, resulting in fatigue curves or *ergograms* (as in fig. 19.4). It is possible to set up structured, progressive therapeutic exercise programs with this instrument, and so it has found use in physical medicine and rehabilitation work.

Strength-Decrement Index. H. H. Clarke (6) and his associates have demonstrated that as heavy work is performed over a sufficient period of time to bring about fatigue, decrements in the strength of the muscles involved can be observed with their cable-tension strength testing procedures. They have suggested the use of the percentage strength loss (of pre-exercise value) as a measure of the level of fatigue. Conversely, the *strength decrement index* (SDI) also provides information relative to muscular endurance.

Electromyographic Evaluation of Fatigue. This method is mentioned at this point not because it has practical use but because it sheds additional light on the physiology of fatigue. It has been shown that as normal human muscles maintain a constant isometric tension, the electrical activity in the muscle increases as the muscle fatigues (12). The most

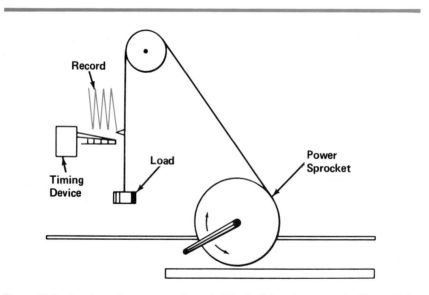

Figure 19-3. A schematic representation of Kelso-Hellebrandt ergograph. (From Hellebrandt, Skowlund, and Kelso. *Archives of Physical Medicine,* 29:21, 1948.)

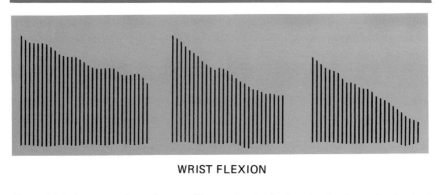

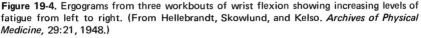

WRIST FLEXION

Figure 19-4. Ergograms from three workbouts of wrist flexion showing increasing levels of fatigue from left to right. (From Hellebrandt, Skowlund, and Kelso. *Archives of Physical Medicine,* 29:21, 1948.)

obvious explanation for this phenomenon is that as the contraction continues and fatigue occurs, each motor unit is able to contribute less force to the contraction, and consequently more and more motor units must be recruited to maintain the same level of tension. The author has found that the rate of increase in electrical activity with time is highly correlated with isometric endurance measured on a hydraulic dynamometer. This relationship may have practical value for estimating muscular endurance in subjects who are unable or unwilling to cooperate fully in testing.

Factors Affecting Muscular Endurance

Age. Relatively little information is available concerning the effect of age. Rich has shown that there seems to be no greater fatigability in young children than in older (high school age) children (24). Evans (14) has shown that older men fatigue more rapidly than young, although the loss of endurance is smaller than expected.

Sex. Most available data seem to agree that there is no significant difference in muscular endurance due to sex, if the strength factor is ruled out.

Temperature. It appears that rate of fatigue and total amount of work done (hand-grip dynamometer) are adversely affected by immersion of the arm for eight minutes in a water bath at 120° F (15). The effects of cold were shown to be advantageous, until an optimum muscle temperature of 80° F was reached. This appears to be an optimal temperature, and temperatures below this produce poorer performance (7).

Cross-education Effect. It has been demonstrated that training one limb brings about changes in its untrained partner (19). When the endurance of the trained limb was increased 966 percent, the untrained contralateral limb improved by 275 percent.

Circulation. Twenty-nine weeks of isometric training have been shown to bring about a decrease in the ratio of blood flow debt per unit of exercise effort (31). This is in agreement with the work of Rohter, Rochelle, and Hyman, who have shown significant improvement in muscle blood flow as the result of the training regimen of college swimmers (25). It seems highly probable that improved peripheral circulation, by virtue of improved vascularization of active muscle tissue, is one of the most important mechanisms in the development of improved muscular endurance levels.

Improvement of Muscular Endurance. In a classic piece of work, with which every student of physical performance should become familiar, Hellebrandt and Houtz provided definitive answers to some of the basic questions that must be answered to place exercise programs upon a scientific, systematized basis (17). Using ergographic procedures, they performed 620 experiments that tested different training procedures on wrist flexion and extension. They used thirty-second work bouts, alternated with thirty-second rest periods, and each bout consisted of twenty-five isotonic contractions.

When experimentation with successively heavier loads are conducted, *work curves* can be plotted in which the work done (kgm) is seen to rise to an *optimum load,* then fall again (fig. 19.5). Thus in figure 19.5 it can be seen that at the initial test, 2.0 kg allowed the best combination of force times distance (distance being the resultant of the number of repetitions and the height lifted for each repetition as recorded on the ergogram). As more weight was loaded in subsequent tests the distance suffered by more than was gained in weight moved and therefore the product of F x D decreased. Resistances less than the value that brings about the optimal load constitute an *underload,* and a greater-than-optimal load constitutes an *overload.* The *initial* and *final curves* of figure 19.5 show the improvement in one of their subjects in six practice periods. It can be seen that strength, power, and endurance improve simultaneously.

Figure 19.6 demonstrates the need for overload conditions in developing muscular endurance. The two groups performed the same number of contractions per day (250), three times a week for eight weeks, the only difference being that one group trained with an underload and one with an overload.

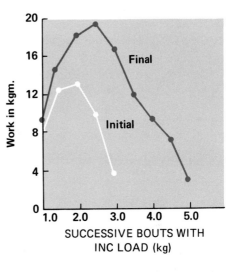

Figure 19-5. Work curve showing the total work done in successive work-bouts as a function of load. (From Hellebrandt and Houtz. *Physical Therapy Review*, 36:371, 1956.)

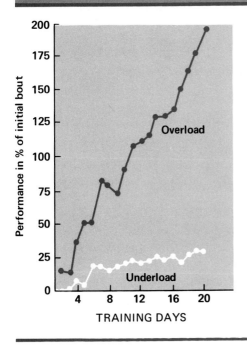

Figure 19-6. Effects of "underload" and "overload" in improving muscular endurance. (From Hellebrandt and Houtz. *Physical Therapy Review*, 36:371, 1956.)

Comparison was also made of two groups that worked with underload and overload conditions when the total work done per day was held constant. In other words, the group that trained with an overload (twenty-five repetitions with the 25 RM) did fewer total bouts than the group that trained with an underload, so that work in terms of force times distance was equal for all subjects. Again, figure 19.7 demonstrates the need for overload conditions.

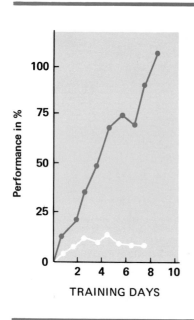

Figure 19-7. Effects of "underload" and "overload" of force overcome at each contraction when the total work done is held constant. Lower curve represents underload; upper curve represents overload. (From Hellebrandt and Houtz. *Physical Therapy Review,* 36:371, 1956.)

It would be very desirable to pursue such avenues of investigation for other muscle groups, and indeed for overall body activity. Only with such systematic investigations can the training and conditioning of athletes become a science.

The results of recent work on the training effects of strength versus endurance oriented workouts is of interest. Clarke and Stull (5, 30) conducted two series of training experiments, one of which used low resistance and high repetitions, a combination which is ordinarily considered to be *endurance type training.* In the other experiment they used the De Lorme technique of heavy resistance and low repetitions (*strength type training*). Surprisingly, the gains in strength were as great from endurance training as from strength training and the gains in absolute endurance were also similar in the two training experiments although relative endurance did not change. Two other investigations support their findings (11, 28) which lead to the conclusion that the first order of business in improving an athlete's muscular endurance is to optimize his strength. Since heavy resistance training such as weight training is more efficient in the use of time this would seem to be the method of choice.

SUMMARY

1. An optimal level of strength should be developed in the endurance training program. This allows a muscle group to work at lower percentages of its all-out capacity, and thus significantly increases endurance (*absolute endurance*).
2. The *overload principle* applies to muscular endurance as well as to strength. Repetitions with easy work loads do not bring about optimal improvement in muscular endurance.
3. In general, suitable overload training brings about improvement in strength and muscular endurance simultaneously.
4. If either the duration of work load or the *total work* is held constant, overload training brings about far greater improvement than underload training, in strength and in endurance.
5. Overload training should not reach the point where the range of motion is curtailed.
6. The *power* (work per unit time) of muscular contraction seems to be more important than the total amount of work in bringing about a training effect.

GENERAL OR CIRCULORESPIRATORY ENDURANCE

When we change our frame of reference from a localized movement, such as elbow flexion or leg extension, to an activity that involves gross body movement, such as running or swimming, the problem changes from local involvement of a small percentage of the body's musculature to one that involves a large percentage with many muscle groups working simultaneously. In local situations, muscle endurance is limited by a combination of energy supply and peripheral vascularization; the central systems of supply are never extended to a large degree. In gross body activity, it is the central systems of respiration, circulation, and heat dissipation, and the nervous system and the homeostatic mechanisms that are likely to establish the outer limits of performance.

Aerobic Versus Anaerobic Work. When work begins, anaerobic energy sources are used during the transition to *steady state* as was described in chapter nine. If the work load is greater than aerobic capacity, anaerobic mechanisms continue to contribute until maximum O_2 debt is achieved, at which point the exercise must end or slow down. The percentual contribution of aerobic and anaerobic energy depends upon the nature of the exercise as shown in figure 16.4, page 329.

Margaria and his associates (1964), who furnished some of the original data on O_2 debt, recently defined the limitations of each of the three processes of energy supply (22). Table 19.1 shows their results.

TABLE 19.1

Capacity and Power of Energetic Processes in Muscle

Processes	Total Energy (cal/kg)	Maximum Power (kcal/kg/hr)
Aerobic	------	15.0
"Alactacid" O_2 debt (fast component)	95	45.0
"Lactacid" O_2 debt (slow component)	220	21.5

From R. Margaria, P. Cerretelli, and F. Mangili, "Balance and Kinetics of Anaerobic Energy Release during Strenuous Exercise in Man," *Journal of Applied Physiology* 19:627, 1964.

The alactacid debt, according to their figures, can be completely utilized in an explosive effort, in as little as a fraction of a second, and the process is completed in less demanding exercise in less than twenty seconds. When a subject exercises at a maximal rate (as in running events, up to the 440) both anaerobic processes are exhausted in about forty seconds, and exercise can continue only on a "pay as you go" basis.

In reality, most athletic events involve both aerobic and anaerobic energy sources, the proportions depending upon the speed and duration of the event. It can be estimated, for example, that sprints are about ninety percent anaerobic and distance runs are about ninety percent aerobic; other athletic events fall in between (see fig. 16.4, p. 329).

The importance of all this in our discussion of endurance is that again, different factors are involved, even for a gross body activity, which depend upon the speed and duration of an athletic event. It can readily be seen that sprint events, and in general, athletic events that last less than one minute, depend largely upon the factors discussed in the first half of this chapter for their endurance element. The remainder of this chapter, then, will be directed toward athletic events in which the energy supply is largely aerobic (events of several minutes' duration or longer).

Determinants of Circulorespiratory Endurance

Energy Substrate. As was discussed in chapter two, exhaustion in lengthy, severe bicycle ergometer rides seems to occur when muscle biopsy techniques show muscle glycogen to be depleted. Thus, there seems little doubt that muscle glycogen depletion is one factor which *can* set the limits of endurance. However, it must be recognized that bicycle exercise places most of the load upon relatively few muscles. Costill et al. (9, 10) have raised the interesting question of whether glycogen depletion is also a factor under conditions of endurance type *running events* where the load is distributed over a greater muscle mass. Since substantial amounts of muscle glycogen were found after both prolonged (ten miles) and short (maximal O_2 consumption test) exhaustive runs on the treadmill, glycogen depletion is an unlikely explanation for the fatigue at exhaustion in such efforts. Furthermore, in a subsequent study, they also found that in an experiment involving three consecutive days of such efforts, the subjects were able to initiate the ten mile run on the third day with leg muscle glycogen concentrations lower than those measured after termination of running on the first day.

Pernow and Saltin (23) have shown the importance of *free fatty acids* (FFA) as an energy substrate. When subjects performed bicycle ergometer work to exhaustion (1 to 1.5 hours duration) it was shown that when the glycogen stores are reduced, prolonged work can still be performed by the same muscles, but only if the intensity of the work is less than sixty to seventy percent maximum VO_2 and if the supply of FFA is adequate. Elimination of both muscle glycogen and FFA seriously impairs the ability for prolonged work.

Maximum O_2 Consumption (Aerobic Capacity). Except in a marathon run lasting several hours, or in athletic events which overload limited muscle masses (as the bicycle ergometer) the limiting factor in endurance is probably O_2 supply rather than oxidizable substrate. We may think of the possible limiting factors for O_2 supply as (1) external respiration, (2) gas transport, or (3) tissue respiration. The available evidence suggests that the limiting factor for high level athletic performance is *gas transport*.

Gas transport, in turn, can be limited by (1) cardiac output, (2) vascular dynamics, and (3) O_2 carrying capacity of the blood (hemoglobin concentration and number of erythrocytes per unit of blood). All of these factors, operating in concert, can be evaluated by the maximal O_2 consumption test, as described earlier in this book. This test is undoubtedly the best single predictive measure of success in endurance-type athletic events. High correlations have been demonstrated between aerobic capacity and time on 4.7 mile run ($r = 0.83$) (8) and endurance time on a bicycle test ($r = 0.78$) (33).

Genetic Factor. As was discussed in chapter nine, training can bring about substantial improvement in aerobic capacity and thus markedly improve performance, but genetic factors set the ultimate ceiling. That is to say that record breaking performance is not to be expected unless the genetic endowment for O_2 transport has been considerably better than average to begin with.

Motivation. In an interesting experiment on the influence of motivation on physiological parameters limiting work capacity, Wilmore (32) tested the PWC of twenty-two college age males on a bicycle ergometer on three occasions, two control and one experimental. On the experimental test the subjects were motivated by competition. As might be expected, the performances were significantly better in the competitive situation, but there were *no significant differences* in the maximum *physiological responses* such as heart rate, maximum ventilation, or O_2 consumption. It may be concluded that the maximal values for the physiological variables are essentially fixed for a given individual at a given time at a given training level and that the supramaximal performances elicited by motivation were the result of increased anaerobic rather than aerobic capacity which may be the result of reduced psychological inhibitions allowing greater tolerance to anaerobic metabolites.

Physiological Changes Resulting from Training. Continual, methodical stressing of the human organism by subjecting it to progressively increasing work loads results in responses that are seemingly directed toward making its reaction to the challenges of increased metabolic rates ever more successful. The physiological changes brought about by training can be summarized as follows:

1. Lower resting heart rate
2. Lower heart rate for any submaximal work load
3. Greater maximal stroke volume
4. Lower ventilation equivalent (less ventilation required per unit O_2 utilized)
5. Greater maximal O_2 consumption
6. Less utilization of anaerobic energy sources for a given work load
7. Capacity for greater O_2 debt (probably due to a combination of improved alkaline reserve and greater willingness to bear pain)
8. Less displacement of physiological function by any given level of work load, and faster recovery to baseline values after completion of exercise

Threshold for Endurance Training Effect. In the light of what has been said of the need for overcoming overload conditions to achieve a training effect for local musculatures, one of the most pertinent and practical questions we can ask at this point seems to be: must a definite degree of loading of the circulorespiratory system occur before improvement in function (training effects) can be expected to occur? In other words, is there a threshold value below which no training effect is seen?

The work of Karvonen answers this question affirmatively (21). His work with treadmill running indicates that the heart rate must be increased at least sixty percent of the way from resting to maximal during workouts before improvement occurs. His work has since been supported by the work of Sharkey and Holleman (27) who also found no training effect from work at heart rates below 150. However, it should be pointed out that for older or sedentary young subjects, lower work loads may provide some, though not optimal, training stimulus.

Various rules of thumb have been advocated and used by coaches in track and swimming. Doherty, an authority in track and field training, suggests that in mature, trained runners the heart rate should go up to 160 or more while running (in interval training) and that the rest interval can be ended when it drops to 120 (13). Roughly similar values are commonly used in training swimmers. The most practical method of applying this rule is to time fifteen beats by stop watch: immediately after the workbout, time should be under 5.6 seconds; when the time for fifteen beats goes up to 7.5 seconds, the next work bout can be started.

Why Interval Training? In years past, much of the training of endurance athletes (in the USA at least) consisted of "grinding out" laps in running or swimming, frequently at a considerably slower pace than that of the competitive event, although some underdistance work was also done.

It is usually difficult, if not impossible, to credit an individual with originating a training system because this is ordinarily more a matter of evolution than invention. Thus many coaches and athletes have contributed to the method of *interval training;* however, its formulation into a structured system that is based on physiological observations can probably be attributed to the coach Gerschler and the physiologist Reindell, whose collaboration resulted in the great performances in the late thirties of the German runner, Harbig. It was the middle fifties before interval training made its way across the ocean and found a place in American athletic programs.

Interval training consists of short periods of work alternating with short rest intervals as distinct from workbouts which are continuous in nature. Thus an individual training for a 1500-meter swim instead of swimming long distances continuously might be trained largely on repeats of 100-meter swims which can be swum faster and the endurance (or training) factor would be gained through manipulation of (1) the speed at which the 100s are negotiated and (2) total number of 100s accomplished, and (3) the duration of the rest interval.

From the standpoint of the exercise physiologist, interval training makes very good sense indeed. Obviously, one of the primary goals of a conditioning program is to achieve the greatest possible work load with the smallest physiological strain (fatigue), and that this can best be achieved through the methods of interval training is supported on physiological bases. Astrand et al. (2) found that a work load (2,160 kgm/min) that could be tolerated for an hour when done intermittently resulted in exhaustion in nine minutes when done continuously. Thus the total work done continuously was 19,400 kilogram-meters while the work done intermittently was 64,800 kilogram-meters.

The level of physiological stress can be evaluated best by the heart rates and blood lactates achieved. In the continuous work the heart rate reached 204 beats per minute and blood lactate rose to 150 milligram percent. In the intermittent work, by contrast, although more than three times as much work was done, heart rate did not exceed 150 and blood lactate was twenty milligram percent, which indicates that very little of the work was done anaerobically.

This work also sheds light on what constitutes desirable intervals. The same work load when done in alternating three-minute intervals of work and rest required heart rates of 188 and blood lactate of 120 milligram percent, but alternating intervals of thirty seconds raised these values to only 150 and twenty, respectively. The thirty-second work interval, which is often recommended, is thus borne out on experimental bases.

As an extension of this work, the effect of changing the length of the rest interval was also investigated (3). It was shown that the physiological stressfulness of the training is not highly related to the duration of the rest interval. Only small increases in blood lactate were observed when the rest interval was decreased from four minutes to thirty seconds, although the total work done increased fourfold.

Although maximal training effect on the circulatory system probably demands maximal loading of the O_2 transport system, this does not necessarily mean that the athletes performance must be maximal in terms of *speed* of running or swimming, etc. Karlsson, Astrand and Ekblom (20) have shown that as an athlete approaches his maximum performance (speeds) there is a considerable range, possibly from eighty to 100 percent of his maximum performance capability (speed of running, etc.) at which O_2 consumption is at its maximum, although the production of lactic acid rises rapidly over this same range. Since they also found a declining O_2 pulse at the highest levels of work, the data suggest that training the O_2 transport system is best carried out at a work rate short of maximal performance but which will still fully load the O_2 transport system. Such a small reduction in speed would imply less fatigue (lower levels of lactate) and thus permit an increase in training volume.

To summarize, interval training for events which are largely *aerobic* can be developed around work intervals ranging from thirty seconds to five minutes with alternating rest intervals of approximately the same duration. It must be realized that the shorter the interval, the greater the training effect on anaerobic capacity and the longer the interval, the more effective for aerobic capacity, so that the selection of interval depends to a large extent on the exact nature of the event trained for. It must also be remembered that the shorter intervals allow very large total work loads to be handled. It is the author's experience with swimmers that such workouts should be reserved for bringing athletes to peak performance. Using intervals of thirty to sixty second swims can bring high school and college swimmers to a peak in four to six weeks. If such workouts are used too early in the season or over too long a period, staleness may well be the result.

Analysis of Pace as an Indicator of Training Needs. In middle-distance and distance athletic events, where pace is established on a voluntary basis, considerable insight can be gained into training needs by comparing *split times* with those of championship performances in the same event. If an athlete's split times, for example, are in the same proportion as those of championship performance but slower for each split, further improvement probably depends upon increased power or better technique. In this case, off-season weight training and interval training, with rate as the variable for progression, should be utilized.

On the other hand, if an athlete meets the championship pace on the first splits but fades badly late in the race, the fault probably stems from circulorespiratory factors, and endurance work is indicated (such as increasing the number of repeats of an interval training workout).

SUMMARY

1. The limits of human circulorespiratory endurance are set by such psychological factors as motivation and willingness to take pain, and by many physiological factors. The most important physiological factors are oxygen transport and the ability to carry an oxygen debt.

2. Both psychological and physiological factors can be greatly improved by training that utilizes the overload principle.

3. Rate of improvement in endurance varies directly with the intensity, frequency, and duration of the overload effort.

4. There is a threshold value for work intensity below which no improvement in endurance occurs. Heart rate must be raised from the resting rate to sixty percent of the maximal value for improvement to take place. As a rule of thumb, double the resting heart rate may be used as the threshold value.

5. Interval training concepts rest on sound experimental evidence. More work can be done per workout for any given physiological stressfulness if it is done intermittently rather than continuously.

6. Thirty-second workbouts are most advantageous, and the rest interval is probably best set by physiological stress as measured by heart rate. The rest interval has been adequate when the resting heart rate has returned to 120 beats per minute.

7. Endurance as a function of muscular strength or power is best improved by progressive increases in the rate of each workbout (intensity); improvement of the circulorespiratory function is best improved by progressive increases in number of workbouts per workout (duration).

8. Training progress can be hampered by exercising to complete exhaustion. Workouts should not exceed intensity and duration levels that allow recovery from fatigue in several hours.

9. Athletes should not be brought along too fast early in the season for fear of hitting peak performances before championship events are scheduled. In general, the early season workout progressions should gradually increase the number of repetitions; late in the season the rate for each repetition is the important variable.

10. If split times are proportional to record performances, further improvement probably depends upon improvement of strength (power) or technique. If split times fade badly in comparison with record performances, circulorespiratory endurance needs improvement.

REFERENCES

1. Ahlborg, B.; Ekelund, L. G.; Guarnieri, G.; Harris, R. C.; Hultman, E.; and Nordesjo, L-O. 1972. Muscle metabolism during isometric exercise performed at constant force. *Journal of Applied Physiology* 33:224-28.

2. Astrand, I.; Astrand, P. O.; Christensen, E. H.; and Hedman, R. 1960a. Intermittent muscular work. *Acta Physiologica Scandinavica* 48:448-53.

3. ————. 1960b. Myohemoglobin as an oxygen store in man. *Acta Physiologica Scandinavica* 48:454-60.

4. Caldwell, L. S. 1963. Relative muscle loading and endurance. *Journal of Engineering Psychology* 2:155-61.

5. Clarke, D. H., and Stull, G. A. 1970. Endurance training as a determinant of strength and fatiguability. *Research Quarterly* 41:19-26.

6. Clarke, H. H.; Shay, C. T.; and Mathews, D. K. 1955. Strength decrement index: a new test of muscle fatigue. *Archives of Physical Medicine and Rehabilitation* 36:376-78.

7. Clarke, R. S. J.; Hellon, R. F.; and Lind, A. R. 1958. The duration of sustained contractions of the human forearm at different muscle temperatures. *Journal of Physiology* 143:454-73.

8. Costill, D. L. 1967. The relationship between selected physiological variables and distance running performance. *Journal of Sports Medicine* 7:61-66.

9. Costill, D. L.; Sparks, K.; Gregor, R.; and Turner, C. 1971a. Muscle glycogen utilization during exhaustive running. *Journal of Applied Physiology* 31:353-56.

10. Costill, D. L.; Bowers, R.; Branam, G.; and Sparks, K. 1971b. Muscle glycogen utilization during prolonged exercise on successive days. *Journal of Applied Physiology* 31:353-56.

11. De Lateur, B. J.; Lehman, J. F.; and Fordyce, W. E. 1968. A test of the De Lorme axiom. *Archives of Physical Medicine and Rehabilitation* 49:245-48.

12. deVries, H. A. 1968. Method for evaluation of muscle fatigue and endurance from electromyographic fatigue curves. *American Journal of Physical Medicine* 47:125-35.

13. Doherty, J. K. 1964. The nature of endurance in running. *Journal of Health, Physical Education and Recreation* 35:29.

14. Evans, S. J. 1971. An electromyographic analysis of skeletal neuromuscular fatigue with special reference to age. Doctoral dissertation, USC (physical education).

15. Grose, J. E. 1958. Depression of muscle fatigue curves by heat and cold. *Research Quarterly* 29:19-31.

16. Hellebrandt, F. A.; Skowlund, H. V.; and Kelso, L. E. A. 1948. New devices for disability evaluation. *Archives of Physical Medicine and Rehabilitation* 29:21-28.

17. Hellebrandt, F. A., and Houtz, S. J. 1956. Mechanisms of muscle training in man. *Physical Therapy Review* 36:371-83.

18. Hermansen, L., and Osnes, J. B. 1972. Blood and muscle pH after maximal exercise in man. *Journal of Applied Physiology* 32:304-8.

19. Hodgkins, J. 1961. Influence of unilateral endurance training on contralateral limb. *Journal of Applied Physiology* 16:991-93.

20. Karlsson, J.; Astrand, P. O.; Ekblom, B. 1967. Training of the oxygen transport system in man. *Journal of Applied Physiology* 22:1061-65.

21. Karvonen, M. J. 1959. Effects of vigorous exercise on the heart. In *Work and the heart*, eds. F. F. Rosenbaum and E. L. Belknap. New York: Paul B. Hoeber, Inc.

22. Margaria, R.; Cerratelli, P.; and Mangili, F. 1964. Balance and kinetics of anaerobic energy release during strenuous exercise in man. *Journal of Applied Physiology* 19:623-28.

23. Pernow, B., and Saltin, B. 1971. Availability of substrates and capacity for prolonged heavy exercise in man. *Journal of Applied Physiology* 31: 416-422.

24. Rich, G. Q. 1960. Muscular fatigue curves in boys and girls. *Research Quarterly* 31:485-98.

25. Rohter, F. D.; Rochelle, R. H.; and Hyman, C. 1963. Exercise blood flow changes in the human forearm during physical training. *Journal of Applied Physiology* 18:789-93.

26. Royce, J. 1958. Isometric fatigue curves in human muscle with normal and occluded circulation. *Research Quarterly* 29:204-12.

27. Sharkey, B. J., and Holleman, J. P. 1967. Cardiorespiratory adaptations to training at specified intensities. *Research Quarterly* 38:698-704.

28. Shaver, L. G. 1970. Effects of training on relative muscular endurance in ipsilateral and contralateral arms. *Medicine and Science in Sports* 2:165-71.

29. Start, K. B., and Graham, J. S. 1964. Relationship between the relative and absolute isometric endurance of an isolated muscle group. *Research Quarterly* 35:193-204.

30. Stull, G. A., and Clarke, D. H. 1970. High resistance, low repetition training as a determiner of strength and fatiguability. *Research Quarterly* 41: 189-93.

31. Vanderhoof, E. R.; Imig, C. J.; and Hines, H. M. 1961. Effect of muscle strength and endurance development on blood flow. *Journal of Applied Physiology* 16:873-77.

32. Wilmore, J. H. 1968. Influence of motivation on physical work capacity and performance. *Journal of Applied Physiology* 24:459-463.

33. ———. 1969. Maximal oxygen intake and its relationship to endurance capacity on a bicycle ergometer. *Research Quarterly* 40:203-10.

20 Efficiency of Muscular Activity

For the engineer and the physicist, definition of the efficiency of a machine is quite simple.

$$\text{Efficiency} = \frac{\text{Output}}{\text{Input}} = \frac{\text{Work done by machine}}{\text{Work done on the machine}}$$

The physiologist usually uses the same concept in the following terms.

$$\text{Efficiency} = \frac{\text{Work output}}{\text{Energy input}}$$

In practice, energy input is measured indirectly by oxygen consumption, which is converted into heat units (calories), and the work output in foot-pounds (or kgm) is also converted into heat units (3,087 ft-lb = 1 kcal) in order to work with similar units. This is a simple procedure for activities in which the work output is easily measured as force times distance, such as riding a bicycle ergometer or lifting the body weight in bench-stepping. This concept, however, is difficult to apply to such activities as walking and running, where large proportions of the working forces are dissipated in reciprocal movements of the arms and legs.

Fenn (20) has demonstrated that even the more difficult problems are capable of solution through application of motion picture recording and subsequent analysis of the forces involved in accelerating and decelerating the various body segments. His analysis, as shown below, of the forces and energy involved in running is of interest.

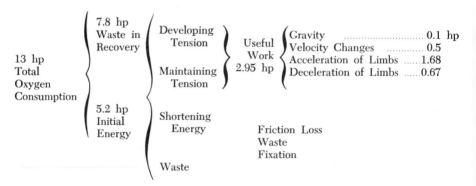

The efficiency of machines varies between ten and twenty percent in steam engines, twenty and thirty percent in gasoline engines, and eighty and ninety percent in electric motors. The mechanical efficiency of man varies from less than ten percent to thirty or even forty percent, depending upon the activity and many other factors.

It would be well at this point to consider in which athletic activities efficiency plays an important role. Obviously, any event that involves endurance will be very much influenced by the factor of muscle efficiency. Thus we are talking largely about running events greater than a quarter mile and swimming events beyond 100 yards. In the events where a single explosive effort is required such as the shot put, power rather than efficiency is the critical factor. In sprint events efficiency of movement is of some importance but is probably secondary to the need for power.

An analogy from the automotive world seems appropriate. In an acceleration contest, one does not care how many miles per gallon of gas (efficiency) the machine achieves; *power* is all-important. For an economy run, however, power is unimportant; miles per gallon determines the winner.

Thus this chapter may be considered a continuation of the last chapter in that it also is mainly concerned with endurance. The maximum speed at which a man can run a quarter mile (or more) depends very largely upon the rate at which he can supply energy (limited by maximal O_2 consumption) and his efficiency in using this energy.

AEROBIC VERSUS ANAEROBIC EFFICIENCY

The efficiency of work done at the expense of incurring lactacid oxygen debt is only about half that of work done aerobically (5, 12, 13). This fact has important implications for athletics, and will be referred to from time to time in the following discussions.

EFFECT OF SPEED ON EFFICIENCY

Simple Movements. In a classic experiment (1922) of muscle physiology, A. V. Hill (24) provided evidence of an optimum speed of movement below which efficiency falls slowly and above which it falls rapidly. It must be cautioned, however, that this work was done on a simple contraction of isolated muscle groups.

Running. In another important experiment, Sargent (1926) determined the oxygen consumption of a subject who ran 120 yards at varying rates of speed, up to an all-out sprint (30). His results indicated that O_2 consumption increased as the 3.8th power of speed. This would mean that O_2 consumption is increased almost sixteen times when speed is doubled. This would also mean a tremendous loss of efficiency as running speed increases, and many theories of pace, etc., have been built on this concept.

Sargent's subject, however, ran anaerobically, and his O_2 consumption was calculated as O_2 debt based on the O_2 consumption after the race; from this was subtracted the resting rate measured *before* the run. It has, however, been demonstrated that resting consumption after exercise remains considerably higher for six to eight hours after exercise, and this higher metabolism is not related to the O_2 debt incurred during the run. Consequently, Sargent's calculations resulted in erroneously high O_2 consumptions because he had subtracted too low a baseline value from the recovery O_2 consumption rates.

More recent work (18, 19, 28) shows that—at least for rates of speed at which no O_2 debt occurs—the rate of increase in energy demand is only *proportional* to increases in speed. Thus efficiency remains constant in spite of changes in speed for all distance events (these are run almost entirely aerobically). Moreover, even decreased efficiency due to anaerobic conditions is probably much less than that predicted by the 3.8th power law. A loss of approximately fifty percent in efficiency, as described above, is probably realistic.

There are large differences in the efficiency of running from individual to individual. Figure 20.1 shows the differences in O_2 consumption for runners of varying skill as studied by Dill, Talbot and Edwards in 1930. It is seen that the famous marathoner of that time, Clarence De Mar had the lowest O_2 consumption at 26 ml/kg/min while the less skilled runners went fifty-four percent higher, requiring as much as 40 ml/kg/min for the same run. This classic study demonstrates the importance of skill in running although we still do not fully understand the methods required to optimize this factor.

Walking. The most economical rate of walking has been found to be four kilometers per hour (2.4 mph) (8) at which the energy consumption is about one-half kilocalorie per kilometer walked per kilogram of body weight. The energy consumption for aerobic running is about twice that value, regardless of speed.

In walking more slowly than four kilometers per hour, energy is apparently wasted in static components of muscle activity because weight is supported too long in respect to the useful work. In walking faster, energy consumption increases faster than the useful work done, and efficiency again falls off, presumably because of a disproportionate increase of energy wasted in accelerating and decelerating body parts.

As a result of the increasing inefficiency at increasing rates, energy consumption of walking at about 8 km/hr (4.8 mph) becomes greater than that required for running, so that running is more efficient than walking above 8 km/hr.

Cycling. Using total work loads on bicycle ergometers that were equated for energy cost, Henry (21) found that at 69 rpm this resulted in work output of 620 kilogram meters per minute while a rate of 116 rpm produced only ninety-five kilogram meters per minute. The differ-

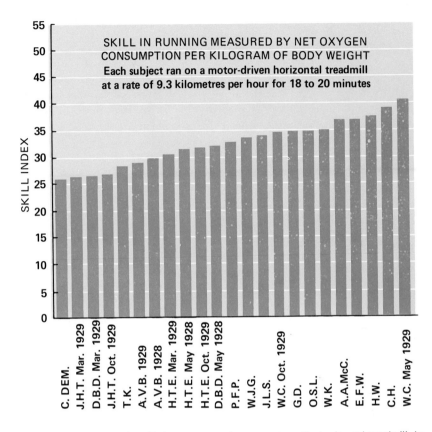

Figure 20-1. Skill in running. Each man ran at the same rate on the horizontal treadmill. In contrast with the relatively uniform cost of walking at ninety m/min the cost varied widely. The most efficient was Clarence DeMar, the famous marathoner of that time, 1929. (From Dill, Talbot, and Edwards. *J. Physiol.* 69:267, 1930.)

ence in efficiency is obvious. Earlier workers had already demonstrated that 70 rpm is the most efficient pedaling rate.

Storage of Elastic Energy. At this point an explanation seems called for to rationalize the fact that many forms of physical activity have an optimum rate, above which increased speed demands disproportionately greater energy expenditure. The efficiency of running, on the other hand, seems to be unaffected by speed, at least until anaerobiosis occurs.

Early workers, such as Fenn (20) and Hubbard (26), discussed the possibility of the storage of mechanical energy in the muscles and tendons. The extension of a muscle and tendon that are antagonistic in one phase of reciprocating movement might store the kinetic energy of the protagonist as potential energy, which is released when the antagonist contracts.

It has been demonstrated in a laboratory preparation that such a storage of energy can and does occur (10). When a contracted muscle was forcibly stretched, a substantial amount of the work done in stretching the muscle appeared to be available in the work done in the subsequent contraction. Furthermore, the sooner the contraction followed the forced stretch the greater was the increase in work performed. It must be realized that this phenomenon could bring about considerable economy in quickly reciprocating movements, as in running, but the economy would be less as the rate slows because of the greater length of time during which the contracted muscle exerts tension (uses energy) against the stretching. It has been calculated by the same investigators that this elastic work may contribute as much as half of the total mechanical work performed in running (9). More recent work from the same laboratory has corroborated this concept and extended it into the realm of human arm and leg movement (11, 32). Using an electronic force platform Thys, Farragiana, and Margaria (32) studied subjects in deep knee bending exercise under two conditions, (1) rebounding where they bounced back up immediately after the full squat position thus using the elastic energy stored in stretching the leg extensors in the subsequent contraction, and (2) nonrebounding exercise identical except that the exercise stopped for a fraction of a second in the full squat position, thus allowing the elastic energy to be dissipated as heat. They found the rebounding movement to have faster maximum speed of movement (twenty percent), more power (twenty-nine percent), and better efficiency (thirty-seven percent). This appears to be an important factor to be applied in athletics wherever pertinent. These facts would seem to offer the best explanation for the failure of the efficiency of running to decrease with increasing speed.

EFFECT OF WORK LOAD ON EFFICIENCY

If speed is held constant, work load (or the force overcome) probably affects efficiency only to the extent that the work load requires energy from anaerobic sources (22). In other words, efficiency probably remains constant as long as a steady state can be maintained, as determined by other factors; and it declines only when the work is done anaerobically.

EFFECT OF FATIGUE ON EFFICIENCY

It has been pointed out that the electrical activity of a muscle increases with time even though it maintains constant tension; Figure 20.2 illustrates this fact. The best explanation for this is that, as fatigue occurs, more and more motor units are required to do the same piece of work. It is obvious that the recruitment of more units should result in greater energy consumption. Since the work *output* remains constant, the increased energy *input* must result in lowered efficiency. This will be important to our discussion of pace and efficiency.

DIET AND EFFICIENCY

There appears to be agreement among various investigators that the efficiency of muscular work is greatest when carbohydrate supplies the energy for muscular contraction; however, the differences due to this factor are small, and probably not more than five percent.

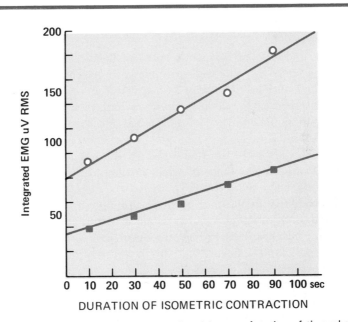

Figure 20-2. Illustration of increased electrical activity as a function of time when forty percent of maximal voluntary contraction strength is maintained isometrically in the elbow flexors. Open circles represent data for a subject whose maximal duration was 127 seconds; squares represent subject with duration of 338 seconds.

EFFECTS OF ENVIRONMENTAL TEMPERATURE

It has been shown that moderate work performed at 100° F requires an average 13.3 percent higher metabolic rate than at 85° F. When the work was heavy, the increase was 11.7 percent (14). The difference between work loads is probably not significant.

This decreased efficiency is undoubtedly the result of the increased load upon the circulatory system for meeting the demand for increased peripheral circulation to transport heat from the core to the skin (increased heart rate, etc.).

EFFECT OF OBESITY ON EFFICIENCY

Dempsey et al. (15) compared the exercise responses of fourteen normal young men with fourteen obese young men. It was shown that the obese required 2.01 l/min of O_2 at a work load of 650 kgM/min while the normals used only 1.54 l/min for a slightly larger work load. Thus the obese required thirty percent more energy to do the same job.

THE LOOSENESS FACTOR IN ATHLETICS

Athletes and coaches frequently speak of being *loose* or *tight* in such activities as sprint running and swimming. It has been suggested that a tight runner may be thought of as one whose movements are impeded by the resistance of antagonistic muscles and their connective tissues due to a lack of flexibility. The author has investigated this possibility by controlled experiments in which four subjects ran ten 100-yard sprints. Five of the sprints were run under normal conditions of flexibility, and five were run after flexibility of trunk flexion, ankle flexion, and ankle extension had been significantly improved by static stretching. No significant differences in speed or oxygen consumption were found (17).

In the light of much personal experience with the looseness factor by athletes and coaches, it is difficult to reject its existence; however, the author's experiments indicate that this factor is probably not a simple matter of increased or decreased static flexibility. More likely it is a matter of changes in neuromuscular coordination. There is also the possibility that it is a psychological illusion.

ACCELERATION-DECELERATION VERSUS SMOOTH MOVEMENT

In some activities (such as swimming) the smoothness of movement is important in determining efficiency. In swimming the butterfly stroke, for example, if constant velocity could be maintained throughout the various events of the single-stroke cycle (the pull, the arm recovery, and the leg drive), maximum efficiency would be achieved. This is so because at a constant speed a constant amount of energy is required to overcome the resistance of the body's movement through the water. This resistance is called *drag*. If the stroke is coordinated so that the leg drive sustains the velocity achieved by the arm pull during the recovery phase of the arms, only the force of drag must be overcome. If the coordination is such that the swimmer comes to a virtual standstill during arm recovery, then, in addition, the body must be *accelerated* by each arm pull. The energy required for acceleration is very costly because it varies as the square of the velocity. To double the velocity, then, requires four times the energy output.

To illustrate this concept, table 20.1 was prepared from an experiment in which the author measured the velocity of outstanding butterfly swimmers for each 0.10 second within their stroke cycles (16). For the sake of comparison, arbitrary energy units were calculated for (1) an

TABLE 20.1

Comparison of Energy Requirements for
One Stroke (in Arbitrary Units)
(V = Velocity in ft/sec; V^2 is an Estimate of Energy Consumption)

Consecutive 1/10-second Periods	Ideal Swimmer		National Record-holder		Inexperienced Swimmer	
	V	V^2	V	V^2	V	V^2
0-0.1	6.07	36.54	8.00	64.00	11.10	123.21
0.1-0.2	6.07	36.54	6.72	45.13	8.63	74.48
0.2-0.3	6.07	36.54	6.63	43.96	6.12	37.45
0.3-0.4	6.07	36.54	4.92	24.21	3.08	9.49
0.4-0.5	6.07	36.54	4.42	19.54	1.00	1.00
0.5-0.6	6.07	36.54	6.22	38.69	5.76	33.18
0.6-0.7	6.07	36.54	5.33	28.41	4.35	18.92
0.7-0.8	6.07	36.54	4.92	24.21	3.21	10.30
0.8-0.9	6.07	36.54	4.84	23.43	2.42	5.86
0.9-1.0	6.07	36.54	6.22	38.69	6.55	42.90
1.0-1.1	6.07	36.54	8.52	72.59	14.52	210.83
Mean	6.07		6.07		6.07	
Total energy units used for 1 stroke		405.24		422.86		567.62

ideal swimmer, swimming so smoothly that no acceleration-deceleration occurs, (2) a national record-holder, whose highest velocity was 1.94 times his slowest velocity, and (3) an inexperienced swimmer, whose highest velocity was 14.52 times his slowest velocity (not unusual).

Although all three swimmers achieved an *average* velocity of 6.07 feet per second for the stroke that was analyzed, even the champion used four percent more energy than was necessary, and the inexperienced swimmer used forty percent more. Furthermore, it has been shown that drag increases disproportionately above five or six feet per second, so that the actual differences in efficiency would be even greater than those predicted (4).

PACE AND EFFICIENCY

The question of how best to pace an endurance event cannot be answered simply. First, we have seen that efficiency for most activities (but apparently not running) falls off beyond some optimum rate of speed. Second, efficiency decreases as a lactacid oxygen debt is incurred. Third, the fatigue level must be considered inasmuch as efficiency falls off rapidly as fatigue brings about greater recruitment of muscle fibers to do the same job and possibly interferes with neuromuscular coordination.

In events that are largely aerobic (two-mile or more run), a constant rate is probably the most efficient. This is true even in running in which efficiency does not seem to vary with speed (aerobic condition); even though the varying rates may be equally efficient, the *changes in rate* cost additional energy.

Constant rate does not necessarily mean running or swimming equal split times. For example, it is typical in distance swimming that the number of strokes per minute remains constant throughout the 1500-meter swim, but each successive 100 meters shows a small decrement in speed—2 or 3 seconds, or more, depending on the swimmer. This is the result of the fatigue process; even though cadence remains the same, the force developed—and consequently the *distance per stroke*—decreases.

For middle-distance running events, some very interesting evidence *against* the constant rate has been presented by Robinson et al. (29), who ran two men on three different pace plans. Each man ran one trial at constant speed, one trial with a fast first minute and slower remainder, and one trial with a slow first minute and faster remainder. In both men, it was found, the slow start and faster finish resulted in slightly less O_2 consumption than the constant rate, and in considerably less than the fast start and slower remainder. The overall time for the three pace plans was kept constant on the treadmill.

They also showed that when three men (in another experiment) ran to exhaustion in from 2.58 to 3.37 minutes, each man's O_2 consumption increased from sixty percent to 143 percent during the last half minute, as the lactic acid rose to high levels.

Thus the explanation for the results in the pace experiment would seem to be that starting out fast results in an earlier accumulation of lactic acid, and thus more of the race is run inefficiently. On this basis, it would seem wise to run middle-distance races in which high O_2 debts are encountered on a pace plan that postpones the O_2 debt until late in the race. However more recent studies which measured O_2 consumption to compare similar pace plans did not entirely support Robinson's data. Adams and Bernauer found the steady pace to be significantly less demanding (3) and Kollias et al. found no difference between steady state and slow-fast pace but the fast-slow pace required significantly greater O_2 consumption than either (27). Summarizing the evidence from these three metabolic studies with two radiotelemetry studies on the cardiac cost of similar pace plans (7, 31) leaves us with complete agreement only on the fact that the fast-slow pacing creates greater physiological demands for middle distance runs. Whether the slow-fast pace is better than steady pace will be finally resolved only by further investigation.

EFFICIENCY OF POSITIVE AND NEGATIVE WORK

Positive work is done when muscle contraction provides force that works through a distance, and this is associated with the concentric contraction of muscle. Negative work results when an extrinsic force overcomes the force developed by muscular contraction, and thus the muscle lengthens during contraction (eccentric contraction). By definition, positive work lifts a weight; negative work lowers a weight to its resting place. These definitions are not altogether satisfactory, however, for if we continue increasing the velocity with which we lower the weight until we accelerate its lowering to 32 ft/sec², all of the work would be done by gravitational force. A very slow lowering, on the other hand, could require a large degree of effort in a physiological sense. Undoubtedly, increasing efforts by biophysicists will improve our definitions of these terms; in the meantime, some very interesting findings revolve about these definitions.

A. V. Hill and his co-workers have recently discovered the surprising fact that application of external mechanical work to a living muscle cell can reverse the normal biochemical processes (1, 25). Their experiments leave no doubt that an absorption of energy by muscle tissue occurs during the forced extension of the contractile component when the muscle is in isometric contraction, and experiments on intact human muscles have supported these findings.

Asmussen (6) studied a man's energy expenditure in riding a bicycle uphill and downhill on a treadmill. He found it required from three to nine times as much energy to pedal uphill (positive work) as it did to resist the force of gravity in backpedaling downhill (negative work).

Abbott, Bigland, and Ritchie (2) found similar results. They used a pair of subjects on two bicycle ergometers, coupled in opposition (back to back) so that all the positive work of one subject was dissipated as negative work in the other. Although the subjects used the same leg muscles in similar movements at identical speeds, at 35 rpm the O_2 consumption for positive work was 3.7 times that of negative work. This ratio increased with the speed of pedaling.

PRINCIPLES FOR IMPROVEMENT OF EFFICIENCY

1. Improve the skills involved first.
   a. Eliminate *unnecessary movements.*
   b. Eliminate *unnecessary muscle activity*—within even the necessary movement.
      (1) Maintain relaxation in antagonistic muscles.
      (2) Relax even the prime movers when possible; for example, convert tension movements into ballistic movements wherever possible; thus even the prime movers can relax during a large portion of the movement.
   c. Make all movements in the *correct directions;* for example, an arm pull that moves laterally from the body in swimming the crawl wastes a considerable component of its total force.
   d. Apply only the *necessary amount of power;* too forceful an effort is usually wasteful.
   e. Use *muscles that are best suited to the activity;* for example, use the larger leg muscles in lifting heavy weights rather than the weaker back muscles.
   f. Use the *optimum speed* if time is not a factor.
2. Improve physical condition so that a given level of work requires less energy from anaerobic sources, which are inefficient. Better condition also delays fatigue; and fatigue increases energy cost.
3. Avoid costly acceleration. Maintain a constant cadence if possible, even though fatigue may result in progressively slower split times.
4. Use a high carbohydrate, low fat, normal protein diet.
5. Pace (for a distance event) should adhere to principle three. For

middle-distance events that incur large oxygen debts, a gradually accelerating pace may have advantages.

REFERENCES

1. Abbott, B. C.; Aubert, V. M.; and Hill, A. V. 1951. Absorption of work by muscle stretched during single twitch or short tetanus. *Procedures of Royal Society* (London) 139:86-104.
2. Abbott, B. C.; Bigland, B.; and Ritchie, J. M. 1952. Physiological cost of negative work. *Journal of Physiology* 117:380-90.
3. Adams, W. C., and Bernauer, E. M. 1968. The effect of selected pace variations on the oxygen requirement of running a 4:37 mile. *Research Quarterly* 39:837-46.
4. Alley, L. E. 1952. An analysis of water resistance and propulsion in swimming the crawl stroke. *Research Quarterly* 23:253-70.
5. Asmussen, E. 1946. Aerobic recovery after anaerobiosis in rest and work. *Acta Physiologica Scandinavica* 11:197-210.
6. ———. 1953. Experiments on positive and negative work. In *Fatigue*, eds. W. F. Floyd and A. T. Welford. London: H. K. Lewis & Co.
7. Bowles, C. J., and Sigerseth, P. O. 1968. Telemetered heart rate responses to pace patterns in the one mile run. *Research Quarterly* 39:36-46.
8. Cavagna, G. A.; Saibene, F. P.; and Margaria, R. 1963. External work in walking. *Journal of Applied Physiology* 18:1-9.
9. ———. 1964. Mechanical work in running. *Journal of Applied Physiology* 19:249-56.
10. ———. 1956. Effect of negative work on the amount of positive work performed by an isolated muscle. *Journal of Applied Physiology* 20:157-58.
11. Cavagna, G. A.; Dusman, B.; and Margaria, R. 1968. Positive work done by a previously stretched muscle. *Journal of Applied Physiology* 24:21-32.
12. Christensen, E. H., and Hogberg, P. 1950. The efficiency of anaerobical work. *Arbeitsphysiologie* 14:249-50.
13. ———. 1950. Steady state, O_2 deficit and O_2 debt at severe work. *Arbeitsphysiologie* 14:251-54.
14. Consolazio, C. F.; Matoush, L. D.; Nelson, R. A.; Torres, J. B.; and Isaac, G. J. 1963. Environmental temperature and energy expenditure. *Journal of Applied Physiology* 18:65-68.
15. Dempsey, J. A.; Reddan, W.; Balke, B.; and Rankin, J. 1966. Work capacity determinants and physiologic cost of weight supported work in obesity. *Journal of Applied Physiology* 21:1815-20.
16. deVries, H. A. 1959. A cinematographical analysis of the dolphin swimming stroke. *Research Quarterly* 30:413-22.
17. ———. 1963. The "looseness" factor in speed and O_2 consumption of an anaerobic 100-yard dash. *Research Quarterly* 34:305-13.
18. Dill, D. B. 1963. Comparative physiology of oxygen transport. *Journal of Sport, Medicine and Physical Fitness* 3:191-200.

19. ———. 1965. Oxygen used in horizontal and grade walking and running on the treadmill. *Journal of Applied Physiology* 20:19-22.
20. Fenn, W. O. 1930. Frictional and kinetic factors in the work of sprint runners. *American Journal of Physiology* 92:583-610.
21. Henry, F. M. 1951. Individual differences in O_2 metabolism of work at two speeds of movement. *Research Quarterly* 22:324-33.
22. Henry, F. M., and De Moor, J. 1950. Metabolic efficiency of exercise in relation to workload at constant speed. *Journal of Applied Physiology* 2: 481-87.
23. Henry, F. M., and Trafton, I. R. 1951. The velocity curve of sprint running with some observations on the muscle viscosity factor. *Research Quarterly* 22:409-22.
24. Hill, A. V. 1922. The maximum work and mechanical efficiency of human muscles and their most economical speed. *Journal of Physiology* 56:19-41.
25. ———. 1960. Production and absorption of work by muscle. *Science* 131: 897-903.
26. Hubbard, A. W. 1939. An experimental analysis of running and a certain fundamental difference between trained and untrained runners. *Research Quarterly* 10:28-38.
27. Kollias, J.; Nicholas, W. C.; Buskirk, E. R.; and Mendez, J. 1970. Oxygen requirements for running at moderate altitude. *Journal of Sport Medicine* 10:27-35.
28. Margaria, R.; Cerretelli, P.; Aghemo, P.; and Sassi, G. Energy cost of running. *Journal of Applied Physiology* 18:367-70.
29. Robinson, S.; Robinson, D. L.; Mountjoy, R. J.; and Bullard, R. W. 1958. Fatigue and efficiency of men during exhauting runs. *Journal of Applied Physiology* 12:197-202.
30. Sargent, R. M. 1926. The relation between O_2 requirement and speed in running. *Procedures of the Royal Society* (London) 100:10-22.
31. Sorani, R. P. 1967. The effect of three different pace plans on the cardiac cost of 1320-yard runs. Doctoral dissertation, USC (physical education).
32. Thys, H.; Faraggiana, T.; and Margaria, R. 1972. Utilization of muscle elasticity in exercise. *Journal of Applied Physiology* 32:491-94.

21 Speed

Speed of movement is a very important factor in athletics. As such, it is worthy of careful analysis so that we may better understand this aspect of human performance and thus be in a better position to improve this function in athletes.

First, we must realize that, basically, speed is the result of applying force to a mass. Second, speed usually implies movement at a *constant* rate. The movement of a body (human or otherwise) at a constant rate requires sufficient driving force to balance the forces that resist movement. An airplane must have just enough force to overcome the friction of air drag to maintain a constant speed; if more than this balancing amount of force is applied, acceleration occurs (speed increases with time); if less, the aircraft decelerates.

In the human body the resisting force has several components, and we can think of a balance of positive and negative forces in respect to its propulsion or any of its parts (the same physical laws apply). The positive force that propels the body is provided by muscular contractions, in some cases aided by the storage of elastic energy (see chapter twenty). The negative forces depend upon the nature of the activity.

In running, for example, it was shown that the 2.95 hp of useful work (positive force) developed by the muscles were used to balance the negative forces, as follows: (1) gravity, 0.1 hp, (2) velocity changes, 0.5 hp, (3) acceleration of limbs, 1.68 hp, and (4) deceleration of limbs, 0.67 hp. Had this run been performed on the track instead of on a treadmill, another negative force, air resistance—possibly as much as 0.5 hp—would have had to have been overcome; and the positive or propelling force needed for maintaining a constant rate of speed would have been 3.45 hp.

From the above considerations we might hypothesize that speed may be improved by either increasing the positive or by decreasing the negative factors. In a practical sense, this suggests that improving strength would be the most important positive factor. The negative factors might be reduced through improved neuromuscular coordination (skill) and flexibility, which might conceivably decrease the values of the factors listed above. We shall examine these possibilities in this chapter.

INTRINSIC SPEED OF MUSCLE CONTRACTION

As has been pointed out, muscles differ in their ability to produce fast movement. The postural muscles (red) are relatively slow, and the flexor muscles (pale) usually are relatively fast. Furthermore, speed of contraction varies greatly from one animal species to another, approximately in inverse ratio to size. A. V. Hill (12) has pointed out that this variability in speed of contraction is inherent in the muscle tissue since even isolated muscles that are deprived of innervation differ greatly in speed. The differences in speed of muscle contraction appear to depend on the physicochemical and biochemical properties of the contractile material.

Comparing the intrinsic speeds of different muscles requires that we equate them by fiber length. Obviously, a muscle fiber that is ten times longer than another fiber can shorten at one end ten times as fast, although intrinsic properties are the same (12).

Although evidence is lacking, it seems very likely that ultimate maximal speed capacity is limited by the intrinsic speed of an individual's muscle tissue and by the nicety of his neuromuscular coordination patterns. Neither factor is amenable to changes as large as those that affect strength and endurance.

FORCE-VELOCITY RELATIONSHIP

It has been shown with experimental muscle preparations that the force available from a muscle's shortening decreases as the rate of shortening increases. Figure 21.1 illustrates this relationship, which has important implications for athletics.

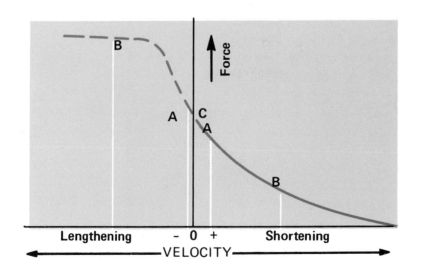

Figure 21-1. Force-velocity relation of contracting muscle: to the right, shortening; to the left, lengthening. C, at zero speed, represents an isometric contraction. A and A are at the same velocity of shortening and lengthening; so are B and B. (From Hill, A.V. *Lancet,* 261:947, 1951.)

The shape of the curve in figure 21.1 also leads us to conclude that there must be an *optimum speed* at which a muscle can produce its greatest *power* and greatest *efficiency*. It has been found that this optimum speed is approximately one-third of the maximum speed at which it can shorten under zero load (13). Kaneko (15) has shown that maximum power is developed when force and velocity are both about thirty-five percent of their maximum values. Data from our laboratory shown in figure 21.2 are in essential agreement.

injury. Hill (12) has pointed out that if a rapid flexor movement is made, and the object is suddenly wrenched in the opposite direction, the muscle or its attachments may be torn. This can happen because the forces of the muscle in the lengthening movement could be increased several times beyond what they were in shortening before a reflex inhibition (from the inverse myotatic reflex) could take place. This sudden increase in the forces, which is predicted from figure 21.1, could well exceed the elastic limits of the tissues.

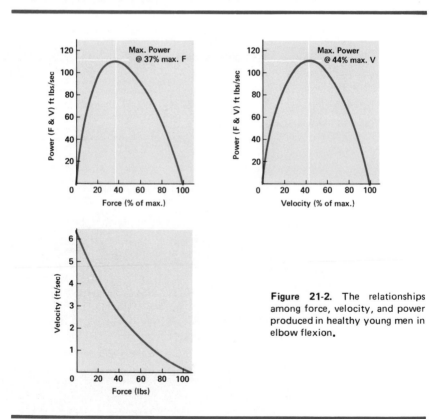

Figure 21-2. The relationships among force, velocity, and power produced in healthy young men in elbow flexion.

From the standpoint of human performance in the intact individual, there are two aspects of speed (10). The first (really acceleration) is related to how fast an athlete can accelerate from a standstill (a football lineman's charge), and this factor is an important determinant of speed for the first five or ten yards. This factor is probably determined by the shape of an individual's force-velocity curve. On the other hand, for distances more than twenty yards, the only important determinant is the maximal movement rate, which is in turn limited by intrinsic speed and neuromuscular coordination.

These two factors are not highly related. Therefore, an individual could conceivably be a slow starter with a good 100-yard speed, or a fast starter with a poor 100-yard time or, indeed be proficient in football, tennis, etc., where quick-starting movements are important, but be a poor 100-yard sprinter.

SPECIFICITY OF SPEED

It is commonplace in physical education and athletics to speak of an individual as fast or slow, but evidence is accumulating that speed has very little generality. Indeed, an individual with a fast arm movement may well have slow leg movement. In fact, this specificity extends even to the type of task and the direction of movement (3, 9, 19).

It has been shown, for example (19) that speed is eighty-seven or eighty-eight percent specific to the limb. Even within a limb, speed is eighty-eight to ninety percent specific to the direction of movement. This means there is practically no correlation between the speeds with which one can perform an arm movement and a leg movement, and that there is only a small relationship between speed of movement in a forward arm swing compared with a backward arm swing. This might lead us to describe an individual as fast in a backward swing of the right leg! Obviously, this makes no sense, but neither does it make sense to speak of a fast or slow individual. We may speak of a fast runner, but we are not justified in assuming the same individual can throw a fast ball in baseball.

STRENGTH AND SPEED

It might be expected from the preceding discussions that strength and speed of movement would be highly related; however, the experimental evidence is controversial. Four different studies have agreed in findings that strength and speed are unrelated (2, 9, 11, 21). However all of these studies were concerned with the same movement pattern, the horizontal adductive arm swing. Nelson and Fahrney (16) have shown rather strong significant and consistent correlations in three experimental subject groups of 0.74, 0.79 and 0.75 between strength and speed of elbow flexion. Thus a final decision on strength-speed relationships must await further research.

Interestingly, if movements are resisted by substantial loads on a tested limb, sizable relationships between strength and speed (up to 0.76) can be demonstrated (21). This leads us to think of speed in terms of the neuromotor specificity that has been demonstrated in so many other aspects of human performance. What we are saying, in effect, is that various speeds of movement against varying loads require different neuromotor coordination patterns. Thus if we measure strength statically, we might expect higher correlations between strength and speed (as we slow the speed (or increase the load) to more closely approximate static contraction. And this, we find, is what happens.

Carrying our discussion further requires that we visualize two strength factors: one a *static strength*, as we usually measure it by dynamometer or cable tensiometer, and the other a dynamic or *strength in action* factor, which must be measured during movement. Each may involve a separate and distinct coordination pattern. Dynamic strength can be described as:

$$F = 2md/t^2$$

where F is the force of contraction, m is the mass moved, d is the distance, and t is the time. This approach has been widely used by F. M. Henry and his collaborators at the University of California. In this approach the mass is measured and the distance moved is timed electrically so that F, the force of contraction (or strength, if a maximal effort is made), can be calculated. Although the relationship between dynamic strength and speed is very close, it is hard to define: in calculating a correlation the results are spurious because distance is usually a constant and mass varies very little. In effect, one would be correlating speed against itself.

Now for the most practical question: Can we improve speed of movement by improving strength? Even though there is no relationship between the static strength level of achievement and speed at any given time, considerable evidence (13, 6, 20) indicates a strong relationship between gain in strength and gain in speed. It has been shown that gains in strength, whether brought about by isometric or isotonic training, are associated with significant gains in speed of movement. The gain in speed has also been demonstrated to result from both strength training that used the same movement as was tested and from training that merely improved the strength of the involved muscles but avoided training in the same movement.

Interestingly, Francis and Tipton (8) found that the knee-jerk reflex time is improved by physical conditioning of the involved muscles. A significant five percent improvement in reflex time was shown after six weeks of weight training, although there appeared to be no correlation between strength and reflex time or between improvement in strength and reflex time. Thus while the mechanism remains obscure, there seems to be good reason to include strength training in a training regimen for speed. Furthermore, it must be realized that in most speed events there is a period of acceleration to attain maximum velocity as in running the 100-yard sprint. Since acceleration of the body's mass is by definition dependent upon strength (force = mass $\times$ acceleration) there can be no question of the importance of optimizing strength (force) in the practical coaching situation.

FLEXIBILITY AND SPEED

As we have pointed out, logic would indicate that improvement of flexibility should decrease the negative forces (resistance) involved in running and thus improve the speed. However, experiments by the author —in which speed and oxygen consumption on a 100-yard dash were measured—failed to confirm this hypothesis (5). Even though range of motion was significantly improved, the short-term effect upon speed was not significant.

In another experiment, in which the long-term effects of supplementing sprint training with flexibility work and weight training were investigated, it was found that neither weight training nor flexibility added to the gains in speed of the sprint training program. When both were used, however, the gains in speed were significantly better than those by sprint training alone (6).

It must be realized that stop-watch errors in timing a 100-yard dash can be one or two percent, and the changes brought about by an improved range of motion are not likely to be much larger than this; so the question can not be considered closed.

BODY MECHANICS AND SPEED IN RUNNING

This area of human performance has not yet been exhaustively investigated, but some experiments have been performed and their results are interesting.

Bringing about many accelerations and decelerations of the limbs at exactly the right time, at exactly the right rate, and with precisely the appropriate amount of force to run well, obviously requires exquisite neuromuscular coordination patterns. One of the basic questions about running: "Is the maximum speed limited by the maximum rate of leg alternation?" was answered by a simple but clever experiment by Slater-Hammel (18), who demonstrated that the rates of leg alternation in sprinting were 3.10 to 4.85 per second. Because considerably higher rates are possible in cycling (5.5 to 7.1), he concluded that speed in running is not limited in this way.

In another interesting kinesiological analysis of running, Hubbard (14) demonstrated that improvement results from increasing the length of stride rather than the rate of movement. Applying the formula for dynamic strength, $F = 2md/t^2$, we see that this requires more dynamic strength because d increases while t, and m remain the same; thus F, the force required (strength), must be greater. Again, we see that strength is a factor in speed.

Photographic analyses have shown that efficient running is also characterized by a high knee lift, a long running stride, and placement of the feet beneath the runner's center of gravity (4).

Use of the electrogoniometer (17) which provides electrical recording of joint angle changes has shown that experienced distance runners increase both stride length and frequency when increasing velocity from that of running a 440 in 2:12 to that of a 440 in 60.9 seconds. Stride length is more important at the lower speeds while frequency becomes more important at the higher speeds. The only joint function which may become limiting appears to be that of hip flexion since it is the only joint angle which increases markedly at the higher speeds. Thus the track coach would be well advised to include flexibility work such as the static stretching techniques described in the following chapter.

SEX DIFFERENCES IN SPEED OF MOVEMENT

In sports such as running and swimming, records for women show their speed to be eighty-five to ninety percent that of men, but that this reflects true differences in speed of movement per se is questionable. First, it has been shown that speed depends to a large extent upon strength, so that the difference in speed may merely reflect the sex differences in strength. Second, the selection of women for sports represents a much smaller population of athletes, and it is possible that the fastest women athletes have not been found.

In controlled experiments, arm speed was found to be seventeen percent slower in women than in men, but when the length of the arm was removed as a factor, the sex difference was only five percent. This is probably a good evaluation of sex differences in speed of movement.

LIMITING FACTORS IN SPEED

Speed of Single-muscle Contraction. In a simple contraction of a muscle, intrinsic speed of the muscle, which depends upon physicochemical properties, is probably most important. Neuromuscular coordination patterns are a smaller, though still important, factor.

A. V. Hill has pointed out the importance of muscle temperature (13). An animal's muscle contraction can be quickened about twenty percent by raising its body temperature 2° C. He suggests that such an increase might be brought about in a sprinter by diathermy, and he raises the interesting question whether an athlete might not then do the 100-yards in 8.0 seconds.

Speed of Gross Motor Movements. Many important factors act and interact in determining gross motor movements. In lightly loaded and simple movements, the limitations are probably similar to those of a single muscle contraction. In lightly loaded movements of greater complexity, it is likely that ability to coordinate neuromotor patterns would set the upper limits.

In heavily loaded but simple movements, the strength factor is probably dominant. In heavily loaded and complex movements, the limits are undoubtedly set by an interaction to strength and neuromotor coordination.

NEW METHODS FOR IMPROVING SPRINT SPEED

In general, the methods for improving sprinting speed fall into one of two categories: (1) *sprint resisted training* in which sprint running is simulated with added resistance, the effort being to improve the dynamic strength factor, and (2) *sprint assisted training* where the effort is directed toward improving the rate of leg alternation. The first method uses devices such as uphill running, and weighted clothing. The second method uses downhill running, towing behind an auto at velocities above maximum unassisted, and treadmill running at supramaximal rates (possible because of decreased air resistance). Dintiman (7) has provided an excellent review of the literature in this area for the interested reader.

SUMMARY OF PRINCIPLES FOR COACHING

1. The strength of the prime and assistant movers used in an activity should be developed to an optimum level, preferably by dynamic movements that are closely related to the skill.
2. If speed is desired, the skill should be practiced at rates at least as fast as those to be used in competition. Faster-than-competition rates

can be practiced by several different methods. For sprinters it can be accomplished by downhill running, auto towing, or treadmill running.

3. Flexibility should be improved until range of motion is such as to ensure that no resistance to movement can occur in the skill under consideration.

4. Warming-up should be long and vigorous enough to bring about increased deep-muscle temperature. Ordinarily this will require sweating.

5. A skill should be analyzed on the basis of kinesiological principles, and all improper applications of positive forces should be corrected. Any unnecessary accelerations-decelerations, or movements in the vertical dimension, should be eliminated.

6. If the speed of movement is greater than that of middle-distance running, air resistance can become an important negative factor, and it should be held whenever possible to a minimum; e.g., the crouch position is used in ice skating and bicycle racing.

REFERENCES

1. Chui, E. F. 1964. Effects of isometric and dynamic weight training exercises upon strength and speed of movement. *Research Quarterly* 35:246-57.
2. Clarke, D. H. 1960. Correlation between strength/mass ratio and the speed of an arm movement. *Research Quarterly* 31:470-74.
3. Clarke, D. H., and Henry, F. M. 1961. Neuromotor specificity and increased speed from strength development. *Research Quarterly* 32:315-25.
4. Deshon, D. E., and Nelson, R. C. 1964. A cinematographical analysis of sprint running. *Research Quarterly* 35:451-55.
5. deVries, H. A. 1963. The "looseness" factor in speed and O_2 consumption of an anaerobic 100-yard dash. *Research Quarterly* 34:305-13.
6. Dintiman, G. B. 1964. Effects of various training programs on running speed. *Research Quarterly* 35:456-63.
7. ———. 1971. Techniques and methods of developing speed in athletic performance. In *Proc. Int. Symp. Art and Science of Coaching*, eds. L. Percival and J. W. Taylor, vol. 1, pp. 97-139. Willowdale, Canada: F. I. Productions.
8. Francis, P. R., and Tipton, C. M. 1969. Influence of a weight training program on quadriceps reflex time. *Medicine and Science in Sports* 1:91-94.
9. Henry, F. M. 1960. Factorial structure of speed and static strength in a lateral arm movement. *Research Quarterly* 31:440-47.
10. Henry, F. M., and Trafton, I. R. 1951. The velocity curve of sprint running with some observations on the muscle viscosity factor. *Research Quarterly* 22:409-22.

11. Henry, F. M., and Whitley, J. D. 1960. Relationships between individual differences in strength, speed and mass in an arm movement. *Research Quarterly* 31:24-33.
12. Hill, A. V. 1951. The mechanics of voluntary muscle. *Lancet* 261:947-51.
13. ———. 1956. The design of muscles. *British Medical Bulletin* 12:165-66.
14. Hubbard, A. W. 1939. An experimental analysis of running and a certain fundamental difference between trained and untrained runners. *Research Quarterly* 10:28-38.
15. Kaneko, M. 1970. The relation between force, velocity and mechanical power in human muscle. *Research Journal in Physical Education* (Japan) 14:141-45.
16. Nelson, R. C., and Fahrney, R. A. 1965. Relationship between strength and speed of elbow flexion. *Research Quarterly* 36:455-63.
17. Sinning, W. E., and Forsyth, H. L. 1970. Lower limb actions while running at different velocities. *Medicine and Science in Sports* 2:28-34.
18. Slater-Hammel, A. 1941. Possible neuromuscular mechanisms as limiting factors for leg movement in sprinting. *Research Quarterly* 12:745-57.
19. Smith, L. E. 1961. Individual differences in strength, reaction latency, mass and length of limbs and their relation to maximal speed of movement. *Research Quarterly* 32:208-20.
20. ———. 1964. Influence of strength training on pre-tensed and free arm speed. *Research Quarterly* 35:554-61.
21. Whitley, J. D., and Smith, L. E. 1963. Velocity curves and static strength-action strength correlations in relation to the mass moved by the arm. *Research Quarterly* 34:379-95.

22 Flexibility

Flexibility can be most simply defined as the range of possible movement in a joint (as in the hip joint) or series of joints (as when the spinal column is involved). The need for flexibility varies with the athletic endeavor but in some activities it is all-important. A hurdler must have the best possible hip flexion-hip extension flexibility. In competitive swimming, shoulder and ankle flexibility can be decisive factors. And a diver who cannot execute a deep pike position will never achieve outstanding success.

Even for the "arm chair athlete," flexibility is important because graceful movement in walking and running are unlikely without it. More importantly, considerable evidence indicates that maintenance of good joint mobility prevents or to a large extent relieves the aches and pains that grow more common with increasing age.

It should be recognized from the outset that flexibility is specific to a given joint or combination of joints. As with speed of movement, an individual is a composite of many joints, some of which may be unusually flexible, some inflexible, and some average. Accordingly, it would be incorrect to speak of a flexible individual (8).

PHYSIOLOGY OF FLEXIBILITY

What Sets the Limits of Flexibility?   For some joints the bony structure sets a very definite limit on range of motion; for example, extension of the elbow joint and the knee joint are limited in this fashion. Also, in a very heavily muscled man it is likely that flexion of his elbow and knee joints is limited by the bulk of the intervening muscle. These are mechanical factors that cannot be greatly modified, and therefore they are only of academic interest.

In such joints as the ankle joint or hip joint, however, the limitation of range of motion is imposed by the soft tissues: (1) muscle and its fascial sheaths; (2) connective tissue, with tendons, ligaments, joint capsules; and (3) the skin. This, then, is where our interest lies, for these factors are modifiable by physical methods and they are important factors in human performance.

If a resting excised muscle is stretched passively (no contraction), the greater the length becomes the greater the force required to hold the stretch. It has been shown that this resistance does not lie in the contractile elements of the muscle but is due almost entirely to the fascial sheath that covers the muscle and the sarcolemma of the muscle fiber (1, 20). Thus it is the fascial investments of muscle tissue with which we are concerned in the pursuit of flexibility.

What are the relative contributions of the various soft tissues (listed above) in limiting our movement? An ingenious experiment by Johns and Wright (9) was directed toward the problem of joint stiffness, and the author has recalculated their data to estimate the percentage contributions of the various tissues in resisting wrist flexion and extension in the cat (they showed that these functions in a cat are very similar to those of man). Table 22.1 shows the results of these calculations. It can be seen that the most important factors limiting free movement are (1) muscles (and their fascial sheaths), (2) the joint capsule, and (3) the tendons. It must be remembered that these data apply directly only to the wrist joint; but in other joints where ligaments play a more prominent role, as in the ankle joint, these structures are no doubt equally important.

TABLE 22.1

Estimated Contribution of Various Tissues in Resisting Wrist Flexion and Extension in the Cat

Tissue	Extension — 48° Torque Required		Flexion + 48° Torque Required	
	gram cm	% total	gram cm	% total
1. Skin	— 70	11.2	— 45*	— 8.7
2. Extensor muscles	— 35	42.4	0	36.9
3. Flexor muscles	— 230		190	
4. Tendon	— 70	11.2	170	33.0
5. Joint capsule	— 220	35.2	200	38.8
Total	625	100	515	100

Calculated from the data of R. J. Johns and V. Wright, "Relative Importance of Various Tissues in Joint Stiffness," *Journal of Applied Physiology* 17:824-28, 1962.
*Skin aided in flexing the joint.

Static Versus Dynamic Flexibility (Stiffness). It is obvious that the ability to flex and extend a joint through a wide range of motion (which is measured virtually in a static position) is not necessarily a good criterion of the stiffness or looseness of that same joint as this applies to the ability to move the joint quickly with little resistance to the movement. Range of motion is one factor; the only one that has been widely investigated at this point. How easily the joint can be moved in the middle of the range of motion, where the speed is necessarily greatest, is quite another factor.

We should therefore consider two separate components of flexibility: (1) *static flexibility,* which is what we ordinarily measure as range of motion, and (2) *dynamic flexibility,* which has been investigated in respect to stiffness in joint disease (25), but has been neglected in physical education. It may be hypothesized that the flexibility of motion may be of much greater importance to physical performance than the ability to achieve an extreme degree of flexion or extension of a joint!

The method for such investigations was developed by Wright and Johns (25) for laboratory work, and with their methods the physical factors that contribute to joint stiffness and therefore limit dynamic flexibility have been identified and their relative contributions measured (in finger and wrist joints only). They investigated the effects of *elasticity, viscosity, inertia, plasticity,* and *friction* in normal and in diseased joints. It was found that inertia and friction were negligible; viscosity accounted for only one-tenth the torque used in moving the joint passively; and elasticity and plasticity were the major factors. These forces are wasted on the stretching of connective tissues.

Stretch Reflexes and Flexibility. The stretch reflexes as they apply to the stretching of body components for improving static flexibility were discussed at length in chapters four and fifteen, but we remind the reader that a muscle that is stretched with a jerky motion responds with a contraction whose amount and rate vary directly with the amount and rate of the movement that causes the stretch. This is the result of the myotatic reflex that originates in the muscle spindle.

On the other hand, a firm steady, static stretch invokes the inverse myotatic reflex, which brings about inhibition not only of the muscle whose tendon organ was stretched but of the entire functional group of muscles involved. It has been shown, for example, that the amount of *tension increase* for a given amount of stretch is more than doubled by a quick stretch, as compared to slow stretch (22), when the degree of stretching is the same.

MEASURING FLEXIBILITY

Static Flexibility. In general, this quality can be measured by two approaches: (1) by *goniometry,* the *direct measurement* of the angle of the joint in its extremes of movement, and (2) by *indirect measurement* of the joint angles, which measures how closely a body part can be brought into opposition with another body part or some other reference point.

Goniometry, in its classic form, uses a protractor-like device to measure the angle of the joint at both ends of its movement range, but it suffers from the serious disadvantage that body parts are not regular geometric forms and a good deal of subjectivity is introduced into the measurements in deciding where the axis of a bony lever may be. A simple but ingenious device, Leighton's *flexometer,* overcomes this disadvantage to a large extent (fig. 22.1); it is a small instrument that is strapped onto a body part and records range of motion in respect to a perpendicular established by gravity. Reliability coefficients well above 0.90 have been reported (12, 13).

An indirect method has been devised by Cureton (5) for measuring four types of flexibility: (1) trunk flexion forward, (2) trunk extension backward, (3) shoulder elevation, and (4) average ankle flexibility; and the method can be exemplified by a description of the measurement of trunk flexion forward. A subject assumes the long sitting position, with hands behind the neck and feet eighteen inches apart; he then bends downward and forward to place his forehead as close as possible to the floor. The distance from forehead to floor is the score on flexibility for this measure.

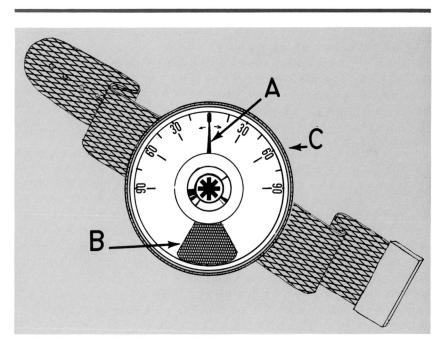

Figure 22-1. Drawing illustrating the principle of the "Leighton flexometer." A indicates needle; B indicates weight that keeps needle vertical; C indicates housing that rotates in respect to needle with movement of body part. (From Leighton. *Archives of Physical Medicine* 36:571, 1955.)

The sit and reach test of Wells and Dillon has been widely used as a test of back and leg flexibility (24). In the long sitting position, the subject slides his hands forward on a table (approximately of shoulder height) to the limit of his reach. The distance reached by the fingertips is the score on this test, and a reliability of 0.98 has been reported.

Dynamic Flexibility. This method, developed by Wright and Johns (25) to measure the stiffness of normal and diseased joints, uses laboratory devices to measure the forces (torque) needed to move a joint through various ranges of motion at varying speeds. Although this method has not yet been applied to research in physical performance, it seems to have distinct possibilities for such use. It seems highly probable that this measurement can tell us more about potential performance in speed events than can static flexibility.

Effects of Anthropometric Measurements upon Measurement of Flexibility. One of the criticisms leveled at tests that use the indirect principle for measurement of static flexibility is that the measurement depends too heavily on anthropometric measurements. For example, it can be argued that an individual with a long upper body and arms and with short legs might have little trouble with such trunk flexion tests as touching the floor with the fingertips.

Several investigators have attacked this problem with respect to (1) men (23), (2) women (7, 16), and (3) elementary school boys (17) but have found no meaningful relationships between static flexibility and various measurements and ratios of body parts. It appears that static flexibility can be measured indirectly, with no undue interference by varying anthropometric measurements.

METHODS FOR IMPROVING RANGE OF MOTION

The question of which methods are most advantageous for improving range of motion has received very little attention. The conventional calisthenic exercises used for this purpose have usually involved bobbing, bouncing, or jerky movements in which one body segment is put in movement by active contraction of a muscle group, and the momentum is then arrested by the antagonists at the end of the range of motion. Thus the antagonists are stretched by the dynamic movements of the agonists. Because momentum is involved, this may be called the *ballistic method.*

On the other hand, Rathbone has suggested the use of the methods of Hatha yoga for the improvement of muscle tone and flexibility (21, p. 242). These methods involve holding a static position (posture or *asana*) for a period of time, and locking the joints involved into a position, which places the muscles and connective tissues at their greatest possible length. The author will refer to this method as *static stretching*.

It has been shown that both slow and fast stretching are effective, and that there is no significant difference between them (14). Since the neurophysiology of the stretch reflexes suggests advantages in static stretching procedures, a study was undertaken in the author's laboratory to compare the ballistic and static methods (6). The difference in the two stretching methods is illustrated by figures 22.2 and 22.3. The ballistic exercises were taken—to a large extent—from Kiphuth's exercises for stretching swimmers (10). The static exercises were developed to best utilize the inverse myotatic reflex and were designed to parallel the ballistic exercises in the affected muscles and joints.

It was found that both methods resulted in significant gains in static flexibility (in seven thirty-minute training periods) in trunk flexion, trunk extension, and shoulder elevation; there was no significant difference between methods. We may therefore conclude that static stretching is just as effective as the conventional ballistic methods, but the former offers three distinct advantages: (1) there is less danger of exceeding the extensibility limits of the tissues involved; (2) energy requirements are lower; (3) although ballistic stretching is apt to cause muscular soreness, static stretching will not; in fact, the latter relieves soreness (see chapter fifteen).

It is also of interest that the changes brought about by stretching exercises persist for a considerable period of time (eight weeks or more) after stretching is discontinued (18).

Chapman has shown that dynamic as well as static flexibility can be significantly improved by exercise in old men as well as in the young (4). This finding would appear to have some importance in gerontology since declining joint mobility creates many problems for the elderly.

WEIGHT TRAINING AND FLEXIBILITY

Many investigators have shown that weight training has no harmful effects upon either speed or range of movement when properly pursued; but an interesting study by Massey and Chaudet (15), which supports these findings, indicates the need for capable guidance. In an experiment designed to evaluate the effects of weight training on range of movement they found no appreciable effects in general, but they did find a significant decrease in ability to hyperextend the arms at the shoulder joint, a movement for which no exercise had been included. It is very probable that inclusion of an exercise for hyperextension would have prevented this decrease in mobility.

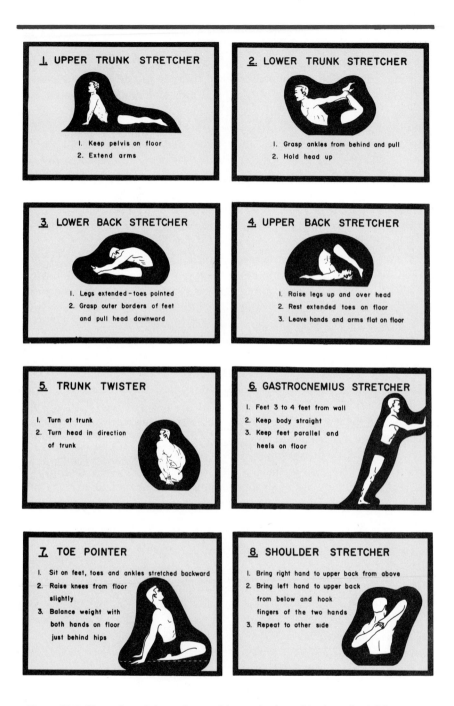

Figure 22-2. Illustration of the static stretching methods used in the author's laboratory.

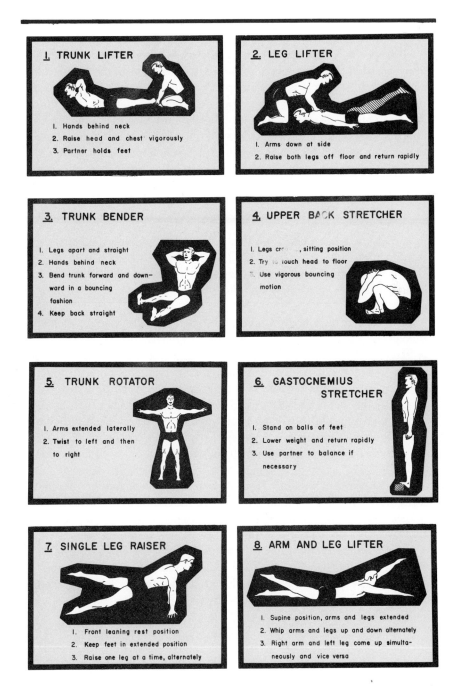

Figure 22-3. Illustration of the "ballistic stretching" exercises against which the static stretching method was compared experimentally.

It is well to recognize the fact that very heavy resistance exercise can, under certain circumstances, result in a restriction of range of motion. This factor, however, is not inherent in weight training, and it can be prevented by inclusion of the proper exercises and performance throughout the full range of motion. As Massey and Chaudet pointed out, it appears that weight lifting increases range of movement in the joints that are exercised but may result in a restriction in the areas not exercised. Therefore, a well-rounded workout is indicated when heavy resistance methods are used.

FACTORS AFFECTING FLEXIBILITY

Activity. It has been found that active individuals tend to be more flexible than inactive individuals (18). This is in accord with the well-known fact that connective tissues tend to shorten when they are maintained in a shortened position (as when a broken limb is placed in a plaster cast).

Sex. The results of two investigations agree that among elementary school age children girls are superior to boys in flexibility (11, 19). It is likely that this difference exists at all ages and throughout adult life.

Age. The results of many tests indicate that elementary school age children become less flexible as they grow older, reaching a low point in flexibility between ten and twelve years of age (3, 11, 19). From this age upward, flexibility seems to improve toward young adulthood, but it never again achieves the levels of early childhood. Dynamic flexibility apparently grows steadily poorer, from childhood on, with increasing age (25).

Temperature. Dynamic flexibility is improved twenty percent by local warming of a joint to 113° F, and it is decreased ten to twenty percent by cooling to 65° F (23). Experience indicates that static flexibility is probably similarly affected by temperature changes.

Ischemia. Dynamic flexibility is markedly reduced by arterial occlusion for twenty-five minutes (25). The physiology underlying this phenomenon has not been elucidated, but would appear to have important implications for the study of joint diseases.

SUMMARY

1. Two types of flexibility should be recognized: (1) *static flexibility*, a measure of range of motion, and (2) *dynamic flexibility*, a measure of the resistance to motion offered by a joint. (The following principles apply to static flexibility only because dynamic flexibility has not yet received the attention of physical educators.)

2. Flexibility can be limited by bone structure or by the soft tissues. When it is limited by soft tissues, great improvements can be brought about by the proper stretching methods.
3. After improvements have been brought about, cessation of the exercise program is not immediately accompanied by regression of flexibility. The effects of a stretching program are relatively long-lasting (at least eight weeks).
4. Stretching by jerking, bobbing, or bouncing methods invokes the stretch reflexes, which actually oppose the desired stretching.
5. Stretching by static methods invokes the inverse myotatic reflex, which helps relax the muscles to be stretched.
6. Static stretching methods have been shown to be just as effective as the ballistic methods.
7. Static stretching is safer than ballistic methods because it does not impose sudden strains upon the tissues involved.
8. Ballistic stretching methods frequently cause severe soreness in muscles. Static stretching does not usually cause soreness; it may, indeed, relieve soreness when it has occurred.

REFERENCES

1. Banus, M. G., and Zetlin, A. M. 1938. The relation of isometric tension to length in skeletal muscle. *Journal of Cellular and Comparative Physiology* 12:403-20.
2. Broer, M. R., and Galles, N. R. G. 1958. Importance of relationship between various body measurements in performance of toe-touch test. *Research Quarterly* 29:253-63.
3. Buxton, D. 1957. Extension of the Kraus-Weber test. *Research Quarterly* 28:210-17.
4. Chapman, E. A.; deVries, H. A.; and Swezey, R. 1972. Joint stiffness: effects of exercise on young and old men. *Journal of Gerontology* 27:218-21.
5. Cureton, T. K. 1941. Flexibility as an aspect of physical fitness. *Research Quarterly* 12:381-90.
6. deVries, H. A. 1962. Evaluation of static stretching procedures for improvement of flexibility. *Research Quarterly* 33:222-29.
7. Harvey, V. P., and Scott, G. D. 1967. Reliability of a measure of forward flexibility and its relationship to physical dimensions of college women. *Research Quarterly* 38:28-33.
8. Hupperich, F. L., and Sigerseth, P. O. 1950. The specificity of flexibility in girls. *Research Quarterly* 21:25.
9. Johns, R. J., and Wright, V. 1962. Relative importance of various tissues in joint stiffness. *Journal of Applied Physiology* 17:824-28.
10. Kiphuth, R. J. H. 1942. *Swimming.* New York: A. G. Barnes & Co.

11. Kirchner, G., and Glines, D. 1957. Comparative analysis of Eugene, Oregon, elementary school children using the Kraus-Weber test of minimum muscular fitness. *Research Quarterly* 28:16-25.

12. Leighton, J. R. 1942. A simple objective and reliable measure of flexibility. *Research Quarterly* 13:205-16.

13. ———. 1955. An instrument and technic for the measurement of range of joint motion. *Archives of Physical Medicine and Rehabilitation* 36:571.

14. Logan, G., and Egstrom, G. H. 1961. The effects of slow and fast stretching on the sacrofemoral angle. *Journal of the Association for Physical and Mental Rehabilitation* 15:85-89.

15. Massey, B. H., and Chaudet, N. L. 1956. Effects of systematic heavy resistance exercise on range of joint movement in young male adults. *Research Quarterly* 27:41-51.

16. Mathews, D. K.; Shaw, V.; and Bohnen, M. 1957. Hip flexibility of college women as related to length of body segments. *Research Quarterly* 28:352-56.

17. Mathews, D. K.; Shaw, V.; and Woods, J. B. 1959. Hip flexibility of elementary school boys as related to body segments. *Research Quarterly* 30: 297-302.

18. McCue, B. F. 1953. Flexibility of college women. *Research Quarterly* 24:316.

19. Phillips, M. 1955. Analysis of results from the Kraus-Weber test of minimum muscular fitness in children. *Research Quarterly* 26:314-23.

20. Ramsey, R. W., and Street, S. 1940. The isometric length tension diagram of isolated skeletal muscle fibers of the frog. *Journal of Cellular and Comparative Physiology* 15:11.

21. Rathbone, J. L. 1959. *Corrective physical education*. Philadelphia: W. B. Saunders Co.

22. Walker, S. M. 1961. Delay of twitch relaxation induced by stress and stress relaxation. *Journal of Applied Physiology* 16:801-6.

23. Wear, C. L. 1963. Relationships of flexibility measurements to length of body segments. *Research Quarterly* 34:234-38.

24. Wells, K. F., and Dillon, E. K. 1952. Sit and reach, a test of back and leg flexibility. *Research Quarterly* 23:115-18.

25. Wright, V., and Johns, R. J. 1960. Physical factors concerned with the stiffness of normal and diseased joints. *Johns Hopkins Hospital Bulletin* 106:215-31.

23 Warming-up

Until relatively recently the value of warming-up had not been challenged. On the basis of theoretical concepts, warming-up was accepted by virtually all coaches and athletes; however, much scientific interest has lately been directed toward (1) its value in athletics, (2) elucidation of its physiological nature, and (3) comparisons of the effectiveness of various warm-up procedures.

Unfortunately, the various investigators have used differing methods, so that the type, intensity, and duration of the warm-ups have varied, as well as the physical activity whose level of performance was to be affected. Consequently, the work of the investigators can seldom be compared, and a welter of confusion has resulted. Some investigations have been equivocal, some poorly controlled, and still others have used so little warm-up activity (in terms of intensity and duration) that no conceivable physiological changes could have been brought about. On the other hand, because some of the experiments have been properly conducted and are quite definitive in certain respects, we will try to provide some principles upon which physical educators and coaches can guide their professional activities.

PRACTICE EFFECT VERSUS PHYSIOLOGICAL WARM-UP

A great source of confusion is the fact that the effects of practice in improving a skill are frequently confounded with the actual warming-up in which physiological changes are brought about. Unquestionably, if skill and accuracy are important factors in a physical activity, practice can bring about improvement in performance. The question considered in this chapter has to do with the physiological aspects of warming-up.

PHYSIOLOGY OF WARMING-UP

On theoretical grounds it might be expected that a warming-up that resulted in increased blood and muscle temperatures should improve performance through the following mechanisms: (1) increased speed of contraction and relaxation of muscles, (2) greater efficiency because of lowered viscous resistance in the muscles, (3) hemoglobin gives up more oxygen at higher temperatures and also dissociates much more rapidly, (4) myoglobin shows temperature effects similar to those of hemoglobin, (5) metabolic processes increase their rate with increasing temperature, and (6) decreased resistance of the vascular bed can be brought about by increased temperature.

General Versus Local Heating. Three well-controlled investigations agree in finding substantial and significant improvements in performance (one to eight percent) when the entire body is heated so that rectal and muscle temperatures are increased (1, 4, 15). This heating can be accomplished actively by vigorous exercise of various kinds, or passively by hot baths, showers, Turkish baths, or diathermy. However, the local heating of only the involved limb has been shown to result in earlier fatigue and lessened work output in that limb (5, 9). It has also been shown that in local heating the factor of major importance is probably the distribution of blood between the skin and the underlying muscles if both are served by the same large artery (16, 17).

It seems likely, then, that the explanation for the different effects of local and general heating lies in the fact that in local heating a large vasodilatation effect is possible in the skin to the detriment of circulation through the underlying muscle. This could well result in the magnitude of decreased performance actually observed. On the other hand, general heating of the entire body must exert some, or all, of the beneficial effects enumerated above—while the vasodilatation effect on the skin cannot be nearly so large, and may not occur to any great extent when a large proportion of the musculature is active.

There seems little doubt, on the basis of all the available evidence, that general heating of the body that results in increased core (rectal) and muscle temperatures improves performance.

Rectal Versus Muscle Temperature. Figure 23.1 illustrates the changes in muscle and rectal temperature that occur as the result of warming-up

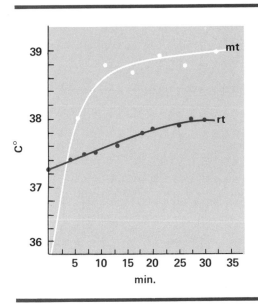

Figure 23-1. Temperature measured in lateral vastus muscle (mt) and in rectum (rt) during a work of 660 kgm/min. (From Asmussen and Boje. *Acta Physiologica Scandinavica* 10:1, 1945.)

by riding the bicycle ergometer at a moderate load. It can be seen that the greatest part of the increase in muscle temperature occurs in the first five minutes, and rectal temperature increases more gradually and steadily for thirty minutes.

Figure 23.2 shows the same temperature data and relates the two temperatures to performance time for a sprint on the bicycle ergometer. On the basis of the fact that performance has shown its greatest improvement during the time that muscle temperature has increased markedly and rectal temperature has increased very little. Asmussen and Boje (1) consider muscle temperature to be the more important factor. This contention has been supported by Carlile (4), who found no positive relationships between rectal temperature and swimming times.

On the other hand, it has been shown that if a subject is warmed-up in such a fashion as to raise rectal temperature, and his muscle tem-

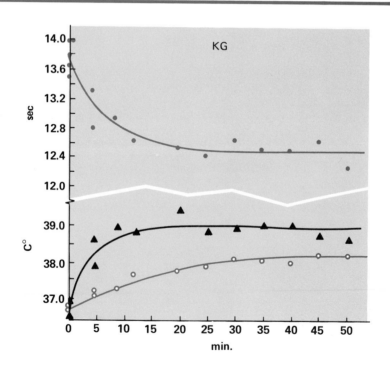

Figure 23-2. Effect of the *duration* of warm-up on performance time: ●————● is performance time for sprint, △————△ is muscle temperature, ○————○ is rectal temperature. (From Asmussen and Boje. *Acta Physiologica Scandinavica* 10:1, 1945.)

perature is allowed to return to normal while rectal temperature is still elevated (rectal temperature returns to normal much more slowly), performance is still somewhat improved over control conditions (15). Thus we must say that muscle and blood temperatures are important, but which is the more important cannot yet be answered conclusively.

O₂ Consumption and Warm-up. It has been shown that maximal oxygen uptake is slighty higher after warming-up, compared with cold conditions, but that the O_2 necessary for a given amount of work is reduced (1, 25). This would seem to indicate efficiency is improved as a result of warming-up.

The author has attempted to separate the effects of temperature from those of increased mobility (flexibility) in warming-up for 100-yard dashes. When flexibility was improved by static stretching, so as to eliminate the temperature and circulatory factors, no improvement in efficiency could be demonstrated (7). Thus it seems that the improvement in efficiency is probably temperature-related.

Blood Flow through the Lungs. An investigation of the effects of exercise on pulmonary blood flow showed that a period of moderate exercise, such as might be used for warming-up, results in a decrease of total pulmonary resistance of about thirteen percent (28). This decrease was highly significant. The reduced resistance to blood flow and its concomitant improvement of lung circulation could make an important contribution to the warm-up phenomenon.

VARIOUS TYPES OF WARM-UP

Passive Versus Active. In regard to whole-body warm-up and large-muscle activity, there seems little doubt that any procedure that increases rectal and muscle temperatures will improve subsequent athletic performance. This warm-up effect has been demonstrated for active warm-up brought about by such diverse activities as running, bicycle riding, bench-stepping, or calisthenics. Passive heating by hot baths, hot showers, Turkish baths, or diathermy has also been found effective.

Related and Unrelated Methods. *Related warm-up* is any procedure that involves the athletic activity itself, or something close to it; *unrelated warm-up* is any procedure designed to bring about the desired physiological changes without involving the actual movement itself. Investigations in this area are somewhat inconclusive, but it can be assumed on the basis of common sense that if the desired physiological changes can be achieved by use of related warm-up procedures, these would be preferable in that a practice effect would also be gained. In many athletic events, however, the activity is not well suited to warming-up (jumping, etc.), or it is too fatiguing.

Intensity and Duration of Warm-up.   Burke (3) has demonstrated that optimal combinations of intensity and duration are needed to bring about the desired warm-up effect. Too little work does not achieve optimal levels of temperature, etc., and too much warm-up can result in impaired performance due to fatigue. The interaction of the effects of warm-up and fatigue in untrained young girls is shown clearly in the work of Richards in figure 23.3. The girls warmed up with varying duraitons (one to six minutes) of bench-stepping prior to a vertical jump test. It can be seen that the warm-up effect is greater than the fatigue effect when the warm-up is carried out for one to three minutes. Longer warm-up results in more loss to fatigue than is gained in warm-up benefit (21). However, figure 23.4 shows that in a *well-conditioned* athlete a very heavy load can be used for as long as thirty minutes, with ever-increasing muscle temperature and constantly improving performance. It should be pointed out that for the average schoolboy or a poorly conditioned athlete a thirty-minute warm-up with an intensity of 1,600 kilogram-meters per minute (fig. 23.4) would result in complete exhaustion.

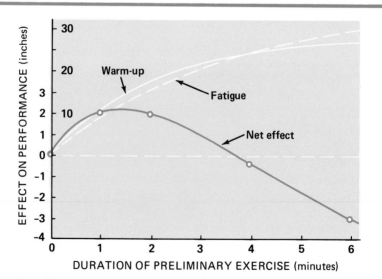

Figure 23-3. Effect of *length* of preliminary exercise on jumping performance. The inner numbers refer to the magnitude of the exponential factors. (From Richards, D.K. *Research Quarterly* 39:668, 1968.)

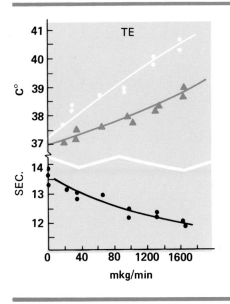

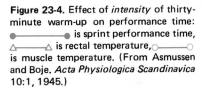

Figure 23-4. Effect of *intensity* of thirty-minute warm-up on performance time: ●————● is sprint performance time, △————△ is rectal temperature,○————○ is muscle temperature. (From Asmussen and Boje. *Acta Physiologica Scandinavica* 10:1, 1945.)

Obviously, the intensity and duration of warm-up must be adjusted to the individual athlete. As a rule of thumb, one may look for signs of development of heat from within, and in normal environment this is indicated by perspiration. For those who wish to be more scientific, an increase in rectal temperature of 1 or 2° F appears desirable.

Overload Warm-up. Common practice in baseball is to swing two or three bats in preparation for a turn at bat. Although this is more a practice effect than a true warm-up, it has interesting implications in a practical and in a scientifc sense. It has been shown that throwing an eleven-ounce baseball for a warm-up results in significantly improved velocity in subsequent tests with a ball of regulation weight (27). The neurophysiology of this phenomenon has not yet been elucidated, and it is also possible that psychological effects are important.

EFFECT OF WARM-UP ON VARIOUS ATHLETIC ACTIVITIES

Speed. Various investigators have shown various types of warm-up to be effective in improving the speed of running (2, 25), cycling (1), and arm speed (20). Other investigators, however, have found no improvement from various warm-up procedures in these activities (3, 10, 11, 12). This conflicting evidence leaves the picture rather unclear. Unfortunately, none of the investigators who found no improvement had measured muscle or rectal temperature; so we cannot be sure that a true physiological warm-up had occurred.

On the other hand, the only study that attempted psychological control over the subjects found no improvement; and it is possible that the improvements the other investigators found were caused by psychological factors. Final conclusions must await further research.

Strength. An interesting picture emerges in respect to strength. The two investigators who used whole-body warm-up found significant increases in strength after warm-up (1, 3), while the three investigators who applied only local heat found no improvement after warm-up (5, 9, 24). It is therefore tempting to hypothesize that strength changes depend upon central nervous system changes that are brought about by temperature change, or circulatory change, or both.

On the basis of this evidence, plus evidence related to jumping and swimming, it seems that strength can be improved by a general body warm-up; but the explanation of the underlying physiology awaits further investigation.

Muscular Endurance. Asmussen and Boje (1), using whole-body heating, found that increased muscle temperature brought about improvement in times for riding a stationary bicycle. The work load of 9,860 kilogram-meters would take about five minutes, and it must therefore be considered to have an element of muscular endurance.

All other investigators have used only local-muscle warm-up. Their results agree that increasing the local-muscle temperature by warming-up, either actively or passively, results in no improvement (23, 24) or in a decrement in endurance (5, 9, 16, 17).

There is also good agreement on the finding that local cooling that reduces skin temperature results in better endurance for the underlying muscle groups (5, 9, 16, 17). The rationale for this improvement was discussed earlier in this chapter.

Circulorespiratory Endurance. Grodjinovsky and Magel (8) found that only a vigorous warm-up consisting of five minutes of jogging, eight calisthenic exercises plus a tenth mile sprint improved time in the one mile run. Warm-up without the sprint had no significant effect.

Power. One of the best measures of human power is the vertical jump, and complete agreement exists among the four investigations on warming-up for jumping (13, 18, 19, 21). Significant improvements, ranging from 2.6 to 20.0 percent, were found to result from the following warm-ups: massage, running in place, isometric stretching, deep knee bends and stool-stepping. These findings moreover, could be predicted on the basis of the strength findings, for power is really the expression of strength (force) per unit of time.

Throwing. Because throwing can be considered to have a strength factor (dynamic strength), this activity would also be expected to show improvement as the result of warming-up, and the three investigations in this area support this contention. Improvement was shown to result from overload warm-up (27), related warm-up (14, 22) and unrelated warm-up (14).

Swimming. All of the investigations in this area show that swimming times can be improved by warming-up. Hot showers of eight minutes' duration resulted in about 1.0 percent improvement in forty-yard times and 1.5 percent improvement in 220-yard times (4). Hot baths of from fifteen to eighteen minutes improved performance in the 400-meter free style and the 200-meter breast stroke by 2.1 to 3.9 percent, and in the 50-meter free style by as much as 2.0 percent (15).

Jogging and bicycle ergometer work improved subsequent swim times by 0.6 to 2.2 percent (15). Short wave diathermy improved swimming times by 1.3 to 1.9 percent, and cold baths caused decreased performances by 3.6 to 6.3 percent (15). One investigator found improvement from a related warm-up (swimming) but not from an unrelated warm-up (26).

The author has attempted to compare the values of various commonly used warm-up procedures for highly skilled varsity university swimmers for 100-yard times in their specialty strokes. It was found that a 500-yard swim was the only warm-up that brought about significant improvement for the group as a whole (1.0 percent). It was also found that calisthenic warm-ups produced the best improvement (2.0 percent) for the butterfly and breast stroke men and that it impaired the performance of the free stylers and backstrokers (6). This phenomenon would seem to point up the need for *individualizing* warm-up procedures.

DURATION OF THE WARM-UP EFFECT

In some athletic events it is not possible to warm-up after the program has begun—swimming meets in which there is only one pool. A very practical question, then, is how long a warm-up effect persists. This question cannot be answered for the practice effect, but for temperature changes in muscle tissue it has been shown that this effect persists for forty-five to eighty minutes (15, 16).

WARM-UP AND PREVENTION OF MUSCLE INJURY

Although there is much uncertainty about the value of warm-up in improving performance, warming-up has been retained as standard practice on the grounds that if it has no other value it might nevertheless prevent injury to muscles; however, there is no evidence to support this contention. The lack of evidence is understandable: no investigator would intentionally subject his subjects to experiments designed to bring about injury.

Quite unintentionally, objective evidence has become available in the author's laboratory. In an unrelated study, four college-age male subjects ran 100-yard dashes (against time) to measure metabolic efficiency (7). When the subjects ran without warming-up (control procedure), two of them developed muscular soreness that might have become severe in the absence of appropriate preventive measures. Thus it seems that muscle injury is indeed a real possibility when vigorous exercise is not preceded by proper warming-up to bring about increased body temperatures.

SUMMARY

Although all the results are not yet in for the warming-up phenomenon, an intelligent coach and athlete uses the best available evidence to govern his activities, and the best available evidence justifies the following principles for warming-up.

1. Whole-body warm-up that raises muscle and blood (rectal) temperatures can significantly improve athletic performance.
2. Wherever possible, a *related warm-up* (which raises muscle and blood temperatures) is preferable so that a practice effect may be simultaneously achieved.
3. Warming-up is important for preventing muscle soreness or injury.
4. Warming-up procedures must be suited to the individual.
5. Warming-up procedures must be suited to the athletic event.
6. A combination of intensity and duration of warm-up must be achieved that results in temperature increases in the deep tissues without undue fatigue. Sweating is an indication of increased internal temperature. For high-level competitive performances, the additional effort of taking the rectal temperature appears worthwhile; an increase of 1 or 2° F is desirable.
7. If active, related warm-up is impossible, passive heating can be used effectively.
8. Warming-up appears to be most important (makes the greatest contribution) in activities that directly involve strength, and indirectly in events that have a large element of power or acceleration of body weight.

9. Overload warm-up may be valuable for events in which neuromuscular coordination patterns are of major importance.
10. Tissue temperature changes brought about by warming-up probably persist for forty-five to eighty minutes.

REFERENCES

1. Asmussen, E., and Boje, O. 1945. Body temperature and capacity for work. *Acta Physiologica Scandinavica* 10:1-22.
2. Blank, L. B. 1955. Effects of warm-up on speed. *Athletic Journal* 10:45-46.
3. Burke, R. K. 1957. Relationships between physical performance and warm-up procedures of varying intensity and duration. Doctoral dissertation, USC.
4. Carlile, F. 1956. Effect of preliminary passive warming-up on swimming performance. *Research Quarterly* 27:143-51.
5. Clarke, R. S. J.; Hellon, R. F.; and Lind, A. R. 1958. The duration of sustained contractions of the human forearm at different muscle temperatures. *Journal of Physiology* 143:454-73.
6. deVries, H. A. 1959. Effects of various warm-up procedures on 100-yard times of competitive swimmers. *Research Quarterly* 30:11-20.
7. ———. 1963. The looseness factor in speed and O_2 Consumption of an anaerobic 100-yard dash. *Research Quarterly* 34:305-13.
8. Grodjinovsky, A., and Magel, J. R. 1970. Effect of warm-up on running performance. *Research Quarterly* 41:116-19.
9. Grose, J. E. 1958. Depression of muscle fatigue curves by heat and cold. *Research Quarterly* 29:19-31.
10. Hipple, J. 1955. Warm-up and fatigue in junior high school sprints. *Research Quarterly* 26:246-47.
11. Lotter, W. S. 1959. Effects of fatigue and warm-up on speed of arm movements. *Research Quarterly* 30:57-65.
12. Massey, B.; Johnson, W. R.; and Kramer, G. F. 1961. Effect of warm-up exercise upon muscular performance using hypnosis to control the psychological variable. *Research Quarterly* 32:63-71.
13. Merlino, L. 1959. Influence of massage on jumping performance. *Research Quarterly* 30:66-74.
14. Michael, E.; Skubic, V.; and Rochelle, R. 1957. Effect of warm-up on softball throw for distance. *Research Quarterly* 28:357-63.
15. Muido, L. 1946. The influence of body temperature on performances in swimming. *Acta Physiologica Scandinavica* 12:102-9.
16. Nukada, A. 1955. Hauttemperatur und Leistungsfahigkeit in Extremitaten bei Statischer Haltearbeit. *Arbeitsphysiologie* 16:74-80.
17. Nukada, A., and Muller, E. A. 1955. Hauttemperatur und Leistungsfahigkeit in Extremitaten bei Dynamischer Arbeit. *Arbeitsphysiologie* 16:61-73.

18. Pacheco, B. A. 1957. Improvement in jumping performance due to preliminary exercise. *Research Quarterly* 28:55-63.
19. ———. 1959. Effectiveness of warm-up on exercise in junior high school girls. *Research Quarterly* 30:202-13.
20. Phillips, W. H. 1963. Influence of fatiguing warm-up exercises on speed of movement and reaction latency. *Research Quarterly* 34:370-78.
21. Richards, D. K. 1968. A two factor theory of the warm-up effect in jumping performance. *Research Quarterly* 39:668-73.
22. Rochelle, R. H.; Skubic, V.; and Michael, E. 1960. Performance as affected by incentive and preliminary warm-up. *Research Quarterly* 31:499-504.
23. Sedgewick, A. W. 1964. Effect of actively increased muscle temperature on local muscular endurance. *Research Quarterly* 35:532-38.
24. Sedgewick, A. W., and Whalen, H. R. 1964. Effect of passive warm-up on muscular strength and endurance. *Research Quarterly* 35:45-59.
25. Simonson, E.; Teslenko, N.; and Gorkin, M. 1936. Einfluss von Vorubungen auf die Leistung beim 100 m. Lauf. *Arbeitsphysiologie* 9:152-65.
26. Thompson, H. 1958. Effect of warm-up upon physical performance in selected activities. *Research Quarterly* 29:231-46.
27. Van Huss, W. D.; Albrecht, L.; Nelson, R.; and Hagerman, R. 1962. Effect of overload warm-up on the velocity and accuracy of throwing. *Research Quarterly* 33:472-75.
28. Widimsky, J.; Berglund, E.; and Malmberg, R. 1963. Effect of repeated exercise on the lesser circulation. *Journal of Applied Physiology* 18:983-86.

24 Nutrition for Athletes

Dietary Considerations and Requirements (Long-term)
Suggested Training Rules for Good Nutrition
Principles Involved in Pre-game Nutrition
Pre-game Procedure

In recent years, with ever-improving levels of competition, athletes and coaches have developed considerable interest in nutrition, but this, unfortunately, is an area in which the scientific efforts of trained nutritionists (and biochemists, who are the experts in this field) have often been obscured by clouds of misinformation generated by faddists and self-proclaimed experts.

Furthermore, athletes seem to be too easily influnced by the success of other athletes whose training regimen may have included such dietary fads as royal honey, kelp, blackstrap molasses, or other substance thought to have "miraculous" properties for improving athletic performance. More often than not, when these potions are tested by scientific methods in controlled experiments, it turns out that an athlete's success was achieved in spite of—not because of—his unusual dietary modifications.

Let it be clearly stated from the outset: *There is no scientific evidence at the present time to indicate that athletic performance can be improved by modifying a basically sound diet.* Furthermore, there are many different ways in which a nutritious diet can be obtained, and the best diet for one athlete will seldom be the best diet for all athletes. Individual differences exist in our senses of taste as well as in our enzyme systems, which are so necessary for digestion and absorption. In other words, "one man's meat may be another man's poison."

It should also be recognized, in the total scheme of things, that for explosive or short-duration events skill is the all-important factor. Even in endurance events, where the total energy supply and the rate of energy supply are very important, the role of conditioning is infinitely more important than diet (if a diet is nutritionally sound). Still, in all athletic events psychological as well as physiological factors affect performance, and there is no way to evaluate the psychological importance of eating steak when less expensive protein foods are just as nutritious. When ego and prestige factors enter the picture, science may fade into the background.

Although we may not be able to modify a sound diet to improve performance, an athlete can go downhill very rapidly if his diet is less than optimum. Thus diet is still a very important consideration.

DIETARY CONSIDERATIONS AND REQUIREMENTS (LONG-TERM)

Caloric Intake. Because this factor was discussed in chapter twelve, it is enough at this point to say that an athlete must consume enough food daily to meet the energy demands of his training program. If he eats less than this, he will burn his body tissues to make up the deficit, and will approach "staleness" more rapidly. If he consumes more food than he needs, the result will be an increase in body weight with its accompanying mechanical disadvantages.

Proportion of Foodstuffs Ingested (Long-term Diet). There are many opinions of what constitutes the proper proportion of carbohydrate, fat, and protein in human diet. None of the opinions, however, is supported by acceptable experimental evidence. In lieu of such evidence, we must apply theory and common sense.

As for theory, it is well known that in steady-state exercise the respiratory quotient goes up gradually from an average resting value of 0.85 to something like 0.90 or 0.95. This is interpreted as meaning that the organism prefers to burn carbohydrate for energy purposes during muscular activity, although it is also capable of utilizing fat. Furthermore, although fat produces more than twice as much energy per gram as carbohydrate, it requires more oxygen for each calorie (213 milliliters per calorie of fat compared with 198 milliliters per calorie of carbohydrate). In any athletic event where the work of the respiratory muscles is an important factor, there would seem to be an advantage of some 7.5 percent in favor of carbohydrate. In this regard, increased overall muscular efficiency of up to ten percent has been shown experimentally for high carbohydrate diets (11). It has also been experimentally shown that fatigue occurs earlier on high fat diets (8).

The end products of protein metabolism are excreted in the urine, and by measuring the urinary nitrogen an estimate of protein metabolism can be made. Because urinary nitrogen increases very little with exercise under normal conditions, it is not considered an important source of energy. Only under conditions of starvation, when the carbohydrate and fat stores have been completely utilized, is the protein of body tissue consumed for energy. Protein is needed mainly for building new body tissue. Thus for growing children, and for athletes whose training is severe enough to result in increased muscle mass, the demands for protein are increased. This is not true of course, for mature endurance athletes.

On the basis of these theoretical considerations, the proportions shown in table 24.1 seem to be sensible when the energy expenditure is not excessive—up to 3,000 kilocalories daily (5, p. 776).

If energy requirements rise to very high values, where muscle mass is also likely to increase, it would seem reasonable to increase the percentage of protein to as much as twenty percent with a proportional decrease in the fat consumed. In this regard it is interesting to note that Abrahams (1) reports that Schenk, who studied the diet of 4,700 competitors at the 1936 Olympic games, found an average daily consumption of over 7,000 kilocalories (see table 24.2).

TABLE 24.1

Suggested Proportion of Basic Foodstuffs

	Grams	Kcal	Percentage of Total Kcal
Carbohydrate	380	1,440	48
Fat	133	1,200	40
Protein	70	360	12

TABLE 24.2

Proportion of Basic Foodstuffs in Diet of 4,700 Olympic Athletes

	Grams	Kcal	Percentage of Total Kcal
Carbohydrate	800	3,280	46
Fat	270	2,510	35
Protein	320	1,320	19

Importance of Glycogen Storage in Preparation for Endurance Type Competition. The theoretical basis for the importance of glycogen storage in endurance type exercise was laid in chapter two. When work loads greater than about seventy percent of aerobic capacity must be born for thirty to sixty minutes or more the *rate* of work is limited by aerobic capacity but the *duration* over which the load can be maintained depends very largely on the level of glycogen storage in the involved muscles since the muscle cell apparently cannot use other energy substrates to any great extent at these high levels of work. When glycogen depletion occurs work can be continued on other energy substrates but only at work loads considerably below seventy percent.

Karlsson and Saltin (10) demonstrated this effect quite clearly when they had ten subjects run the same 30 Km race twice, three weeks apart, once after a carbohydrate enriched diet and once after a mixed diet. They found the muscle glycogen level in the quadriceps to be doubled after the high carbohydrate diet compared to the mixed diet and every subject turned in his best performance after the high carbohydrate diet.

Interestingly, identical pace was maintained after both diets in the early part of the race when glycogen content was high, but pace fell off earlier after the mixed diet as glycogen depots were emptied.

The work of the original investigators in this area, Bergstrom et al. (4) also provides clear cut data for modifying the diet to best prepare for prolonged endurance type events. To achieve the highest possible level of muscle glycogen for such events, the athlete must work the same muscles to exhaustion about one week prior to the event. For the next three days, the diet should be almost exclusively fat and protein since it was shown that low carbohydrate diet followed by high carbohydrate diet results in the greatest possible glycogen storage. About three days should now be left for a carbohydrate rich diet with only very light workouts to result in the maximum possible glycogen storage in the muscles. The low carbohydrate diet consisted of 1,500 Kcal protein and 1,300 Kcal fat for a total daily energy expenditure estimated at 2,800 Kcal. The high carbohydrate diet made up the same total with 2,300 Kcal of carbohydrate and 500 Kcal of protein (4).

Long-term data on such diet modifications are not available and it is questionable if such procedures would be wise to follow where weekly endurance competitions are held since high protein-high fat diets may have adverse long-term effects due to their lowering pH and slowing gastrointestinal tract emptying. It would seem that the best course would be that of following a basically well-balanced diet throughout most of the competitive season, reserving this modification for the one or two most important competitions of the season. In any event, the exhaustion of the involved musculature early in the week followed by relatively high carbohydrate diet and relatively lighter workouts is sound procedure.

Quality of Protein. We have so far concerned ourselves only with the total quantity and with the proportions of the basic foodstuffs within that total. In regard to protein, the quality is also very important. All proteins break down to amino acids during the digestive processes, so that these may be considered the units or building blocks for the synthesis of the proteins found in the human body. Of the twenty-three amino acids normally present in animal protein, only thirteen can be synthesized in the cells. The other ten must be supplied in the diet, and they are therefore called *essential amino acids*.

Supplying the essential amino acids is no problem for those who eat meat and animal products. The use of complete proteins (those that include all the essential amino acids), from milk and eggs and a generous and varied use of meat, solves the problem quite easily. For those who for religious or other reasons do not eat animal products, the problem is more complicated, but vegetarians can be well-nourished if they include all the essential amino acids in their diet. This can be done by including a diversity of vegetable products in their diet: leaves, seeds, roots, and fruits (14, p. 41).

Vitamins. The need for vitamins in the human diet is well established and needs no comment here, but a question of recurring interest is whether an athlete needs vitamin supplementation of his normal diet. It was at one time thought that the requirements for vitamins increased much more rapidly than the increase in metabolism due to exercise, but recent work (6) indicates that vitamin needs increase only in approximate proportion to metabolic activity. Thus ingestion of larger amounts of food as daily workout levels increase automatically provides the needed increase in vitamins (if the diet is sound to begin with).

Some investigators have claimed that vitamin supplementation has improved athletic performance in their subjects. However, when the proper controls are instituted, assuring that subjects were on an adequate diet *before starting the experiment,* these improvements in performance can no longer be demonstrated. Thus in all likelihood the reported improvements in performance because of vitamin supplementation were the result of having improved previously inadequate diets.

One point should be made before we leave this subject. Trace quantities of mineral elements seem to be intimately connected with the body's proper use of certain vitamins (6, p. 628). Furthermore, it seems likely that several unknown factors affect nutrition. For these reasons, common sense dictates that, wherever possible, vitamins should be obtained from their natural sources rather than from purified, synthetic sources.

Minerals. Table 24.3 shows the suggested minimum daily requirements for mineral constituents (5, 14). As with vitamins, there is no evidence that the need for minerals is increased in exercise (in comfortable climates) beyond the increase brought about by the increased daily food consumption needed for metabolic demands.

SUGGESTED TRAINING RULES FOR GOOD NUTRITION

It is obviously impossible, as well as undesirable, to belabor athletes with the specifics of diet; it is also unnecessary because a relatively simple set of rules will result in good nutrition without making a dietitian (and possibly a hypochondriac) of each athlete. The author has found the following set of rules to be workable and effective, not only for good athletic conditioning but also for forming sound, life-long dietary habits.

TABLE 24.3

Suggested Minimum Daily Requirements of
Mineral Constituents in the Diet

Element	Amount	Source
Calcium	1.0 gr	Milk and other dairy products
Phosphorus (PO₄)	1.5 gr	Most proteins
Iron	15.0 mg	Eggs, meat, certain nuts, vegetables
Sodium (Na Cl)	10.0 gr	Cereals, fruits, vegetables, table salt
Potassium	1.0 gr	Cereals, fruits, vegetables, table salt
Magnesium	250.0 mg	Cereals, fruits, vegetables, table salt
Iodine	0.1 mg	Seafoods and iodized salt
Cobalt	0.1 mg	If diet is otherwise adequate,
Copper	2.0 mg	these trace elements will
Manganese	5.0 mg	probably be supplied.
Zinc	10.0 mg	

1. Distribute the daily consumption of food over three regularly spaced meals. If weight gain (or prevention of weight loss) is desirable, an evening snack can be added.
2. Eliminate from the diet (as much as possible) the foods that furnish only calories without contributing their share of vitamins and minerals (candy, cake, carbonated beverages, etc.). Use fruit and fruit juices for desserts and snacks.
3. Eliminate tea, coffee, and alcohol. Not only do these drinks usurp the place of more nutritious food, they may cause undesirable pharmacological effects (such as decreased muscular efficiency).
4. Avoid fatty foods; they slow peristalsis and therefore gastic emptying.
5. Eat two servings daily of fresh fruit (one to be citrus fruit or tomatoes).
6. Eat four servings daily of vegetables, including leafy green vegetables (salads) and roots and tubers (turnips, beets, potatoes, etc.).
7. Eat at least three slices of whole-grain bread daily.
8. Eat enough butter (or fortified margarine) to supplement the bread in item seven.
9. Drink at least three glasses of milk daily.

A study of twenty-eight athletes (7) from varsity teams of three "Big Ten" universities showed that only ten of the athletes followed sound diets. The foods most commonly omitted were the green and yellow vegetables, citrus fruits, eggs and milk. This indicated that their diets were probably low in vitamins A and C and in calcium. If these dietary habits can be accepted as typical of American athletes, then coaches would be well advised to provide vitamin supplementation for their athletes in the form of a multiple vitamin and mineral pill in spite of the earlier discussion to the effect that athletes (on a well-balanced diet) do not require vitamin or mineral supplementation because of the heavy workouts.

In situations that involve mature athletes, a coach may have to compromise his principles if firmly held dietary beliefs are in evidence. But, individual differences being what they are, it is conceivable that some individuals will thrive on diets that would be totally unsatisfactory for most athletes. Furthermore, it is all-important to maintain harmonious relationships and undisturbed psychological equilibrium for successful athletic efforts.

PRINCIPLES INVOLVED IN PRE-GAME NUTRITION

The digestive functions of the stomach can be divided into two components: secretory and motor functions. The secretory function consists of the elaboration and discharge into the stomach of hydrochloric acid, digestive enzymes, and alkaline mucus. The motor function consists of the maintenance of a degree of tonus plus the peristaltic contractions found during digestive processes. In some individuals there are, in addition, muscular contractions related to hunger pangs. Any factor which interferes with either secretory or motor function may of course cause nausea in the athlete.

The most definitive work on the effects of exercise on these functions of the stomach (in the human) has been provided by Hellebrandt and co-workers (9). For the secretory cycle it was found that severe exercise results in inhibition of the secretory response, and that the resulting hypoacidity lasted as long as one hour. In mild activity, the acidity (secretory activity) was either unchanged or only slightly increased.

In respect to stomach motility, they found that mild exercise during the digestion of a meal seemed advantageous in hastening the final emptying time. Violent or exhaustive exercise, however, was found to inhibit gastric peristalsis, although this inhibition was followed (after exercise was ended) by augmented activity that resulted in little alteration of the final emptying time of the stomach.

Some evidence for a psychic effect was provided in their series of experiments in that repetition generally decreased a subject's response to the same exercise stressor.

Experimental evidence for the effects of exercise on the other portions of the digestive tract is lacking, inconclusive, or has been performed only on animals under conditions that do not justify extrapolation of the conclusions to humans.

The objectives to be attained in the twenty-four to forty-eight-hour period preceding competition are as follows.

1. Attaining the largest possible storage of carbohydrate in the liver and musculature.
2. Entering competition with the smallest possible stomach volume, so that the diaphragm may descend as far as possible in inhalation.
3. Preventing gastric disturbances from occurring during a competition.
4. Maintaining an optimum psychological attitude in the athlete while accomplishing the first three items.

PRE-GAME PROCEDURE

Liver and muscle glycogen can be increased by the methods discussed above.

Breakfast on the day of competition may be relatively larger if the event is scheduled for the afternoon, and breakfast and lunch may be larger if the event is in the evening.

In any event the pre-event meal should be light, and the two meals that immediately precede competition should be high-carbohydrate meals: cereals such as oatmeal, toast with jam, honey, etc.

The final pre-event meal has usually preceded competition by three or four hours, but there is evidence that if it consists of cereal and milk of no more than 500 kilocalories, no adverse effects are suffered if it is taken up to thirty minutes before competition (2, 3, 12, 13).

The Pre-game Meal. Theory and common sense dictate that the following precautions be observed for the pre-game meal.

1. Avoid foods that are even mildly distasteful to an individual athlete— no matter how well they may serve nutritional objectives. An athlete may get sick even though the food is excellent.
2. Avoid irritating foods, such as highly spiced foods and roughage.
3. Avoid gas-forming foods: onions, cabbage, apples, baked beans, etc.
4. Avoid fatty foods; they slow peristalsis and therefore gastric emptying.

5. Hold protein foods to a minimum because their metabolism results in fixed acids; in large quantities, this could result in an undesirable acidosis.

6. Fluid can best be supplied by boullion (which supplies sodium, which is excreted in perspiration during an event). Many athletes will prefer milk or juices, and if experience shows no ill effects it is probably wise to accede to this preference.

REFERENCES

1. Abrahams, A. 1948. The nutrition of athletes. *British Journal of Nutrition* 2:266-69.

2. Asprey, G. M.; Alley, L. E.; and Tuttle, W. W. 1963. Effect of eating at various times on subsequent performances in the 440-yard dash and half-mile run. *Research Quarterly* 34:267-70.

3. ———. 1964. Effect of eating at various times upon subsequent performance in the one-mile run. *Research Quarterly* 35:227-30.

4. Bergestrom, J.; Hermansen, L.; Hultman, E.; and Saltin, B. 1967. Diet, muscle glycogen and physical performance. *Acta Physiologica Scandinavica* 71:140-50.

5. Best, C. H., and Taylor, N. B. 1955. *The physiological basis of medical practice*. Baltimore: Williams & Wilkins Co.

6. Bicknell, F., and Prescott, F. 1953. *The vitamins in medicine*. New York: Grune & Stratton.

7. Bobb, A.; Pringle, D.; and Ryan, A. J. 1969. A brief study of the diet of athletes. *Journal of Sports Medicine* 9:255-62.

8. Christensen, E. H. 1931. Beitrage zur Physiologie Schwerer Korperlicher Arbeit I-IX. *Arbeitsphysiologie* 4:453-503.

9. Hellebrandt, F. A., and Hooper, S. L. 1934. Studies in the influence of exercise on the digestive work of the stomach. *American Journal of Physiology* 107:348, 355, 364, 370.

10. Karlsson, J., and Saltin, B. 1971. Diet, muscle glycogen, and endurance performance. *Journal of Applied Physiology* 31:203-206.

11. Krogh, A., and Lindhard, J. 1920. The relative value of fats and carbo-hydrates as sources of muscular energy. *Biochemistry Journal* 14:290.

12. Singer, R. N., and Neeves, R. E. 1968. Effect of food consumption on 200-yard freestyle swim performance. *Research Quarterly* 39:355-60.

13. White, J. R. 1968. Effects of eating a liquid meal at specific times upon subsequent performances in the one-mile run. *Research Quarterly* 39:206-10.

14. Williams, R. J. 1962. *Nutrition in a nutshell*. New York: Doubleday & Co.

25 Special Aids to Athletic Performance

Very small improvements in athletic performance can make the difference between mediocre and championship achievement. Differences of one or two percent may have large meaning. An improvement of only two percent in a four-minute mile brings the time down to 3:55.2.

Because of the importance of small improvements, which are very difficult to obtain by normal training methods when performance approaches record times or championship levels, coaches and athletes have cast about for special aids to performance, sometimes called *ergogenic aids*. Manipulation of diet, use of various drugs, use of "miracle" foods, etc., have all been areas of interest at various times. This search for methods to improve athletic achievement can be considered wholesome as long as (1) special aids are used to supplement, not to supplant, excellence in training and conditioning, and (2) the special aids constitute no hazard to the athletes.

Ergogenic aids can function in one of two ways: (1) by improving the capacity of the muscles to do work or (2) by removing or reducing inhibitory mechanisms in order to allow use of previously untapped reserves. The first function must be considered the sounder approach because the second function must inevitably reduce the safety factor with which the organism has been provided.

In general, the use of drugs falls into the second category; furthermore, the use of any drugs to improve athletic performance is cause for disqualification by the International Amateur Athletic Federation, the Amateur Athletic Union, and the US Olympic Association as being contrary to the highest ideals of sportsmanship. Even more important, some of the drugs that have reportedly been used by athletes (such as the amphetamines) can be habituating and can have other harmful effects (34). Although the ergogenic effects of some drugs are discussed in this chapter, this should in no way be construed as support for their use; this discussion is included for academic purposes only.

ALKALINIZERS

The amount of oxygen debt attainable by an athlete is a very important factor in heavy endurance work. The size of the O_2 debt, in turn, is very likely limited by the blood pH, which depends upon the alkaline reserve (the capacity for buffering the lactic acid formed during work).

Early workers in this area established the feasibility of displacing the pH of the blood upward (prior to exercise) by the ingestion of alkaline salts, so that a heavy workout resulted only in a return to the normal pH value instead of a displacement toward more acidic values, which usually occurs (32). Dennig et al. (9), working at the Harvard Fatigue

Laboratory, demonstrated a decreased ability to accumulate O_2 debt in acidosis brought about by ingestion of acid salts; and it was inferred from this that alkalosis should improve the possibility for buffering an increased O_2 debt. Dill et al. (11) demonstrated this increased O_2 debt capability; a runner in an alkaline state ran 6:04 minutes to exhaustion (on a treadmill), compared with 5:22 minutes from a normal state. The O_2 debt was about twenty percent greater in the first case, which agrees roughly with the increased time of running.

Dennig (10) continued this line of experimentation in Germany with a well-controlled study on ten subjects who worked to exhaustion on a treadmill and bicycle ergometer. In all cases, his subjects were able to increase their endurance by thirty to 100 percent when they started in an alkaline state. His procedure, after many experiments, consisted of ingestion of a mixture of sodium citrate (5.0 gm), sodium bicarbonate (3.5 gm), and potassium citrate (1.5 gm), in two to four doses per day taken after mealtime. (This procedure should start two days before an event and should cease at least five hours before the event.) Dennig pointed out that the effect will be lost over longer periods because the organism adjusts to the artificial alkalinization (it would also be undesirable from a health standpoint). Some of his subjects experienced moderate side effects, such as stomach gas and loose bowels.

Dennig's experiments furnish strong evidence for the value of alkaline salts in *his* subjects, who were only moderately trained. Whether this effect can be demonstrated on highly trained athletes, who might have already improved their alkaline reserve through their training, is questionable. Only one study has been conducted subsequently on highly trained runners; and in this case no significant changes were found (22). The salt mixture was given four hours before the event, however, and this timing was shown by Dennig to be ineffective. Further work seems justified.

AMPHETAMINE (BENZEDRINE)

This drug, in all its various forms (primarily d-amphetamine sulfate and its European relative Pervitin) is a sympathomimetic amine, and it is used by the medical profession as a central nervous system stimulant. Pharmacology texts warn against its use as a remedy for sleepiness or fatigue, or to increase capacity for work, because (1) there is a danger of addiction, (2) it removes the warning of impending overstrain, (3) its vasopressor effects are undesirable, and (4) cases of collapse have been reported. Obviously, this discussion is academic, as the use of such drugs by athletes is to be strongly discouraged.

The literature contains evidence that amphetamine sulfate inhibits fatigue as measured by voluntary contractions on an ergograph (1), improves hand and arm coordination (29), improves the strength of forearm flexion (21), and handgrip (20, 29), and improves the athletic performance of swimmers, runners and weight throwers (37). Pervitin was found to increase work output on a bicycle ergometer (27).

On the other hand, some investigators have been unable to verify these results (18, 25), and we must conclude that the ergogenic effects are—at best—debatable and that the dangers involved are considerable. Dr. A. J. Ryan, an expert in sports medicine, recommended in an editorial in the *Journal of the American Medical Association*: Because these drugs can be obtained legally only on prescription, a serious obligation devolves on physicians to help prevent such usage [in athletes] by prescribing them only for well-recognized medical indications. It is acknowledged there is an illegal traffic in the amphetamines in the United States and that problems of its control still remain to be solved (34).

ANABOLIC STEROIDS

Evidence has been offered to suggest that administering testosterone (a male sex hormone) to animals (31) and humans (35) results in an increase in muscle weight (hypertrophy) and strength. Testosterone is a steroid that has both androgenic (producing masculine characteristics) and anabolic (nitrogen retention-protein building) qualities. Recently steroids have been synthetically developed that are chemically related to testosterone, but in which structural changes in the molecule have increased the anabolic effects while decreasing the androgenic effects (16). It has come to the author's attention that various commercial preparations of the *anabolic steroids* are in vogue among strength athletes. This, again is a drug of considerable physiological potency, with many undesirable side effects, and thus it must be prescribed by a physician.

As a matter of academic interest, investigations have been made of the effectiveness of this drug for young athletes in whom secretion of male hormones is presumably still at a high level. An experiment by Fowler, Gardner, and Egstrom at UCLA failed to substantiate the claims made for these anabolic steroids by the weight trainers (14). Another study, performed independently on another anabolic steroid at Long Beach State College, also failed to demonstrate any significant differences in either weight gain or strength gain (28). It is of interest that, in the LBSC study, clinical laboratory analyses showed no abnormal findings in the experimental group that had been on anabolic steroids for six weeks. However, a follow-up study on a subject who continued on anabolic steroids for twelve weeks showed a significant rise in serum glutamic-oxalacetic transaminase (SGOT) that approached the upper limit of normal values. High values of SGOT are related to liver damage.

The strongest evidence to support strength and body weight gains from anabolic steroids has been recently provided by Johnson and co-workers (23, 24). However, other good recent evidence tends to refute their findings. Cosner, et al. (3), who also found significantly better weight gains after anabolic steroids than in controls, provided evidence that the weight gain resulted from water retention (a detriment not a benefit) rather than muscle hypertrophy. They found no significant changes in strength.

The use of large doses of anabolic steroids can have serious medical side effects such as:

1. Suppressed secretion of gonadotropin
2. Atrophy of tubules and interstitial tissue of the testes
3. Occasional prostatic hypertrophy
4. Cholestatic hepatitis
5. Excessive erythrocyte formation resulting in polycythemia

For a more complete discussion of the medical side effects the reader is referred to the review by Fowler (15).

The conclusion is inescapable. These are very dangerous drugs and the likelihood of athletic gains is far from proven.

ASPARTATES

Aspartic acid is a dicarboxylic amino acid that is known to form one of the links between protein and carbohydrate metabolism. Its conversion to oxalacetic acid places it in the citric acid cycle, which provides energy from carbohydrate breakdown (chapter two). It has been shown that the respiration of a minced pigeon breast muscle can be increased by the addition of aspartic acid.

These well-known facts of biochemistry led to experimentation by the medical profession with aspartic acid salts for the relief of fatigue. In a group of 200 patients, all of whom complained of fatigue (post-influenza, neurosis, gastrointestinal problems, menopause, old age, etc.), administration of potassium and magnesium aspartates resulted in subjective relief in a large percentage of cases (26). A more objective study on rats showed that the swim time to complete exhaustion was increased fifteen percent in a group of thirty-six on aspartates, compared with a similar control group (33). It is of interest that in this experiment the improvement was seen most clearly in the low-endurance group of rats; the "athletic" rats were very little altered.

In an investigation of fatigue in 163 subjects that comprised a blind study (subjects did not know whether they were on aspartates or placebo) and a double blind crossover trial (neither subjects nor investigator knew, and each group had a course of aspartates and placebo), subjective and objective evidence of relief of fatigue were presented (36).

On the other hand, Consolazio and his co-workers at the US Army Medical Research and Nutrition Laboratory were unable to verify these results on animals or on men (4, 30). Fallis et al. (13) ran an experiment on twenty-six penitentiary-inmate weight lifters who regularly engaged in athletic activities; and they reported no significant differences in eight different measures that involved weight lifting and endurance. It is of interest, however, that in six of the seven events that could be considered as having a muscular endurance factor, the results favored the aspartate trials. The lack of statistical significance of the differences could conceivably be the result of a real difference, which was obscured by a large variability and the small number of subjects.

Since the aspartic acid salts can be considered as foods rather than drugs, there would be no danger (with sensible doses) in further experimentation; and this seems advisable in view of the lack of agreement.

CAFFEINE

Caffeine is used in medicine as a central nervous system stimulant, particularly for psychical functions; it is also used as a diuretic. Medicinal dosage ranges from 100 to 500 milligrams. A cup of coffee usually contains 100 to 150 mgm and tea contains slightly less.

Graf (19) has reported on experiments in Germany during World War II, to find stimulants suitable for improving physical and mental efficiency in combatting the stressful conditions of war. It was found that, although caffeine was a strong mental stimulant, it resulted in a very undesirable impairment of motor coordination (in target shooting, writing, and simulated auto driving). There was also a hangover effect, in which mental efficiency, after having been improved, fell off below normal values from one to three hours after taking the stimulant.

A combination of caffeine and metrazol was found to provide the best long-term stimulation and the least interference with sleep. Ganzlen et al. (17) found an increase in work capacity and in maximal oxygen consumption as a result of this combination of drugs, which would seem to indicate a degree of usefulness for caffeine-metrazol for aerospace emergencies. Metrazol, however, is a dangerous drug; its main use has been to bring about epileptiform convulsions in psychiatric disorders, and it is of course totally unsuited (as well as illegal) for use as an ergogenic aid.

It should also be mentioned that investigative work (in Germany) indicates that caffeine can interfere with carbohydrate and protein metabolism, and may also cause a lowering of blood chloride, thus adversely effecting the cardiovascular function (2). Far from being an ergogenic aid, caffeine should be excluded from an athlete's diet if this can be accomplished without psychic trauma!

DISINHIBITION BY PAVLOVIAN PROCEDURES

Ikai and Steinhaus (21) performed a very interesting series of experiments to study the factors that may modify the *expression* of human strength. They used the cable tensiometer, and measured the force of elbow flexion at one-minute intervals while the subject was exposed to the following experimental conditions:

1. A pistol shot at two to ten seconds before each pull
2. Pull with subject's shout
3. Varying stages of hypnosis
4. Ingestion of alcohol
5. Adrenalin injection
6. Amphetamine sulfate (oral)

They found significant improvements, of 7.4 to 26.5 percent for all conditions except four and five. Ikai and Steinhaus concluded that the *true* maximum limit of human performance is always established by structure and the physiological state of the performing muscles, but that the maximum that is usually observed is the result of acquired inhibitions, which are subject to disinhibition by Pavlovian procedures. This very interesting concept deserves further investigation as a practical and ethical approach to providing ergogenic aids for athletes.

OXYGEN AND VITAMINS

The use of oxygen to improve athletic performance was discussed in chapter eight. Vitamin supplementation as an ergogenic aid has also been discussed; the reader is referred to chapter 24, pp. ??.

WHEAT-GERM OIL

Wheat-germ oil (WGO) contains several factors that seem to have biological activity: (1) vitamin E (alpha, beta, and gamma tocopherols),

(2) fatty acids, such as linoleic acid, and (3) octacosanol, an alcohol that can be synthetically prepared. Cureton and his co-workers have provided evidence of an improved training effect on middle-age men when the physical training was supplemented by WGO (6, 7); however, a later study by Cureton on young men provided only statistically nonsignificant differences (8).

In a dietary study on guinea pigs that lasted twenty-eight days and ended with a swim test to exhaustion, it was found that all animals on a natural (control) diet drowned within ten minutes; twenty-five to thirty-three percent of those on a corn oil (vitamin E) supplemented diet were still swimming at sixty minutes; and sixty percent of those fed WGO were still swimming at sixty minutes. Weanling rats who were fed on WGO showed no difference in swimming ability from those supplemented with corn oil (12).

In another study on swimming rats, no differences in performance were observed between those on WGO, vitamin E, or octacosanol as compared with controls (5).

It must be concluded that neither an ergogenic principle in WGO nor an ergogenic effect of the whole oil has been conclusively established. Cureton's early work (6, 7) is persuasive, and the failure to achieve significant differences in the later work might be explained on the basis of age differences in the subject populations. Further experimentation seems justified.

SUMMARY

1. A survey of the literature on ergogenic aids leaves the distinct impression that even if "doping" with drugs were legal, ethical, and nonhazardous, their use could not be based on experimental evidence. On the other hand, use of some of the proposed ergogenic aids that are nonhazardous and that can be considered normal hygienic procedures to aid an athlete gain an extra one or two percent improvement in performance may be justified if every effort has been exerted to bring the training and conditioning to a peak.

2. A further disadvantage of ergogenic acids is that an athlete may become psychologically addicted, and if at a critical moment the aid is unavailable, a decrement from normal performance can occur.

3. In interpretation of research data, the finding of no positive results can never be conclusive because a single experiment is never capable of seeing all the possible changes that may occur. For example, an investigator using a simple magnifying glass might deny the existence of bacteria, which are clearly seen under a high-power microscope; similarly, a research design is not omnipotent.

4. In some experiments the differences that favor the working hypothesis were disregarded because they did not achieve statistical significance. This is as it should be, but the rigor of our method must not obscure the fact that even a real difference may remain statistically non-significant if (1) the difference is small, (2) the number of subjects is small, and (3) the variability within or between subjects on the parameter of interest is large.

This concept was clearly demonstrated in a study that showed the advantage of using expert swimmers instead of non-experts for evaluation of the effects of ergogenic aids (38). Obtaining as much precision with non-experts as was provided by the fifteen experts would have necessitated (because of greater intrasubject variability) an increase of the non-expert sample size from fifteen to about eighty.

5. In view of the experiments cited, it seems that further experimentation is justified for such ergogenic aids as the alkalinizers, aspartates, disinhibition, and wheat-germ oil. Used judiciously, none of these should be hazardous; and further research is needed.

REFERENCES

1. Alles, G. A., and Feigen, G. A. 1942. The influence of benzedrine on work decrement and patellar reflex. *American Journal of Physiology* 136:392-400.

2. Atzler, E.; Lehman, G.; and Szakall, A. 1939. Ueber die Wirkung des Caffeins auf den Kohlehydrat und Eiweiss-Stoffwechsel. *Arbetisphysiologie* 10:30-56.

3. Casner, S. W.; Early, R. G.; and Carlson, B. R. 1971. Anabolic steroid effects on body composition in normal young men. *Journal of Sports Medicine* 11:98-103.

4. Consolazio, C. F.; Nelson, R. A.; Matoush, L. O.; and Isaac, G. J. 1964. Effects of aspartic acid salts (Mg + K) on physical performance of men. *Journal of Applied Physiology* 19:257-61.

5. Consolazio, C. F.; Matoush, L. O.; Nelson, R. A.; Isaac, G. J.; and Hursh, L. M. Effects of octacosanol, wheat germ oil, and vitamin E on performance of swimming rats. *Journal of Applied Physiology* 19:265-67.

6. Cureton, T. K. 1954. Effects of wheat germ oil and vitamin E on normal human subjects in physical training programs. *American Journal of Physiology* 179:628.

7. Cureton, T. K., and Pohndorf, R. 1955. Influence of wheat germ oil as a dietary supplement in a program of conditioning exercises with middle-aged subjects. *Research Quarterly* 26:391-407.

8. ----. 1963. Improvements in physical fitness associated with a course of US Navy underwater trainees with and without dietary supplements. *Research Quarterly* 34:440-53.

9. Dennig, H.; Talbot, J. H.; Edwards, H. T.; and Dill, D. B. 1931. Effect of acidosis and alkalosis upon capacity for work. *Journal of Clinical Investigation* 9:601-13.

10. ———. 1937. Ueber Steigerung der Korperlichen Leistungsfahigkeit durch Eingriffe in den Saurebasenhaushalt. *Deutsche Medizinische Wochenschrift* 63:733-36.

11. Dill, D. B.; Edwards, H. T.; and Talbott, J. H. 1932. Alkalosis and the capacity for work. *Journal of Biological Chemistry* 97:58-59.

12. Erschoff, B. H., and Levin, E. 1955. Beneficial effect of an unidentified factor in wheat germ oil on the swimming performance of guinea pigs. *Federation Proceedings* 14:431-32.

13. Fallis, N.; Wilson, W. R.; Tetreault, L. L.; and La Sagna, L. 1963. Effect of potassium and magnesium aspartates on athletic performance. *Journal of the American Medical Association* 185 (2):129.

14. Fowler, W. H., Jr.; Gardner, G. H.; and Egstrom, G. H. 1965. Effect of an anabolic steroid on physical performance of young men. *Journal of Applied Physiology* 20:1038-40.

15. Fowler, W. H., Jr. 1969. The facts about ergogenic aids and sports performance. *Journal of the Association for Health, Physical Education, and Recreation.* Nov.-Dec. 1969, pp. 37-42.

16. Fox, M.; Minot, A. S.; and Liddle, G. W. 1962. Oxandrolone: a potent anabolic steroid of novel chemical configuration. *Journal of Clinical Endocrinology* 22:921-24.

17. Ganzlen, R. V.; Balke, B.; Nagle, F. J.; and Phillips, E. E. 1964. Effects of some tranquilizing analeptic and vasodilating drugs on physical work capacity and orthostatic tolerance. *Aerospace Medicine* 35:630-33.

18. Golding, L. A., and Barnard, J. R. 1963. The effects of d-amphetamine sulfate on physical performance. *Journal of Sports Medicine* 3:221-24.

19. Graf, O. 1950. Increase of efficiency by means of pharmaceutics (stimulants). In *German aviation medicine, W.W. II,* vol. 2, p. 1080. Washington, D. C.: US Government Printing Office.

20. Hurst, P. M.; Radlow, R.; and Bagley, S. K. 1968. The effects of d-amphetamine and chlordiazepoxide upon strength and estimated strength. *Ergonomics* 11:47-52.

21. Ikai, M., and Steinhaus, A. H. 1961. Some factors modifying the expression of human strength. *Journal of Applied Physiology* 16:157-63.

22. Johnson, W. R., and Black, D. H. 1953. Comparison of effects of certain blood alkalinizers and glucose upon competitive endurance performance. *Journal of Applied Physiology* 5:577-78.

23. Johnson, L. C., and O'Shea, J. P. 1969. Anabolic steroids: effects on strength development. *Science* 164:957-59.

24. Johnson, L. C.; Fisher, G;. Silvester, L. J.; and Hofheins, C. C. 1972. Anabolic steroid: effects on strength, body weight, oxygen uptake and spermatogenesis upon mature males. *Medicine and Science in Sports* 4:43-45.

25. Karpovich, P. V. 1959. Effect of amphetamine sulfate on athletic performance. *Journal of the American Medical Association* 170:558-61.

26. Kruse, C. A. 1961. Treatment of fatigue with aspartic acid salts. *Northwest Medicine* 60:597-603.
27. Lehman, G.; Straub, H.; and Szakall, A. 1939. Pervitin als Leistungssteigerndes Mittel. *Arbeitsphysiologie* 10:680-91.
28. Losner, I. 1965. A personal communication on 27 September 1965.
29. Lovingood, B. W.; Blyth, C. S.; Peacock, W. H.; Lindsay, R. B. 1967. Effects of d-amphetamine sulfate, caffeine and high temperature on human performance. *Research Quarterly* 38:64-71.
30. Matoush, L. O.; Consolazio, C. F.; Nelson, R. A.; Isaac, G. I.; and Torres, J. B. 1964. Effects of aspartic acid salts (Mg $+$ K) on swimming performance of rats and dogs. *Journal of Applied Physiology* 19:262-64.
31. Papanicolaou, G. N., and Falk, E. A. 1938. General muscular hypertrophy induced by androgenic hormone. *Science* 82:238-39.
32. Ronzoni, E. 1926. The effect of exercise on breathing in experimental alkalosis by ingested sodium bicarbonate. *Journal of Biological Chemistry* 67(2):25-27.
33. Rosen, H.; Blumenthal, A.; and Agersborg, H. P. K. 1962. Effects of the potassium and magnesium salts of aspartic acid on metabolic exhaustion. *Journal of Pharmaceutical Science* 51:592-93.
34. Ryan, A. J. 1959. Use of amphetamine in athletics. *Journal of the American Medical Association* 170:562.
35. Simonson, E.; Kearns, W. M.; and Enzer, N. 1944. Effect of methyl testosterone treatment on muscular performance and central nervous system of older men. *Journal of Clinical Endocrinology and Metabolism* 10:528-34.
36. Shaw, D. L., Jr.; Chesney, M. A.; Tullis, I. F.; and Agersborg, H. P. K. 1962. Management of fatigue: a physiologic approach. *American Journal of Medical Science* 243:758-69.
37. Smith, G. M., and Beecher, H. K. 1959. Amphetamine sulfate and athletic performance. *Journal of the American Medical Association* 170:542-57.
38. Weitzner, M., and Beecher, H. K. 1963. Increased sensitivity of measurements of drug effects in expert swimmers. *Journal of Pharmacology* 139:114-19.

26 The Female in Athletics

Athletic competition at the higher levels for women is a fairly recent development; it awaited the emancipation of the fair sex from its enslavement to puritan concepts and from clothes unsuited for comfortable movement, let alone athletic performances. It is indeed amusing to attempt to visualize present-day performances in swimming or running in the athletic costumes of the nineteenth century. Women's athletics—worthy of the name—did not exist prior to World War I, and women began Olympic competition only in 1928.

As a consequence we are only beginning to learn the specialized physiology involved in the reaction of the female at different ages to the various stressors in athletic competition. Furthermore, women's athletics have developed around modifications of existing men's sports, and whether these activities are best suited to the unique interests and the physiological, psychological, and sociological needs of girls and women has not really been investigated. Nevertheless, participation by girls and women in competitive athletics is increasing, and every physical educator and coach should be aware of the available knowledge about the special problems of the female in competitive sports. Obviously, girls' athletics should be directed and supervised by professional physical educators because the problems require even greater concern for the principles of anatomy, physiology, and kinesiology than do men's sports.

STRUCTURAL SEX DIFFERENCES

One of the most obvious and most important differences between the sexes in regard to sports performance is the ratio of strength to weight, which (after puberty) is normally much greater in the male. This factor is most important in activities in which the weight is supported by the relatively smaller muscles of the arms and shoulder girdle, as in gymnastics. It is also a consideration wherever the mass of the body must be accelerated rapidly, as in jumping.

The reason for the poorer strength-weight ratio is, of course, the smaller proportion of muscle in relation to the considerably larger amount of adipose tissue (chapter twelve) in the female. The larger stores of fatty tissue are not an unmitigated disadvantage, however; in swimming, for example, this results in better buoyancy and less heat losses to cold water.

Not only are the proportions of various tissues different in the female, even the chemical constituents within each tissue are different. The female tissues, for example, contain much greater amounts of sulfer (twenty-three percent more in skeletal muscle), and the creatinine coefficients are also different. More research is required to establish the significance of these facts.

A structural difference that has very significant physiological implications for athletic performance is the difference in the ratio of heart weight to body weight in the sexes. From the age of ten to the age of sixty, the average value for women is only eighty-five to ninety percent of the value for men (4). After age sixty, however, the ratio is similar for men and women.

PHYSIOLOGICAL SEX DIFFERENCES

Although there are many physiological differences that have general significance, only those that apply directly to athletic performance will be considered here.

Basal Metabolic Rate. From just before puberty, and through the rest of the lifespan, BMR (as customarily measured and normalized for body surface area) is higher for the male than for the female. When BMR is evaluated in relationship to muscle mass instead of to surface area, however, the sex difference disappears (4). Thus this difference would have significance only in respect to resting heat dissipation, not for the efficiency of muscular activtiy.

Blood Constituents. On the average in the age group twenty to thirty, men have approximately fifteen percent more hemoglobin per 100 milliliters of blood and about six percent more erythrocytes per cubic millimeter (4). The combination of these two factors should militate toward a greater oxygen-carrying capacity for men.

Microcirculation. When the reddening of skin in reaction to ultraviolet radiation was used as a measure of capillary function, men were found superior through the entire age range (4). The resistance of the capillary wall to breakdown from mechanical manipulation was also found to be greater in the male. This very likely is the reason for the greater susceptibility to bruises in the female.

Erholungs Quotient. In German physiology laboratories the relationship of increased oxygen consumption during exercise to the increased oxygen during recovery is used as a measure of physical work capacity, or condition.

$$\text{Erholungs Quotient (EQ)} = \frac{\text{Net } O_2 \text{ during exercise}}{\text{Net } O_2 \text{ in recovery}}$$

Obviously, this is a measure of the degree to which an individual must encroach upon her anaerobic reserves to perform at a given level of work load. EQ values for the female are lower than those for the male throughout all ages (18).

Oxygen Pulse. This is a widely used measure of the efficiency of the heart as a respiratory organ, and it is calculated as the O_2 consumption in milliliters per heart beat. For equal work loads, boys and girls are about equal on this measure for ages twelve to fifteen. It is interesting to note, however, that there is a rapid improvement in the male to a value about twice as high at ages twenty-one to twenty-five, while the female's oxygen pulse remains constant at the twelve to fifteen age value (18). This has implications that will be discussed below.

Cardiac Cost. Cardiac cost provides a measure of the stressfulness of a given work load on the heart (chapter five). Again, the most advantageous age for girls is about twelve or thirteen, and there is no further improvement with increasing age. The male, however, has a cardiac cost for equal work loads only a little more than a third as high at ages thirty-one to thirty-six, compared with his value for ages twelve to thirteen (18).

Maximum O_2 Consumption. The classic work of Astrand (1) has shown that girls reach a high point in their maximum O_2 per unit weight between eight and nine years of age; this figure declines slowly, to about age fifteen, after which it remains constant through young adulthood. Boys reach their peak later, at about fifteen or sixteen years of age, and maintain this peak through young adulthood.

Thus in the younger age groups (seven to thirteen) sex differences grow larger with each increasing year. At ages seven to nine the differences are small and probably not significant. By age twelve or thirteen however differences favoring boys of thirteen to sixteen percent in maximal O_2 consumption normalized for body weight have appeared (27). McNab, Conger and Taylor (15) have shown in a direct comparison of twenty-four male versus twenty-four female college physical education majors that the difference at this age has grown to thirty-two percent when measured as maximal O_2 per Kg as in the data above. Even when the increasing adiposity of the female is taken into consideration by expressing the data as O_2 per unit fat free weight the difference still favors the male by eighteen percent. These differences were, of course, highly significant.

Phenomenal Success of Young Girl Swimmers. In the light of the foregoing facts about EQ, O_2 pulse, and maximum O_2 consumption, the success of young American girl swimmers in national and international competition becomes understandable. It would seem that all physiological functions essential to competitive swimming have achieved peak values by age twelve to fourteen in the female, whereas these are delayed in the male to late high school and college age. When we add to this the factors of (1) very early commencement of training and (2) absence of social pressures, the accomplishment of our young girl swimmers is entirely comprehensible.

Neuromuscular Functions. Thus far we have discussed the physiology of endurance-type sports, and it is time to consider some of the factors that collectively make up the *skill* of motor perforance. It has been reported (from Germany) that women generally have greater manual skill and dexterity than men (13). In the USA, Pierson and Lockhart (21) have shown there is no significant sex difference in reaction time to a visual stimulus, although men have faster movement times.

A review of the literature in this area seems to indicate that there are probably no real sex differences in regard either to motor learning rate or capacity, unless strength is a factor.

PHYSIOLOGICAL ADJUSTMENTS TO HEAVY TRAINING

The physiological adjustments to heavy training in girls and women have not as yet had much attention. The best information at this time comes from Astrand and his co-workers (2) in Stockholm, who studied thirty girl swimmers, twelve to sixteen years of age, for one year. The girls trained from 6,000 to 71,500 yards (six to twenty-eight hours) per week, and were examined extensively—medically and physiologically—during this period. It was shown that large differences existed in such important measures as maximal O_2 consumption when these girls were compared with average, untrained girls. Furthermore, the differences were highly correlated to the volume of training for each girl. More recently Brown, et al. (3) studied the effects of training for competitive cross-country running upon pre-adolescent girls. They found maximal O_2 consumption increased by eighteen percent at six weeks and twenty-six percent at twelve weeks. Heart rate at submaximal loads declined and no detrimental effects were seen. Kilbom (11) studied the effects of conditioning on mature females with the bicycle or walking routines using work loads which represented fifty-two to seventy-seven percent of maximal O_2. In the young group (nineteen to thitry-one years) aerobic capacity improved twelve percent, and cardiac output eleven percent, in the middle-aged the improvements were eleven percent and ten percent, and in the older women (fifty-one to sixty-four), eight percent and ten percent. Systolic blood pressure dropped by fifteen mm in the older group and serum cholesterol declined by ten percent. They saw no orthopedic training complications (ordinarily common with middle-aged men) since they used the bicycle and walking type exercise. However, they did find that serum iron levels declined by twenty-five percent in all groups. This finding is probably due to greater iron usage in the enhanced erythropoeisis which accompanies vigorous exercise, and suggests the need for iron supplementation in all post pubertal females undergoing rigorous physical training. Thus it seems that the female adjusts to heavy training in much the same fashion as the male.

Occasionally girls are concerned about the possibility that heavy training may result in increased growth rates, or that on cessation of activity unseemly weight increases may detract from their appearance. No real evidence has been found to substantiate these fears.

Another factor of great concern to young girls contemplating athletic participation is that of becoming less feminine in appearance because of larger or more bunchy muscles, etc. Klaus and Noack, two of the foremost experts on the effects of athletics and exercise upon the female, feel the available evidence suggests that *properly designed* exercise programs improve rather than hinder femininity (13). The observation that some girl athletes are very muscular is undoubtedly due to the fact that muscular girls are more apt to be successful in such sports as track and field athletics, and therefore they are more likely to elect to participate in such competition.

GYNECOLOGICAL PROBLEMS

The effects of strenuous exercise programs upon the sexual and reproductive functions of the female have been a matter of some concern in the past, although not on the basis of scientific evidence. Observations upon 729 Hungarian female athletes show there is no disturbance of the onset of menarche (7). Nor has there been evidence of dysmenorrhea of any consequence as the result of athletic participation much less from moderate physical exercise (2, 7).

In the case of girl swimmers, however, bacteriological examination disclosed the presence of pathogenic organisms in the vagina of a third of the subjects (2). In spite of this, there were no signs of any infection of reproductive organs, except in one case of colpitis (inflammation of the vagina). In view of these observations, it would seem undesirable from the medical standpoint for girls to train for swimming during the menstrual period, although this is now common practice in this country.

FEMALE LIMITATIONS IN ATHLETICS

Table 26.1 shows a comparison of world records in various activites between male and female competitors. Among other things, the table shows the undesirability of competition between the sexes. Most important, however, is the comparison of how close girls come to men in the various types of activity. For lack of better information at this time, it may be inferred from table 26.1 that those activities in which women approach men's records most closely are those in which women suffer the smallest physiological disadvantage, and thus these activities may be considered more suitable, at least until better evidence is available.

In general, it can be seen that the events that depend upon explosive power (such as the high jump and long jump) show the greatest sex difference. The free style and backstroke swimming events and the short runs seem to be the best suited to the feminine physiology if we can assume that all events attract equal numbers of participants (a rather doubtful assumption).

Trainability of the Female. In relation to strength, Hettinger (10) has shown that the female is much less responsive to training than the male. At the age of greatest trainability, twenty to thirty, women respond to training with only fifty percent the rate of improvement of men.

TABLE 26.1

Comparison of World Records for Men and Women
(July 10, 1963)

Event	Women	Men	Percent
Swimming (meters)			
100 free style	59.5	53.6	90
200 " "	2:11.6	1:58.4	90
400 " "	4:44.5	4:13.4	89
800 " "	9:51.6	8:51.5	90
1,500 " "	18:44.0	17:05.5	91
100 breaststroke	1:18.2	1:07.5	86
200 "	2:48.0	2:29.6	89
100 butterfly stroke	1:06.1	57.0	86
200 " "	2:29.1	2:08.2	86
100 backstroke	1:08.9	1:00.9	88
200 "	2:28.2	2:10.9	88
Running (meters)			
100	11.2	10.0	89
200	22.9	20.5	90
400	53.1	44.9	85
800	2:01.2	1:44.3	86
Field events (meters)			
High jump	1.91	2.28	84
Long jump	6.62	8.31	80

For endurance, the experiments of Klaus and Noack (13) on physical education students showed that at the end of an eighteen-week training program the men's capacity was about one-third better than that of the women. This is to be expected in the light of the physiological measurements discussed above. Klaus and Noack suggest, on the basis of their experiments, that competitive distances for women in running events should not exceed 1000 meters, although training procedures may well go beyond this distance.

On the other hand, the data of table 26.1 seem to indicate that endurance per se is not a factor, since in free style swimming events—where power (strength) is not a large factor, girls do relatively as well at 1500 meters as at 100 meters. In running events, a distinct drop in relative performances is seen between the sprints and the middle distances. Whether this is due to a sex difference or to the lesser number of female participants in the middle distances remains to be demonstrated. In any event, the "pure power" events (high jump and long jump) show the greatest sex difference, which undoubtedly is a reflection of the lesser strength in the female.

Heat Adaptation.   It has been shown that women are probably inherently less able to deal with hot environments (9, 16, 26). The threshold for sweating in women appears to be two or three degrees centigrade above that for men, and the temperature gradient from core to skin seems to be smaller for women. Sweat rates are significantly higher in men at equivalent levels of heat stress especially under high heat conditions whether dry or humid (16). While both men and women acclimatize to work in the heat after repeated exposures, the mechanisms and signs of acclimatization appear to be different. Men exhibit substantial increases in the rate of sweating which are not evident in women. Women on the other hand show a significant decrease in rectal temperature with increasing exposure which is not seen in men (26).

THE MENSTRUAL CYCLE AND ATHLETICS

Participation in Sports during the Period.   It is well known that female athletes in the upper levels of competition seldom allow the menstrual cycle to interfere with their training, but this does not, in itself, justify the practice. There is no unanimity of opinion by medical authorities on this matter. The only scientific evidence available is that of Astrand et al. (2), whose work indicates that swimming training during the period is undesirable because of the presence of pathogenic bacteria in the vagina, and because of the reports of lower abdominal pain in about a third of the girls.

It is probably as unwise to *prohibit* participation in physical education or athletics as it would be to *require* it. In either of these extremes, undue emphasis would be placed on a physiological function that girls should learn to accept as normal. Undoubtedly, the preferred course of action until more scientific evidence is available is to *allow* participation on a voluntary basis, with no undue comments about possible undesirable consequences.

Rhythmicity as a Criterion of Training Progress. Regular, asymptomatic menstruation is usually considered to be a measure of general good health in the female after a regular rhythm has been established. Conversely, medical authorities feel that any deviation from the normal rhythmic pattern may be one of the first indications of overtraining (7, 13). It would be good practice for women coaches and physical educators to advise the members of their teams and classes to maintain accurate records of their menstrual cycles, and they should encourage consultations whenever deviations occur. This practice should result in better health and performance for the girls.

Effect of the Menstrual Cycle on Performance. In spite of the widespread impression of impaired performance during certain periods of the menstrual cycle, there is no agreement among the investigators who have attacked this problem. Some have found no effect of the menstrual cycle upon motor performance (6, 8, 14, 19, 20, 22, 23); others report that performance is best in the post-menstrual phase or inter-menstrual phase, at its worst in the two or three days preceding menstruation (7, 13, 17) or during menstruation (25).

PREGNANCY, CHILDBIRTH, AND ATHLETICS

Participation in athletic competition, training or vigorous sports should obviously be forbidden during pregnancy. The reasons for this have been discussed by Klaus and Noack (13), who point out that the work of the right heart is increased threefold and the work of the left heart is increased twofold, even in the non-pregnant female, by a moderate work load. During pregnancy, such an increase—with the demands of fetal circulation—can be considered hazardous for the right heart and for lung circulation. The danger is especialy great if unrecognized heart defects are present. In addition, it should be recognized that the kidneys and liver function with very little reserve capacity during pregnancy.

Effects of Heavy Exercise Programs upon Labor and Delivery. Although it was once believed that athletic women developed tense (unyielding) abdominal walls that hindered normal delivery, the results of many investigations in more recent years indicate that athletic women have quick and easy deliveries (13). Erdelyi (7), who has studied many Hungarian women athletes, found a smaller incidence of complications (especially toxemia) during pregnancy and fifty percent fewer Caesarian sections performed in women athletes when compared with controls. It was also found that the duration of labor was shorter than the average in 87.2 percent of the women athletes.

It would therefore appear that there is no need for concern about the effects of strenuous exercise upon subsequent pregnancies or childbirth. Indeed, physical conditioning seems to be a valuable prophylactic procedure.

Effect of Pregnancy and Childbirth on Subsequent Athletic Performance. Noack (17) took histories of fifteen German champion women athletes who bore children during their athletic careers. Of the fifteen, five gave up sports because of their new responsibilities; of the remaining ten, two maintained equal performance and eight made definite objective improvements after childbirth. All of the women agreed that after childbirth they were "tougher" and had more strength and endurance.

It has been pointed out that pregnancy, far from being an illness, should be considered an intensive, day and night, nine-month period of physical conditioning because of the increased demands upon metabolism and the entire cardiovascular system (13).

ATHLETIC INJURIES IN WOMEN

Even a cursory study of anatomy reveals a considerable difference in the locomotor structures of the female compared with the male. On the average, bones, muscles, tendons, and ligaments are more delicately constructed, although body weight is not decreased proportionately because of the greater percentage of fatty tissue in the female. On this basis, a sex difference in incidence of athletic injuries is to be expected, and indeed is found.

It has been shown in studies involving comparable groups of men and women that the overall incidence of athletic injuries in women was almost double that in men (12). Furthermore, the incidence of injuries involving *overstrain*—such as contractures, inflammations of tendons, tendon sheaths, bursae, foot deficiencies, and periosteal injuries—was almost four times more common in women than in similarly trained men.

The distribution of injuries according to the sport activity is of interest. In women, by far the greatest percentage of all injuries is found in sports that require explosive efforts: short runs (fifty-three percent) and the long jump (thirty-one percent). It is difficult to avoid the conclusion that such activities are not suited to the female's musculoskeletal system.

EMOTIONAL FACTORS IN WOMEN'S ATHLETICS

The comment is frequently heard that the female is less well suited to competitive sport than her brothers because of a more emotional nature, and that highly competitive situations might elicit unfavorable responses, but there is no acceptable scientific evidence to support this assertion. Ulrich who used eosinophil count and cardiorespiratory response to measure the stressfulness of various competitive situations (24) found that measureable stress reactions occurred not only in response to participation in class, intramural, and interscholastic basketball games but in written test situations as well! She concluded that stress was much more closely related to the psychological than the physiological components of a situation. It is of interest that her study showed lesser levels of stress occurred as the result of experience, which suggests that girls successfully adjust to the stress of competition.

Astrand et al. (2), in a year-long study of girl swimmers of ages twelve to sixteen (a supposedly emotional labile period), could not find a single case of demonstrable nervous symptoms that coud be attributed to training or to participation in competitive events.

SUMMARY

1. Probably one of the best criteria for the value of competitive athletics for women can be gained from the opinions of former female athletes in regard to the participation of their daughters. In regard to swimming competitions, at least, eight-four ex top-level Swedish swimmers had a positive attitude toward this participation (2).

2. The anatomic and physiological differences between the sexes bear directly on physical education and athletics, and these should be carefully considered in planning programs for girls. Excellent guidelines have been prepared by the Division of Girls and Womens Sports (AAHPER) that will aid administrators, coaches, and physical educators in establishing sensible programs for girls and women (5).

3. There seems to be athletic-injury evidence that the interests of girls and women would be best served if sports and competition were selected and designed specifically for the female. The adoption and modification of men's sports for girls has undoubtedly resulted, in some cases, in the latter's participation in activities that are not well suited to the female's body structure.

REFERENCES

1. Astrand, P. O. 1952. *Experimental studies of physical working capacity in relation to sex and age.* Copenhagen: E. Munksgaard.
2. Astrand, P. O.; Engstrom, L.; Eriksson, B.; Karlberg, P.; Nylander, I.; Saltin, B.; and Thoren, C. 1963. Girl swimmers—with special reference to respiratory and circulatory adaptation and gynecological and psychiatric aspects. *Acta Paediatrica* (Stockholm), suppl. 147.
3. Brown, C. H.; Harrower, J. R.; and Deeter, M. F. 1972. The effects of cross country running on preadolescent girls. *Medicine and Science in Sports* 4:1-5.
4. Burger, M. 1955. Zur Pathophysiologie der Geschlechter. *Munchener Medizinischer Wochenschrift* 97:981-88.
5. DGWS 1965. Statement on competition for girls and women. *JOHPER* 36:34-26.
6. Doolittle, T. L., and Engebretsen, J. 1972. Performance variations during the menstrual cycle. *Journal of Sports Medicine* 12:54-58.
7. Erdelyi, G. J. 1962. Gynecological survey of female athletes. *Journal of Sports Medicine* 2:174-79.
8. Garlick, M. A., and Bernauer, E. M. 1968. Exercise during the menstrual cycle: variations in physiological baselines. *Research Quarterly* 39:533-42.
9. Hertig, B. A.; Belding, H. S.; Kraning, K. K.; Batterton, D. L.; Smith, C. R.; and Sargent, F. 1963. Artificial acclimatization of women to heat. *Journal of Applied Physiology* 18:383-86.
10. Hettinger, T. 1961. *Physiology of strength.* Springfield: Charles C Thomas, Publisher.
11. Kilbom, A. 1971. Physical training in women. *Scandinavian Journal of Clinical and Laboratory Investigation* 28:suppl. 119.
12. Klaus, E. J. 1964. The athletic status of women. In *International research in sport and physical education,* eds. E. Jokl and E. Simon. Springfield: Charles C Thomas, Publisher.
13. Klaus, E. J., and Noack, H. 1961. *Frau and sport.* Stuttgart: Georg Thieme Verlag.
14. Loucks, J., and Thompson, H. 1968. Effect of menstruation on reaction time. *Research Quarterly* 39:407-8.
15. MacNab, R. B. J.; Conger, P. R.; and Taylor, P. S. 1969. Differences in maximal and submaximal work capacity in men and women. *Journal of Applied Physiology* 27:644-48.
16. Morimoto, T.; Slabochova, Z.; Sargent, F. II; and Naman, R. K. 1967. Sex differences in physiological reactions to thermal stress. *Journal of Applied Physiology* 22:526-32.
17. Noack, H. 1954. Die Sportliche Leistungsfahigkeit der Frau im Menstrualzyklus. *Deutsche Medizinische Wochenschrift* 79(2):1523-25.
18. Nocker, J., and Bohlau, V. 1955. Abhangigkeit der Leistungsfahigkeit vom Alter und Geschlecht. *Munchener Medizinische Wochenschrift* 97:1517-22.

19. Phillips, M. 1968. Effect of the menstrual cycle on pulse rate and blood pressure before and after exercise. *Research Quarterly* 39:327-33.

20. Pierson, W. R., and Lockhart, A. 1963. Effect of menstruation on simple reaction and movement time. *British Medical Journal* i:796-97.

21. ———. 1964. Fatigue, work decrement, and endurance of women in a simple repetitive task. *Aerospace Medicine* 35:724-25.

22. Sloan, A. W. 1961. Effect of training on physical fitness of women students. *Journal of Applied Physiology* 16:167-69.

23. ———. 1963. Physical fitness of college students in South Africa, USA, and England. *Research Quarterly* 34:244-48.

24. Ulrich, C. 1956. Measurement of stress evidenced by college women in situations involving competition. Doctoral dissertation, USC (physical education).

25. Wearing, M. P.; Yuhasz, M. D.; Campbell, R.; and Love, E. I. 1972. The effect of the menstrual cycle on tests of physical fitness. *Journal of Sport Medicine* 12:38-41.

26. Weinman, K. P.; Slabochova, Z.; Bernauer, E. M.; Morimoto, T.; and Sargent, F. 1967. Reactions of men and women to repeated exposure to humid heat. *Journal of Applied Physiology* 22:533-38.

27. Wilmore, J. H., and Sigerseth, P. O. 1967. Physical work capacity of young girls, 7-13 years of age. *Journal of Applied Physiology* 22:923-28.

27 The Unified Athlete: Monitoring Training Progress

Training, Conditioning, and Stress
Monitoring Training Progress
"Getting It All Together"—Administration
Methods and Record Keeping
Interpretation of Physiological Data
Benefits to be Gained from the Scientific Effort

The scientific method often requires analytical procedures which break down the whole into its component parts for greater ease of study. This is typical of the *systems approach* in physiology and we have quite artificially fragmented the athlete into his many systems and even by elements of performance such as strength, endurance, speed. This analytical approach is of course absolutely essential because the immense complexity of the human organism defies human comprehension on any other basis. However, the analytic process must be followed by a synthetic process to encourage a unification of principles which will allow application of theory to practice in athletics.

For example we need to know the individual contributions of the heart, blood vessels, lungs, muscles, endocrine glands, nervous system, to meeting the increased metabolic demand of an exercise bout. But in reality each response of each system is intricately interwoven into the responses of each other system, affecting the others and being in turn affected by them.

The same may be said for the artificially contrived divisions of the elements of performance. The elements of strength and endurance of muscle tissue for instance, while they do have separate identities are so closely related that one can scarcely train one without affecting the other as experiments have shown.

Thus, having benefitted by the analytical procedure to the extent of better understanding of detail, let us now synthesize and unify our thinking, let's try to "get it all together" for the benefit of the athlete and for athletics.

Basically, the ultimate in human performance depends upon maximizing two factors: (1) state of overall health in the athlete, and (2) capacity for physiological response to the challenge of the game situation. These are not one and the same. For example, it is not uncommon for the young inexperienced coach to pursue the second goal at the expense of the first and ultimately lose out with respect to both. Too great a demand in the training regimen may result in loading up the total stress on the athlete to the point where health suffers and performance goes downhill.

We are often faced with such practical questions as "How long should the practice be?"; "How hard can I work my athletes?"; "How much is enough?" It is the purpose of this last chapter to provide, not ready-made answers, but a *sound approach* based on the knowledge gained in the physiology of exercise laboratory and which is practical and feasible on the field.

TRAINING, CONDITIONING, AND STRESS

At the outset, we must recall the earlier discussion (chapter ten) on the *stress syndrome,* and realize that the whole training-conditioning process is nothing more nor less than devising appropriate levels of stress to bring about the best possible combination of responses (training effect) on the part of the athlete. The problem becomes complex for several reasons:

1. We usually deal with fairly large numbers of athletes in a team situation and their physiological responses differ from athlete to athlete.
2. Each sport has a different combination of demands.
3. Even within one sport, there are differences in demand from one point in the season to the next.

Furthermore, we as coaches must realize that stress is cumulative and the athlete is meeting other stressors in his life beyond that of the athletic conditioning program. Any given athlete may be faced with differing combinations of total stress resulting from a combination of athletics with any one or more of the following:

1. Academic problems
2. Home problems
3. Other extracurricular activities
4. Outside work to help support himself or family
5. Problems of social interaction
6. Sex life

In all likelihood, the athlete who succumbs to every respiratory bug, the athlete whose performance falls off in mid or late season, maybe even the athlete who suffers injury is being overstressed. That is, the sum total of stresses exceeds his adaptational capacity.

In the light of this discussion, it is patently impossible to arrive at any given combination of intensity-duration or any arbitrary length of workout which will be optimal for all athletes on any given team. Obviously we must base physiological demands upon physiological capacities and this is where the art and science of coaching must merge. Science, in this case, physiology of exercise methods, can supply the data on the athletes level of response to stress (his training progress) but only the coaches art (and good common sense) can help him in modifying the demands upon the individual athletes to optimize the rate of improvement in performance.

MONITORING TRAINING PROGRESS

In essence, to get the best possible performance from our athletes the training stress must be optimized on an individual basis. To do this we must keep records of training progress so that we can "see the forest for the trees." The items which are of paramount interest fall into four categories:

1. Performance data in sports when this can be measured
2. Physiological capacities, particularly PWC
3. Nutritional status
4. Sleep and rest habits

Schedule for Monitoring. The frequency at which observations are made and recorded should vary with the variability of the measurement. The following schedule is suggested as a basis:

A. Evaluation once per season
  1. Diet evaluation
  2. *Total effort* in which the athlete is involved
    a. Athletics
    b. Home life
    c. Academic load
    d. Extracurricular load
    e. Outside work (jobs, etc.)
    f. Social problems
    g. Problems related to sex life
  3. Patterns of sleep and rest
B. Once per week
  1. Resting heart rate and blood pressure
  2. Estimate of PWC by Astrand test (chapter eleven)
  3. Blood pressure under load of PWC test
C. Daily record
  1. Weight (nude when suiting up for workout)
  2. Performance data (i.e., time for selected distance, height or distance jumped, etc.)

"GETTING IT ALL TOGETHER"—ADMINISTRATION

Having been involved in ten years of age group coaching, seven years of high school coaching, and seven years of college coaching, the author can well anticipate the question formulating in the reader's mind: "Where in the devil do I find time for all this record keeping?" The answer is: "You don't, you become an efficient administrator, finding and motivating skilled help and delegating responsibilities."

To begin with, the actual data collection should be handled by a student manager. This may entail giving an additional letter to entice a suitable prospect. In the college situation a physical education major with an active interest in physiology of exercise makes the ideal choice. In the high school situation one looks for an individual with a good IQ and a history of responsibility.

Next, comes the matter of training the manager to collect reliable data. The training process should be accomplished by the coach working in conjunction with the most interested health professional available. Ideally, this should be the team physician or school physician. If neither can make the time available, then the school nurse or the athletic trainer may assume this responsibility with the coach. In any event, all of the health professionals mentioned (whether directly involved or not) should be made aware of this aspect of the athletic program. Those who are interested should also be provided with brief summaries of the testing results. On such efforts is rapport with the medical community and the community at large established!

In most situations, the direct supervision of the data collection should be handled by the coach or athletic trainer since no other personnel would be sufficiently available at the necessary time.

METHODS AND RECORD KEEPING

Diet Evaluation.   Each athlete is issued seven copies of the form shown in table 27.1 at a preseason team meeting (1). The group is instructed with respect to filling out the form, one for each day of the one-week sampling period. These are collected and the data transferred to the food selection score card shown in table 27.2. The score card is self-explanatory and should be completed by the most interested of the health professionals available (school dietitcian if available) or the coach himself. At a later team meeting the results of this survey should be discussed and will form an excellent springboard for discussion of "good nutrition and its importance in athletics." Every athlete should shoot for one hundred percent on his diet score.

Total Effort and Sleep-rest Evaluation.   The form shown in table 27.3 is used for this purpose and is largely self-explanatory. The coaches evaluation of this chart cannot be made quantitatively without great difficulty and it is therefore suggested that this form be applied only in a rather informal manner, looking for the individual athlete who may

TABLE 27.1

Record for Meals
Keep a complete record of all food and beverages consumed at and between meals for a seven-day period. Use the following form for your
data. One for each day. Under kind of food, specify whether raw or
cooked, if fruit or vegetable, and how prepared. For example, a vegetable salad may be made of cooked carrots and beans and raw celery;
potatoes may be creamed. Amounts should be expressed as definitely
and accurately as possible, servings of meats in measurements, servings of vegetables in cups, slices of bread in number and size, etc.

Time and place of meal	Food	Kind	Amount	Calories

From Chaney and Ross. *Nutrition*. Seventh ed., 1966; courtesy of Houghton-Mifflin
Co.

be grossly overloaded with respect to the total weeks activity. Such
athletes would be counseled on an individual basis and those for whom
a gross overload is unavoidable should be counseled out of the athletics
picture in the interests of both the health of the individual and the welfare of the team. Such an individual would probably be retrogressing in
performance when the team needs him most—late season.

Once a Week Physiological Testing. This most important testing can
be accomplished in little more than ten minutes per athlete when procedures have become routine. The only equipment required is an inexpensive bicycle ergometer which every corrective or adaptive physical education department should have anyway. Purchase may be more easily
justified in this fashion. Also needed are a stethoscope, metronome, and
two stopwatches. The procedure is briefly described in this text in chapter eleven and described in detail in the lab manual which accompanies
this text (2). In any event, the load should be selected to achieve a heart
rate of 150 beats per minute, plus or minus ten beats, and this same load
should be used on the individual athlete throughout the whole season.
Thus changes in his heart rate and blood pressure response to a standard load can be graphed and trends will become obvious over a period
of weeks. The athlete should report for testing at least fifteen minutes
prior to his actual test so that reasonably representative values of resting heart rate and blood pressure can be obtained after fifteen minutes
rest in the lab and just before the test begins. Resting heart rate and
blood pressure and exercise heart rate and blood pressure are then
recorded on the form as shown in figure 27.1. The athlete should be

TABLE 27.2

Score your diet for each day of the above period and determine your average score for the week. For this purpose, use the following score card.

Food Selection Score Card for the College Student

Food Group	Amounts Recommended	Credits		Your Daily Score
Milk[1]	4 cups or more	4 cups	25	
		3 cups	18	
		2 cups	12	
		1 cup	6	
Meat[2]	2 servings or more	2 servings, including at least 1 of meat, poultry, or fish	25	
		1 serving of any of above	15	
		1 serving of another food in meat group	10	
Vegetable-fruit[3]	4 servings or more	1 serving of citrus fruit	10	
		1 serving of dark-green or deep-yellow vegetable	10	
		2 servings of any fruit or vegetable	10	
Bread-cereal[4]	4 servings or more	4 servings	20	
		3 servings	15	
		2 servings	10	
		1 serving	5	
Total Score			100	

[1]Milk group: **maximal score 25.**
1 cup = 8 oz. of milk.
Equivalents in calcium value:
    1″ cube of cheddar-type cheese = 2/3 cup of milk.
    $\frac{1}{2}$ cup of cottage cheese = 1/3 cup of milk.
    2 tablespoons of cream cheese = 1 tablespoon of milk.
    $\frac{1}{2}$ cup ice cream = $\frac{1}{4}$ cup of milk.

[2]Meat group: **maximal score 25.**
1 serving = 2 to 3 oz. of lean cooked meat, poultry, or fish, all without bone.
1 serving = 2 eggs.
1 serving = 1 cup of cooked dry beans, dry peas, or lentils.
1 serving = 4 tablespoons of peanut butter.

[3]Vegetable-fruit group: **maximal score 30.**
1 serving = $\frac{1}{2}$ cup of vegetable or fruit or an ordinary size serving.

[4]Bread-cereal group: **maximal score 20.**
1 serving = 1 slice bread.
1 serving = 1 oz. ready-to-eat cereal.
1 serving = $\frac{1}{2}$ to $\frac{3}{4}$ cup of cooked cereal, rice, macaroni, or cornmeal.

Note: No more than the maximal score for each group may be credited daily.

From Chaney and Ross. *Nutrition.* Seventh ed., 1966; courtesy of Houghton-Mifflin Co.

TABLE 27.3

Total Effort and Sleep-Rest Patterns

List your weekly activities below including sleeping or resting and eating as accurately as you can estimate them. This form will be used by the coach in getting the best possible results from your training program in terms of your health and athletic achievement.

Time	Mon	Tues	Wed	Thurs	Fri	Sat	Sun
A.M.							
12:00- 1:00							
1:00- 2:00							
2:00- 3:00							
3:00- 4:00							
4:00- 5:00							
5:00- 6:00							
7:00- 8:00							
8:00- 9:00							
9:00-10:00							
10:00-11:00							
11:00-12:00							
P.M.							
12:00- 1:00							
1:00- 2:00							
2:00- 3:00							
3:00- 4:00							
4:00- 5:00							
5:00- 6:00							
6:00- 7:00							
7:00- 8:00							
8:00- 9:00							
9:00-10:00							
10:00-11:00							
11:00-12:00							

encouraged to calculate his own estimated maximal O_2 consumption from a table provided for his use (see chapter eleven, table 11.2 page 235). A copy of the norms for maximal O_2 (table 11.2) should also be posted so that he can evaluate his own status. All of the precautions mentioned in chapter eleven such as temperature control must be closely observed

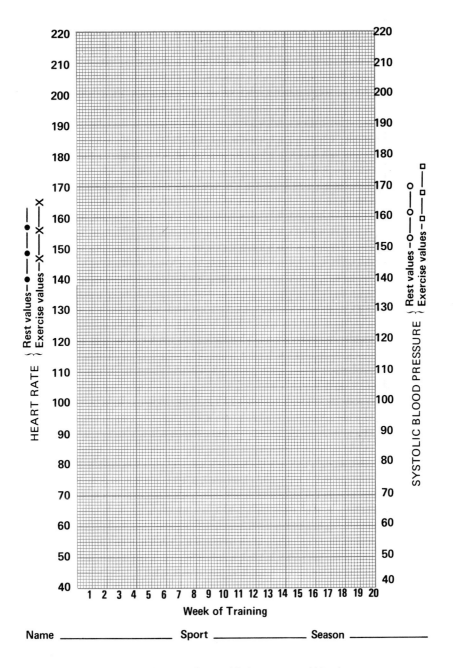

Figure 27-1. Form for recording weekly heart rate and blood pressure.

in order that the data be reliable. Only systolic blood pressure is recorded since diastolic pressure is both difficult to take and notoriously unreliable under exercise conditions. Consequently resting heart rate and blood pressure plus the exercise values can all be entered in one graph (figure 27.1) thus allowing easier visual identification of undesirable trends.

Daily Measurements. Each coach will probably wish to devise his own method of charting performance in accord with his sport and coaching techniques. The suggested form for graphing weight changes is shown in figure 27.2.

INTERPRETATION OF PHYSIOLOGICAL DATA

It must be realized from the outset that all the measurements taken have considerable variability due to unavoidable errors of measurement and due to normal biological variability. This, of course, is the major reason for graphing the data so that meaningful trends will emerge when the data points are connected which would otherwise be lost due to meaningless variability.

In general, a diagnosis of overtraining should not be based on any one measurement of any one parameter alone. The order of importance of the various measurements is as follows:

1. Exercise heart rate
2. Exercise blood pressure
3. Body weight
4. Resting blood pressure
5. Resting heart rate

Furthermore no great importance should be attached to a change observed on only one occasion. Only when a trend is seen over three or more observations are the data likely to be meaningful.

The typical picture seen in overtraining would consist of a rise in exercise heart rate, exercise blood pressure, resting heart rate, and resting blood pressure, combined with a loss in weight. Such a pattern should be considered a clear cut indication for easing up on the training load and the first discernible sign of such a trend should be cause for caution and some lessening of the load.

Obviously, individual counseling is of the utmost importance. For example a continued weight loss over two to three weeks in the absence of other trends would suggest questioning the athlete as to possible changes in diet, etc. *Science* can only supply better data to improve the *art* of personal interactions between coach and athlete!

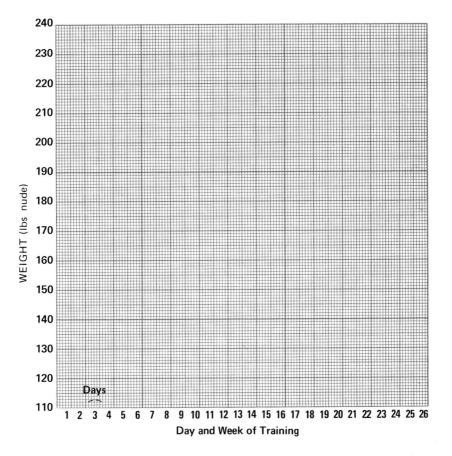

Figure 27-2. Suggested form for recording athletes body weight changes on five day/week basis throughout season.

BENEFITS TO BE GAINED FROM THE SCIENTIFIC EFFORT

No claim is made here to suggest that losers can become winners by the procedures under discussion. However, there is every reason to believe that applying what we know of exercise physiology can make a considerable contribution to better athletic performances. This can be assumed on at least two bases: (1) the *physiological* basis which has been fairly well defined through the course of this text and (2) by virtue of the so called *Hawthorne Effect* which is the name given to performance benefits arising in experiments where the only possible explanation lies in the fact that the subjects have received some change in experimental conditions which is interpreted by them as "concern for their welfare."

There is probably little question but that attention to the details of optimizing the general health of athletes will result in better performances if only due to the lessening of workout time lost to respiratory tract infections, and other "bugs."

Of equal importance is the resulting increased rapport of the coach with the members of the athletes' family, the academic institution, the medical community, and the community at large.

REFERENCES

1. Chaney, M. S., and Ross, M. L. 1966. *Nutrition.* 7th ed. Boston: Houghton Mifflin Co.
2. deVries, H. A. 1971. *Laboratory experiments in physiology of exercise.* Dubuque: William C. Brown Co. Publishers.

Index

503